P9-EET-079

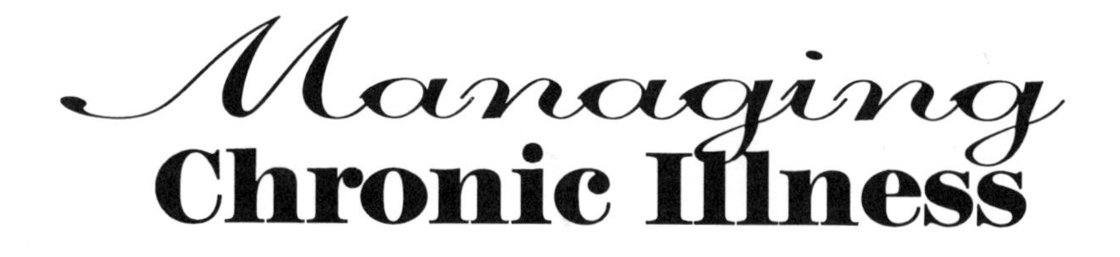
Managing
Chronic Illness

Application and Practice in Health Psychology

Andrew Baum and Margaret Chesney, Series Editors

Series Titles

Managing Chronic Illness: A Biospsychosocial Perspective
Edited by Perry M. Nicassio & Timothy W. Smith

Psychophysiological Disorders: Research and Clinical Applications
Edited by Robert J. Gatchel & Edward B. Blanchard

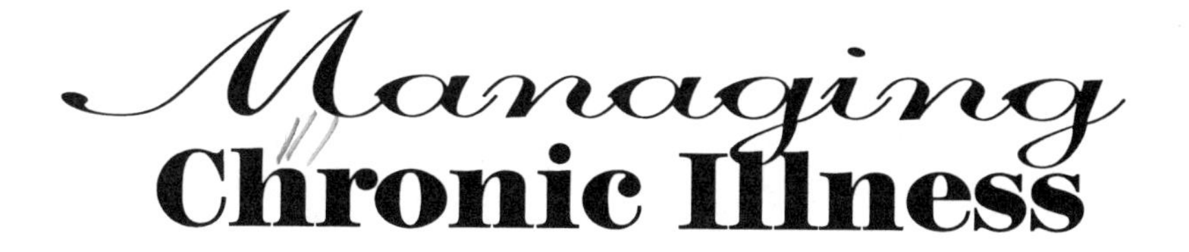

Managing Chronic Illness

A Biopsychosocial Perspective

EDITED BY
Perry M. Nicassio and Timothy W. Smith

AMERICAN PSYCHOLOGICAL ASSOCIATION

WASHINGTON, DC

First printing October 1995
Second printing March 1996

Published by
American Psychological Association
750 First Street, NE
Washington, DC 20002

Copies may be ordered from
APA Order Department
P.O. Box 2710
Hyattsville, MD 20784

In the United Kingdom and Europe, copies may be ordered from
American Psychological Association
3 Henrietta Street
Covent Garden, London
WC2E 8LU England

Typeset in Palatino by PRO-Image Corporation, Techna-Type Div., York, PA

Cover and jacket designer: Minker Design, Bethesda, MD
Printer: Quinn-Woodbine, Inc., Woodbine, NJ
Technical/production editor: Mollie R. McCormick

Library of Congress Cataloging-in-Publication Data
Managing chronic illness: a biopsychosocial perspective / edited by
Perry M. Nicassio and Timothy W. Smith.
p. cm.—(Application and practice in health psychology)
Includes bibliographical references and index.
ISBN 1-55798-300-3 (acid-free paper)
1. Chronic diseases. 2. Clinical health psychology.
I. Nicassio, Perry M. II. Smith, Timothy W. III. Series.
[DNLM: 1. Psychotherapy—methods. 2. Chronic Disease—
psychology.
3. Stress, Psychological—therapy. 4. Psychophysiology. WM 420
M266 1995]
RC108.M365 1995
616'.001'9—dc20
DNLM/DLC
for Library of Congress 95-17909
CIP

British Library Cataloguing-in-Publication Data
A CIP record is available from the British Library.

Printed in the United States of America

Contents

Contributors

Anna Bardone, Department of Psychiatry, School of Medicine, University of California, San Diego

Cynthia D. Belar, College of Health-Related Professions, University of Florida, Gainesville

Lora E. Burke, School of Nursing, University of Pittsburgh

Lynn DellaPietra, Department of Clinical and Health Psychology, Hahnemann University

Leonard R. Derogatis, Clinical Psychometric Research, Baltimore, Maryland

Richard E. Doty, Montebello Hospital, School of Medicine, University of Maryland, Baltimore

Jacqueline Dunbar-Jacob, School of Nursing, University of Pittsburgh

Megan P. Fleming, Department of Clinical and Health Psychology, Hahnemann University, Philadelphia

Michael E. Geisser, University of Michigan Medical Center, Ann Arbor

Mark P. Kelly, Montebello Hospital, Department of Neurology, School of Medicine, University of Maryland, Baltimore

Robert D. Kerns, Veterans Affairs Medical Center, West Haven, Connecticut

Perry M. Nicassio, California School of Professional Psychology, San Diego

Jerry C. Parker, Harry S. Truman Memorial Veterans' Hospital, Columbia, Missouri

Joanna J. Peterkin, Department of Psychiatry, School of Medicine, University of California, San Diego

Sandra Puczynski, School of Nursing, University of Pittsburgh

Peter Salovey, Department of Psychology, Yale University

Stephen R. Shuchter, Department of Psychiatry, School of Medicine, University of California, San Diego

Timothy W. Smith, Department of Psychology, University of Utah, Salt Lake City

Nanette C. Sudler, Department of Clinical and Health Psychology, Hahnemann University

Dennis C. Turk, Pain Evaluation and Treatment Institute, University of Pittsburgh School of Medicine

Kathleen Young, Department of Psychology, University of California, Los Angeles

Nolan Zane, Department of Education, University of California, Santa Barbara

Sidney Zisook, Department of Psychiatry, School of Medicine, University of California, San Diego

Foreword

The Division of Health Psychology (Division 38) of the American Psychological Association presents the second volume in its series highlighting the application and practice of health psychology. One of the driving forces behind the establishment of the division was interest in health promotion and disease prevention and treatment through the application of principles and procedures that were emerging in the research arena. The vitality of health psychology depends on an active dialogue between its researchers and practitioners. One of the important goals of the series is to further expand this dialogue. Attempts to translate research findings into applications and interventions, to test and evaluate the efficacy of these interventions, and to denote important clinical experiences and research needs of the practice of health psychology are the focus of these volumes. Transfer of knowledge; feedback to researchers regarding needs, failures, and successes of clinical interventions; and facilitation and expansion of necessary dialogue between scientist and practitioner are the objectives.

Toward these aims, the volumes in this series are meant to function as vehicles for translating research into practice, with an analysis of issues related to the evaluation, prevention, and treatment of health behaviors and health problems. These goals are met by treating clinical or applied health psychology as broadly as possible, including community and public health assessment and intervention methods and problems of health care use. Issues are considered across a variety of settings, including hospitals, the practitioner's office, community clinics, work-site settings, schools, and managed care settings. Each volume provides direction in areas of need and populations to be served by health psychology intervention; critically examines issues and problems involved in clinical evaluation, prevention, and treatment of specific disorders; and illustrates the effectiveness of novel clinical approaches to diagnosis and treatment that may guide future research and innovation. Each volume focuses on a topic, such as this book's emphasis on chronic illness, and synthesizes research on a range of topics to reinforce the theoretical and scientific rationale for the practice of health psychology and to identify critical issues in the prevention, assessment, and management of health problems.

Andrew Baum

Margaret Chesney

Preface

This book is the result of an initiative adopted by the Executive Committee of Division 38 (Health Psychology) of the American Psychological Association to develop a book series addressing applied and clinical issues in health psychology. As the body of research evidence has grown in the association between psychological processes and health, the demand for the professional application of health psychology principles and methods to various patient populations has expanded as well. Through the series Application and Practice in Health Psychology, Division 38 is attempting to provide practitioners and students with current clinical guidelines based on empirical research in health psychology. This volume, focusing on chronic illness and its management, reflects the growing role that health psychologists have in working with patients taxed by the psychological, social, and physical demands of coping with a chronic medical condition.

In today's health care milieu, it is commonplace for psychologists to render services to patients with chronic illnesses. Although advances in medicine have enabled people to live longer with such illnesses as coronary heart disease, cancer, and diabetes, patients' quality of life often remains limited. The medical specialties are increasingly recognizing the value of psychology for contributing to the overall care of those with chronic illnesses. Currently, psychologists with specialized training in health psychology occupy an important role in the comprehensive care of the medically ill. In the future, they will likely have an even more significant impact as evaluation and treatment strategies are informed by continuing advances in research on how psychological variables both affect and are affected by chronic disease. Through this series of books, Division 38 hopes to facilitate this process by asking leading clinicians and researchers to synthesize the available research and present its clinical implications. This volume provides an overview of the psychology of chronic medical illness that should underscore the large and growing scientific foundation for the psychologist's role in serving those who are chronically ill. It should also demonstrate the many challenges and problems that these professionals will face in their efforts. Such problems will require not only additional research but also the creativity and perseverance of individual professional psychologists working in these settings.

Rather than organizing the book around specific chronic illnesses, we chose to identify themes and issues that are pertinent to clinical work across a broad variety of medical problems. This organizational format was adopted for several reasons. First, patients with different chronic illnesses face many of the same adjustment difficulties and problems. Second, many practicing psychologists must be versatile and flexible in their approaches to generalize their skills across diverse patient groups. Finally, as the field of health psychology becomes more diverse and specialized with regard to the knowledge of specific illnesses, it becomes increasingly important to provide an integrated understanding of its general principles.

The book's chapters thus concentrate on the important themes and problems to be addressed, and the clinical methodologies that the clinician is likely to adopt, in working with diverse patient groups. The chapter authors were asked to address the empirical foundations of the clinical methods they described to convey a sense of the interconnectedness between research and practice. Where appropriate, they have also outlined important areas for future research and clinical inquiry.

We appreciate the contributions of several individuals who provided valuable assistance with this project. First, we thank the members of the Division 38 Executive Committee, who had the vision of developing a book series focusing on clinical and practitioner-related issues in health psychology. Second, we thank Margaret Chesney and Andy Baum, who, as book series coeditors, have provided valuable support and guidance in all phases of development. Third, we thank the chapter authors, who donated their services to the division's mission. Fourth, we acknowledge the production and editorial expertise of Susan Reynolds, Ted Baroody, and other staff members of the Books Department at the American Psychological Association who developed our manuscript into its present form. Furthermore, we are highly grateful to the numerous individuals who provided editorial feedback on drafts of the individual chapters, reviewing each contribution for both content and style. Finally, we thank our families for their continued support and patience throughout all phases of this project.

We dedicate this book to people who have been afflicted with chronic illnesses and their families, as well as to the practitioners charged with the responsibility of providing service to afflicted patients and loved ones.

Introduction

This book provides an overview of a relatively new and increasingly important aspect of professional psychology: the provision of psychological services to adults who have medical illnesses. For several decades, the leading causes of death, disability, and medical expenditures in industrialized nations have included such chronic illnesses as coronary heart disease, stroke, and cancer. Even chronic illnesses with less immediate life-threatening implications (e.g., arthritis, diabetes, and chronic obstructive pulmonary disease) are sources of considerable suffering, disability, and cost. Psychology has become steadily more involved in these medical challenges, for two reasons. First, these medical conditions are, in many cases, diseases of lifestyle. Routine behaviors or habits (e.g., smoking, diet, or activity levels) influence an individual's chances of developing these illnesses. Thus, their prevention involves the modification of behavior.

Second, once developed, chronic medical illness can have a wide-reaching impact on patients' lives. Although medical treatments have produced sometimes dramatic gains in survival rates, cures are still rare. As a result, patients are often left with significant physical distress and limitations in the major roles and activities of their lives. Medical and surgical treatments themselves are often highly stressful for the patient, adding to the already daunting adaptive demands posed by chronic illness. This book presents the clinical implications of this second, major psychological dimension of chronic medical illness. Throughout its chapters, contributors seek (a) to illustrate the extensive advances made to date in scientifically documenting the importance of psychological care in chronic medical illness and (b) to provide an overview of the challenges inherent to applying this knowledge in medical settings.

Clinical and counseling psychologists have much to offer patients suffering from chronic medical illness and can become valuable members of the multidisciplinary teams typically charged with their care. However, traditional psychological techniques and skills—and even the conceptual models guiding their application—cannot be directly applied to these patients and the settings in which they are treated.

There are important differences between medical patients and medical settings and patients and settings of more traditional professional psychological services. This book is a guide for those interested in making the transition to this new role for psychologists.

Plan of the Book

Authors of the individual chapters discuss issues central to applying psychological services in chronic-disease treatment. They have not focused on a single condition, such as heart disease or cancer, but on clinical issues relevant to virtually all chronic medical illnesses. Despite important differences in the nature and implications of major chronic diseases, people in these conditions share many psychological issues. Furthermore, the professional and organizational considerations that shape the delivery of psychological services are similar in the various medical subdisciplines. It is also true that many professional psychologists will not be in a position to specialize in a single chronic disease, and even those who do will profit from an understanding of general issues at the interface of professional psychology and medical care for chronic disease. Thus, the chapters provide overviews of the primary activities and concerns of psychologists who work with patients suffering from any of the common chronic illnesses.

When entering new territory, there are few things as valuable as a good map. The psychology of chronic disease is unfamiliar territory for most professional psychologists and students, so an overview of the primary conceptual map in this area is essential. The provision of psychological services to the chronically medically ill was founded on a relatively new conceptual model of the nature of medical illness and its clinical management. This *biopsychosocial model* (Engel, 1977) recognizes the reciprocal relations among the biological, psychological, and social aspects of patients' lives. This is an abrupt and far-reaching departure from the traditional biomedical model, in which disease and its cure are seen strictly as matters of basic physiological processes. In chapter 1, Smith and Nicassio present the biopsychosocial model and discuss its implications for understanding, assessing, and treating patients with chronic medical illnesses. Current psychiatric diagnostic criteria can be used to articulate much of the biopsychosocial model in individual cases. Yet, adoption of the biopsychosocial model is not simply an intellectual exercise. It has many implications for specific clinical procedures and issues. These implications are illustrated in the chapter through a review of the psychological aspects of clinical care for patients with coronary heart disease.

Often one of the most difficult challenges for psychologists making the transition to the medical setting is understanding the unique culture and organization of medical facilities. Compounding this problem are the personal issues the psychologist faces as a member of an interdisciplinary team dealing with patients who are facing life-threatening conditions. Furthermore, the roles the psychologist assumes in medical settings and the style with which these roles are enacted differ from his or her roles in traditional psychological and psychiatric settings in often confusing ways. A thorough command of the armamentaria of professional psychology is necessary but far from sufficient for psychologists working with the patients who are chronically ill. If psychologists cannot transpose their skills to the unique medical environment, then their usefulness and professional satisfaction are likely to suffer considerably. In chapter 2, Belar and Geisser address these issues and provide an invaluable guide for transitioning into this new role and setting. Their insights will be useful for psychologists in the early stages of training as well as for seasoned professionals considering a move into this newer aspect of the profession.

Psychological assessment is perhaps the most common aspect of psychological services provided to patients with chronic medical illnesses. Although many of the traditional techniques and procedures of psychological assessment are also relevant in the medical setting, there are important differences. Traditional assessment devices must be interpreted differently in many cases, and some devices are unique to chronically ill patients and related issues. Derogatis, Fleming, Sudler, and DellaPietra therefore provide a comprehensive review of this area, in chapter 3. This review should prove useful for shaping the assessment of particular patients and for designing standard assessment protocols with specific populations. In many cases, questions arise about cognitive process and their likely neurological substrates. Many chronic illnesses affect the brain and, therefore, can produce neurological effects with important consequences for patients' functioning. In some cases (e.g., radiation therapy), treatments themselves can influence cognitive functioning. As a result, neuropsychological assessment is an integral feature of the professional services offered to these populations. The clinical health psychologist, at a minimum, must have sufficient skill in cognitive and neuropsychological screening and be able to make informed referrals for more extensive neuropsychological evaluation. In chapter 4, Kelly and Doty thoroughly review these issues.

Each of the issues and topics covered in this text can be influenced by the patient's ethnic and cultural context, especially if it is different from that of the medical team. The psychologist can be uniquely positioned to deal with the problems that this "mismatch" can present. Furthermore, cultural and ethnic factors can be important in the design and implementation of the psychologist's own services for chronically ill patients. Young and Zane (chap. 5) discuss the ways in which culture and ethnicity can influence the nature of problems experienced by these patients, as well as how psychologists can address these factors.

It perhaps goes without saying that chronic illness afflicts not only the patient but the family as well. A chronic illness can create unique adjustive demands among family members, and the illness and its treatment often disrupt family functioning in far-reaching ways. Furthermore, the emotional and behavioral functioning of the patient can be influenced by the family's reaction to the changes put into motion by his or her disease. Standard medical care of chronic illness often fails to take full account of this reciprocal relationship between the illness and family process. In chapter 6, Kerns reviews these issues and their implications for providing psychological services to patients and their families. This is a clear case in which the broader and more complex perspective of the biopsychosocial model leads to more effective patient care.

Chronic medical illness can profoundly affect what patients do. Restrictions in activities resulting from disease are common and are often a primary source of dissatisfaction among patients and their families. Limitations in behavioral functioning can have important economic consequences as well, such as when patients are unable to return to work. Indeed, it has been argued that behavior is the most important indicator of the impact of chronic illness and of the success of related treatments (Kaplan, 1994). However, the effects of chronic illness on subsequent vocational, social, and recreational functioning do not tend to be simple and direct. The impact of illness on levels of disability and functional activity certainly depends, at least in part, on the nature of the disease and its medical or surgical management. But this impact is also mediated in a variety of ways by psychological factors.

Thus, maximizing patient functioning is not only a matter of medical treatment; psychological interventions can have useful effects as well, even in cases where medical and surgical treatments are only somewhat effective. Turk and Salovey (chap. 7) present such a cognitive–behavioral framework for conceptualizing and assessing the psychological determinants of patients' levels of disability or functional activity. They also examine the implications of this framework for designing and implementing cognitive–behavioral interventions intended to maximize patients' adaptive activity.

Patients typically experience chronic medical illness—and often, the related medical and surgical treatments—as quite stressful. In some cases, this stress is not only a potential threat to the patient's emotional quality of life: Stress can also exacerbate the chronic illness itself, through its pathophysiological effects on disease processes (e.g., Smith & Gallo, 1994). For these reasons, stress management procedures are an integral aspect of the services provided by psychologists to those who are chronically ill. In chapter 8, Parker reviews commonly used stress management techniques and their variations, discussing how these techniques are adapted to the special needs of this population.

Many of the most important advances in the medical care of people with chronic illnesses have involved the development of medications. As effective as many of these treatments have proven to be, their success is often limited when patients inconsistently follow prescribed therapeutic regimens. Problems of medical adherence contribute to many referrals of chronic illness patients for psychological consultation. In chapter 9, Dunbar-Jacob, Burke, and Puczynski review the clinical literature on this important topic and present guidelines for evaluating and managing these common and challenging cases. Successful management of such cases is often deeply appreciated by referring physicians and so can ease the psychologist's integration into the medical team.

An inescapable facet of psychological services for chronically ill patients is the issue of terminal care. Death, dying, and bereavement pose difficult personal and professional challenges for the professional psychologist in these settings. In the last chapter, Zisook, Peterkin, Shuchter, and Bardone discuss these issues and present guidelines for appropriate care. Psychological services for chronically ill patients simply cannot be comprehensive if they do not include adequate attention to the final stages of the disease course and the final phase of patients' lives. Despite the difficulty surrounding this aspect of patient care, it is often the source of considerable gratification for professional psychologists working with chronically ill patients.

The necessary separation of each of these topics into individual chapters might suggest a compartmentalization of professional psychological services for patients with chronic medical illness. Nothing could be further from the truth, however. Just as the biopsychosocial model that is so fundamental to this field explicitly recognizes the inherent interplay of several levels of analysis, effective psychological care of these patients involves a comprehensive and integrative approach to the various topics presented in the individual chapters. It would be a rare case that presented a problem of only one type. By separating the field into these topics, we hope to have presented them in sufficient detail as to provide a working introduction to the field. Assembling these components into a flexible and effective package of psychological services is one of the gratifying and continuing challenges of clinical health psychology.

Emerging Themes and Future Challenges

Several issues emerge repeatedly in the chapters of this book. Perhaps most striking of these is that, unlike in traditional mental health services, clinical health psychologists work with other professionals who have dramatically different backgrounds and orientations. On the one hand, this broad array of perspectives on the interdisciplinary team is necessitated by the complexity of chronic illness and the challenges it poses. Thus, interdisciplinary care contains the potential for comprehensive and effective patient care. On the other hand, this presents the possibility that care will be confusing and fractionated. Although rarely vested with the responsibility of coordinating the interdisciplinary teams of physicians, nurses, and other health professionals, psychologists often have the greatest potential for recognizing and managing the demands of this convergence of diverse professional perspectives. A hidden challenge for the psychologist, then, is not only to become skilled and comfortable working in this setting but also to recognize and accept his or her informal role as the biopsychosocial facilitator of integrated patient care.

Other challenges of the interdisciplinary setting are made apparent throughout this book. Psychologists must be sufficiently expert in their own discipline to provide efficient and effective service with difficult cases. However, such psychological expertise alone is not sufficient for their ultimate success. Psychologists must also understand enough about the related disciplines to offer services that mesh well with the overall mission of the specific medical service. Relatedly, they must recognize that it will be essential for them to communicate with their medical colleagues on an ongoing basis about the potential contributions of psychology to patient care. Current medical education contains more psychological material than did medical curricula even a decade ago, but few physicians will have an appreciation of the possible contributions of professional psychology to their mission. Clinical health psychologists must therefore often play the role of continuing medical educator as well as the roles of psychological clinician and informal interdisciplinary coordinator.

This disparate set of formal and informal activities places a considerable burden on the psychologist. This burden is compounded by the enormous amount of information—both within and outside psychology—that the clinical health psychologist must master. In many respects, the psychologist must take the stance of a continual student of medical care. As noted in several places in this book, one of the challenges for clinical health psychologists is to cope with this enormous volume of information without losing their own unique perspective, as opposed to that of a traditional medical professional.

An extremely valuable contribution of the psychologist's unique perspective in the interdisciplinary team is his or her recognition of individual differences. In many ways, traditional medical care obscures individual differences, emphasizing instead common features in diagnosis and standard care. In contrast, the psychologist is the most likely member of the team to attend to the unique and distinguishing aspects of the patient's history, personality, relationships, and culture. To paraphrase Sir William Osler, a nineteenth-century physician and founding figure in modern medicine, although much of traditional medicine is concerned with which disease the patient has, the clinical health psychologist is naturally concerned with which patient has the disease. A hallmark of the biopsychosocial perspective—and perhaps the source of much of professional psychology's potential contribution to the care of chronically ill patients—is this "recontextualizing" of the illness within the patient and of the patient within his or her social and cultural niche.

Medical care is changing rapidly. Unfolding technological advances in medicine (e.g., organ transplantation, genetic screening and therapy, and the use of artificial organs) are likely to create new opportunities for professional psychologists interested in treating chronic disease. The financing of this already expensive health care system is also undergoing great change. As a result, current and future opportunities for psychologists are coupled with an increased need to justify the utility and cost-effectiveness of their contribution to medical care. One likely consequence of these circumstances is a closer coupling of research, practice, and public policy for clinical health psychologists. Few health care services will be reimbursed without clear empirical evidence of efficacy, and research of this type must attend to the nuances of the clinical context to be maximally informative. Given professional psychology's historical adherence to the scientist–practitioner model in training and practice, psychologists should be well-suited to meet these demands in the future of the field.

This book owes a great deal to previous works on the topic (e.g., Burish & Bradley, 1983; Holroyd & Creer, 1986; Moos, 1977). Like these predecessors, we hope to have provided a useful, current overview of the field and its future challenges. The earlier works provided the impetus for a great deal of subsequent research and expansion of clinical services. As a result, the status of clinical health psychology portrayed in this book reflects many significant advances in scientific foundations, theory, and practice over the course of even a few years. It is also our hope to have brought together the elements of a tempting invitation to this growing aspect of professional psychology, in a helpful, initial guide for those students and professional psychologists whose interests are sparked.

REFERENCES

Burish, T. G., & Bradley, L. A. (1983). *Coping with chronic disease: Research and applications.* San Diego, CA: Academic Press.

Engel, G. L. (1977, April 8). The need for a new medical model: A challenge for biomedicine. *Science, 196,* 129–136.

Holroyd, K. A., & Creer, T. L. (1986). *Self-management in chronic disease: Handbook of clinical interventions and research.* San Diego, CA: Academic Press.

Kaplan, R. M. (1994). The Ziggy theorem: Toward an outcomes-focused health psychology. *Health Psychology, 13,* 451–460.
Moos, R. H. (1977). *Coping with physical illness.* New York: Plenum.
Smith, T. W., & Gallo, L. C. (1994). Psychosocial influences on coronary heart disease. *Irish Journal of Psychology, 15,* 8–26.

Chapter

1

Psychological Practice: Clinical Application of the Biopsychosocial Model

Timothy W. Smith and Perry M. Nicassio

Professional psychology has grown dramatically in the latter half of the twentieth century. The number of practicing psychologists has risen rapidly, as has the number of doctoral, internship, and post-doctoral programs offering clinical and research training. During this period, the repertoire of clinical assessment and intervention techniques has been expanded and refined through the accumulation of basic and applied research. The profession serves a growing list of populations and settings. Its maturity is further evident from the establishment of ethical guidelines and self-regulation policies as well as from the legal and political status of psychology in the nation's health care system.

One of professional psychology's greatest challenges also emerged during this period of rapid growth and development—the psychological care of people with chronic medical illnesses. The patterns of physical illness afflicting industrialized nations changed profoundly over the past 50 years, as did the health care systems designed to address these diseases. These changes have altered the conceptual framework for understanding medical illness and have virtually necessitated the expansion of professional psychology into new areas of medicine and health care delivery.

The acute, infectious diseases that were leading causes of death and disability during the first half of the twentieth century have largely been controlled by important advances in biomedical science. Despite the recent resurgence of tuberculosis (Bloom & Murray, 1992), cases of influenza, pneumonia, and other infectious diseases are far less common and lethal now, largely because of developments in antibiotic medications, inoculations, sanitation, and other public health practices. These infectious conditions have been replaced as leading causes of death by chronic illnesses, such as coronary heart disease (CHD), cancer, and cerebrovascular disease. Death rates due to heart disease doubled during the twentieth century, and cancer deaths tripled. As was the case with acute, infectious diseases, biomedical science has produced important advances in the diagnosis, management, and prevention of these conditions. Nonetheless, these "new" diseases continue to take millions of lives prematurely each year, and they account for much of the over $800 billion that Americans spend annually on health care.

Chronic Illness and the Mandate for Psychology

Heart disease, cancer, and stroke share important challenges for professional psychology. Behavior and psychological processes influence the risk of developing these conditions. Diet, physical activity levels, smoking, alcohol consumption, and psychological stress can all significantly affect an individual's chances of developing cancer and cardiovascular diseases. These behaviors and others (e.g., delay in seeking treatment or lack of adherence to medical regimens) also have a significant effect on one's prognosis for surviving heart disease, cancer, and stroke. Thus, the cause and course of major threats to public health include many psychological factors. Psychologists can play an important role in the primary and secondary prevention of these health problems, by acting to modify health-relevant behavior. This is also true with the more recent and troubling public health problems of HIV infection and AIDS. With relatively rare exceptions (e.g., infection from contaminated blood during transfusion), the primary modes of HIV infection are behaviorally influenced (Catania, Kegeles, & Coates, 1990). Psychologists can thus potentially reduce the prevalence of chronic disease by working to prevent or reduce patients' unhealthy behavior (e.g., smoking, inactivity, and unprotected sexual intercourse in the case of cancer, heart disease, and HIV, respectively).

Yet prevention is not the only role for psychologists in dealing with chronic disease. This is because the association between psychological phenomena and chronic illness is not unidirectional: Psychological processes can be either important consequences of chronic disease or contributing causes. Life-threatening conditions often profoundly affect people's emotional, social, vocational, and sexual functioning, as do many other chronic medical conditions. Depression, disrupted marital and family relationships, decreased sexual activity and enjoyment, and decreased ability to work are common among people who are chronically ill. These negative psychosocial consequences of chronic medical illness pose significant threats to the patient's quality of life, tax his or her adaptive resources, and are the source of much of associated health care expenditures. Traditional medical care of people with chronic disease has focused much more on the underlying pathophysiological process than on how the disease affects patients' lives. When seen from a more comprehensive perspective, the care of people with chronic disease includes many psychological issues.

Managing chronic illness and its potential effects on many aspects of the patient's life represents important opportunities for professional psychology. The scope and cost—both in financial terms and in human suffering—provide compelling incentives to develop and implement effective psychological interventions. However, the same rising health care costs that provide incentives for these efforts also increase competition among health care providers for closely scrutinized expenditures. Expert, cost-effective psychological services are needed, and the professional psychologist must be able to justify and provide them in the complex and changing climate of the current health care system. This demands resourcefulness and accountability on the part of the clinician.

The emergence of chronic disease as the leading cause of death and primary source of health expenditures (National Center for Health Statistics, 1992) has prompted reformulation of the conceptual models guiding health services. The resulting biopsychosocial model is an invaluable guide for psychologists who work with people struggling with chronic illness. In this chapter, we introduce the biopsychosocial model and the variety of connections among biological, psychological, and social processes that it articulates. In addition, we present a general outline for the clinical application of the model in cases of chronic medical illness and illustrate this application with a review of the psychological aspects of CHD. We thus provide an overview of the predominant conceptual approach to the interface of psychology and medicine—one that is an essential perspective in clinical work with patients suffering from chronic illness.

The Biopsychosocial Model

The need to consider psychological and social components in health care has been articulated for many years, although this notion has met with some resistance in the traditional medical community. For example, in his landmark 1977 paper, Engel argued that the dominant biomedical model of physical illness was no longer satisfactory, despite the many revolutionary treatments it had produced in the history of medicine. The traditional biomedical model assumes that all illness reflects only biological malfunctions. From this perspective, aberrations in biochemistry or physiology underlie the onset and course of chronic physical illness, and psychological or social factors are generally seen as irrelevant. In emphasizing biological abnormality, the biomedical model espouses a reductionistic philosophy that frequently ignores or minimizes important psychological and social differences between patients who share the same medical diagnosis. The adoption of this model may lead to stereotypes based on the illnesses that patients have (e.g., the "arthritis patient" or the "myocardial infarction patient"), with the result that the person with the illness is not fully recognized, and hence, is neither evaluated nor treated in a comprehensive manner.

In contrast, the biopsychosocial model (Engel, 1977) identifies biological, psychological, and social factors as interrelated influences on health and illness. Under the model, the onset, course, and treatment of physical illness are best understood as involving each of these levels of analysis (Engel, 1980). CHD, cancer, stroke, AIDS, and virtually all other chronic medical illnesses seem to provide clear examples of the relevance and utility of the biopsychosocial model.

The biopsychosocial model provides a broad conceptual framework—rather than a unifying theory—for understanding chronic illness and its management. General systems theory (von Bertalanffy, 1968) has contributed to the development of the biopsychosocial model by affirming that nature is organized in terms of a hierarchy of units reflecting a continuum of complexity. The units range from those that are small and less complex, to those that are large, complex, and superordinate, to those lower in the hierarchy (see Figure 1). Each unit represents a system with its own distinct qualities, organization, and methods of study that are appropriate to that system. For example, the methodology for studying cell metabolism differs dramatically from procedures for evaluating dysfunctional patterns of interaction in families of patients with chronic illness.

Although distinctive, each system is a component of a higher system that can exert both downward and upward effects in the hierarchy. This feature addresses the interdependence between systems and promotes the concept that any system can only be fully characterized by comprehension of the larger system of which it is a part. The application of this concept to the biopsychosocial model is highly relevant

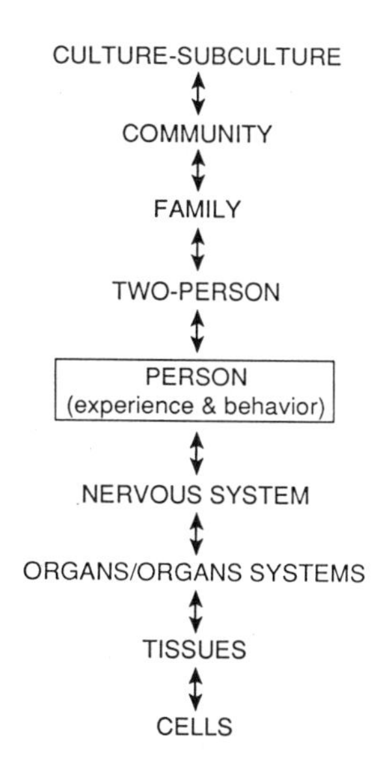

Figure 1. Schema of the interactional nature of systems. From "Clinical Application of the Biopsychosocial Model," by G. L. Engel, 1980, *American Journal of Psychiatry, 137,* p. 537. Copyright 1980 by the American Psychiatric Association. Reprinted with permission.

to the clinician. For instance, when evidence of biological abnormality is found in an organ of the patient, its full meaning and impact on the patient's functioning must be understood in light of the patient's coping resources and relationships with significant others. Similarly, the culture of the patient may affect his or her interpretation of available coping resources and social adjustment. The biopsychosocial model and its foundation in systems theory have long been identified as useful integrative perspectives for behavioral medicine and clinical health psychology (e.g., Schwartz, 1982).

Biopsychosocial Diagnoses

The basic distinguishing feature of the biopsychosocial model—that psychological and social factors can both influence and be influenced by pathophysiological processes—has been acknowledged in the formal psychiatric diagnostic systems for many years. For example, the second edition of the *Diagnostic and Statistical Manual of Mental Disorders* (*DSM-II*) of the American Psychiatric Association (APA, 1968) included the category of Psychophysiological Disorders. This category pertained to a variety of disorders in which psychological stress was presumed to be a contributing and exacerbating factor (e.g., asthma and essential hypertension). This category was replaced in the *DSM-III* (APA, 1980) and *DSM-III-R* (APA, 1987) by the category of Psychological Factors Affecting Physical Condition (316.0). The criteria for the *DSM-III-R* diagnosis are presented in Exhibit 1.

Several important points are evident in these criteria. First, the exclusion of somatoform disorders and specification of actual pathophysiological changes or processes restricts the diagnosis to actual illness, rather than including abnormal illness behaviors in the absence of disease (e.g., hypochondriasis). Identifiable psychological stimuli precede either the onset or exacerbation of this demonstrable condition. The text accompanying these criteria identifies potential examples of "psychologically meaningful environmental stimuli" that are consistent with the spirit of the biopsychosocial model (e.g., interpersonal conflict or loss), and several chronic physical illnesses are listed as examples of relevant physical conditions (e.g., angina, rheumatoid arthritis, and ulcerative colitis).

However, one unfortunate limitation of these criteria is that they are vague. Although they provide the clinician with considerable flexibility for their application, they lack detail in identifying the types of

Exhibit 1

DSM-III-R *Criteria for Psychological Factors Affecting Physical Condition*

A. Psychologically meaningful environmental stimuli are temporally related to the initiation or exacerbation of a specific physical condition or disorder (recorded on Axis III).
B. The physical condition involves either demonstrable organic pathology (e.g., rheumatoid arthritis) or a known pathophysiologic process (e.g., migraine headache).
C. The condition does not meet the criteria for a Somatoform Disorder.

Note. From *Diagnostic and Statistical Manual of Mental Disorders* (3rd ed., revised, p. 334), American Psychiatric Association, 1987, Washington, DC: Author. Copyright 1987 by the American Psychiatric Association. Reprinted with permission.

psychological factors influencing physical conditions and the processes through which these factors exert their effects. Furthermore, the criteria are devoid of operational procedures that would guide the clinician in implementing the diagnostic code in a given case. These limitations were the source of much of the discussion guiding the reformulation of these criteria for the *DSM-IV* (APA, 1994). The criteria for the revised diagnosis are listed in Exhibit 2.

Discerning Relationships Between Psychosocial Processes and Health Outcomes

When applying the diagnostic criteria from this code to a specific case, it is essential for the clinician to consider the various ways in which a psychosocial process may exert influence on the health outcome under evaluation. It is equally important to be cautious in addressing this question, because it has been very difficult to establish causal relationships between psychosocial processes and the onset or exacerbation of medical conditions. Even though the biopsychosocial model promotes the inference of causal influences between systems, in most instances the relevant empirical research is limited.

This problem is further compounded by the difficulty of analyzing causality between systems in a clinical encounter with a single patient.

Exhibit 2

DSM-IV *Criteria for Psychological Factors Affecting Medical Condition*

A. The presence of a general medical condition (coded on Axis III).
B. Psychological factors affect the general medical condition in at least one of the following ways:
   1. the factors have influenced the course of the medical condition as shown by a close temporal association between the development, exacerbation, or delayed recovery from the general medical condition
   2. the factors interfere with treatment of the general medical condition
   3. the factors constitute additional health risks for the individual
   4. stress-related physiological responses precipitate or exacerbate symptoms of a general medical condition.

Note. From *Diagnostic and Statistical Manual of Mental Disorders* (4th ed., p. 678), American Psychiatric Association, 1994, Washington, DC: Author. Copyright 1994 by the American Psychiatric Association. Adapted with permission.

The circumstances of the clinical evaluation can be artificial for the patient, as they are established primarily for the convenience of the health care provider. Most diagnostic interviews, for example, actually take place outside of the social context in which the patient's health-related problems may exist. The evaluation and analysis of these problems typically occurs in a health care setting in which a professional assumes control over all aspects of the process of gathering information. Although the clinical encounter is an important component of the evaluation process, it may only be the first step—that is, the time when the clinician generates hypotheses to be evaluated through other methods of data collection, such as interviewing family members, reviewing patients' daily diaries, or even observing patients at home or work.

But how can a psychosocial factor affect a particular health outcome? The use of models that specify potential linkages between systems may be particularly helpful in guiding clinical decision making. The *DSM-IV* (APA, 1994) criteria include several types of mechanisms linking psychosocial variables and health outcomes. These more specific models vary in complexity depending on the number of factors in the model and the nature of the relationships between factors. The relationships between psychosocial factors and health outcomes may take several forms. Specifically, psychosocial factors may have direct, indirect, or moderating influences on health outcomes.

Direct effects refer to relationships in which some quality of the psychosocial factor (e.g., presence or magnitude) is reliably associated with predicted changes in the health outcome. Direct relationships do not require mediation by other processes and, in essence, describe a closed loop between the psychosocial process and health outcome. The psychosocial process may either precede or follow the health outcome. Figure 2 illustrates two different examples of direct effects. In the first example, anxiety is depicted as contributing to increased muscle tension. In the second example, a patient's verbal report or behavioral expression (e.g., grimace) of pain is followed by social reinforcement from significant others, such as attention, reassurance, or an expression of concern or affection. This reinforcement, in turn, increases the likelihood of further patient reports of pain. In both cases, the psychosocial factor directly influences the health outcome independent of other factors (e.g., underlying tissue pathology) that may potentially contribute to the explanation of the health outcome.

In contrast, *indirect effects* involve more complex relationships between psychosocial factors and health outcomes and require the contribution of mediational processes. In the simplest case, such effects describe sequences of relationships in which an initial factor (Factor A) contributes to another (Factor B), which in turn causes a change in yet another factor (Factor C; Baron & Kenny, 1986). Factor B thus constitutes the mechanism through which Factor A is related to Factor C. Many examples from the health psychology literature attest to the

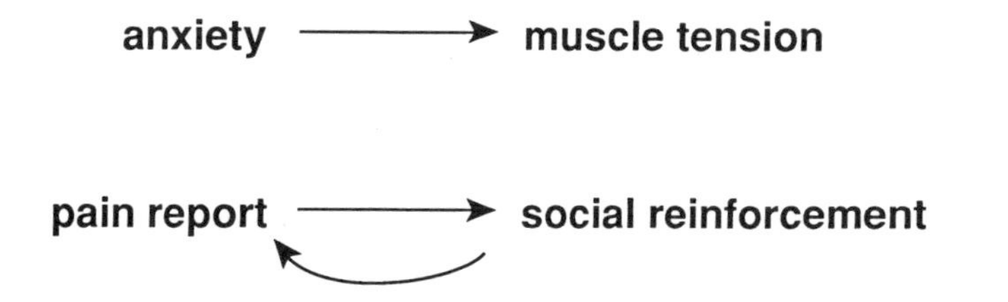

Figure 2. Mechanisms of action: Examples of direct effects of psychosocial processes on health outcomes.

relevance of this type of relationship within the context of the biopsychosocial model. Figure 3 depicts two different forms of mediational processes: one involving physiological mechanisms (A), and the other involving behavioral mechanisms (B). In Example A, peripheral vasoconstriction mediates the relationship between an increase in anxiety, fueled by daily stress and elevation of blood pressure in a patient with essential hypertension. The effect of anxiety on blood pressure is totally accounted for by changes in peripheral vasoconstriction. In contrast, Example B shows a process in which a patient with rheumatoid arthritis who, because he or she excessively denies illness as a coping strategy, does not take anti-inflammatory medication as prescribed and consequently experiences increased inflammation of the joints. The psychosocial factor (denial of illness) is only relevant for explaining the health outcome (joint inflammation) to the extent that it leads to poor compliance with the prescribed medical regimen.

Finally, psychosocial processes may frequently moderate the effects of other variables on health outcomes (i.e., in a *moderator effect*). As opposed to serving as the causal mechanism linking variables, then, moderating factors alter the relationship between a causal factor and a health outcome. Social support from others and patients' coping mechanisms have received extensive research attention as factors that may change the way that adverse life experiences or aspects of illness affect the well-being of people with chronic medical conditions. When exposed to high degrees of life stress, for example, patients who re-

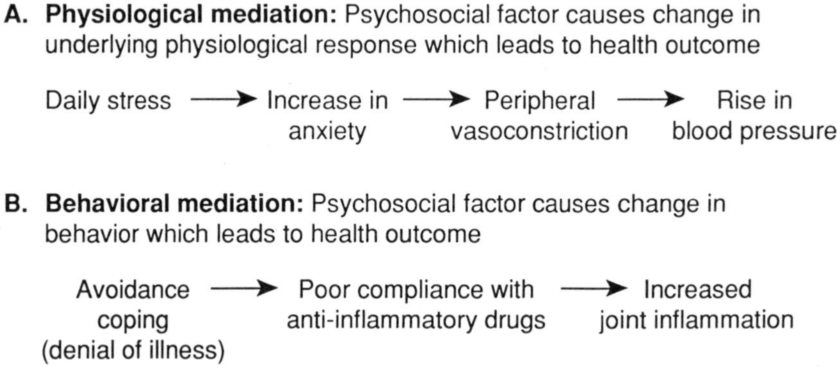

A. Physiological mediation: Psychosocial factor causes change in underlying physiological response which leads to health outcome

Daily stress ⟶ Increase in anxiety ⟶ Peripheral vasoconstriction ⟶ Rise in blood pressure

B. Behavioral mediation: Psychosocial factor causes change in behavior which leads to health outcome

Avoidance coping (denial of illness) ⟶ Poor compliance with anti-inflammatory drugs ⟶ Increased joint inflammation

Figure 3. Mechanisms of action: Examples of indirect effects of psychosocial processes on health outcomes.

ceive low or ineffective social support from others may be more likely to develop depression or to suffer from other adverse health consequences than are patients who receive high or effective support (Cohen, 1988; Cohen & Wills, 1985). Similarly, patients who cope passively with their pain when it is at a high level of intensity may be more vulnerable to becoming depressed than patients who exhibit lower levels of this coping tendency (Brown, Nicassio, & Wallston, 1989). Figure 4 shows these two scenarios. In both instances, the moderating factor alters the relationship between a psychosocial process (i.e., life stress or pain) and the health outcome (i.e., disease activity or depression). The clinical implications of moderating variables can be important. In these examples, greater social support in the face of stress may lead to lower disease activity, whereas a reduction in passive coping in dealing with pain may prevent the development of depressive symptoms.

The functional analysis, borrowed from the behavior therapy literature (Haynes & O'Brien, 1990), provides an important methodology that can be applied to evaluating relationships between psychosocial factors and health outcomes in an individual case. A key feature of the functional analysis is to examine patterns of association between

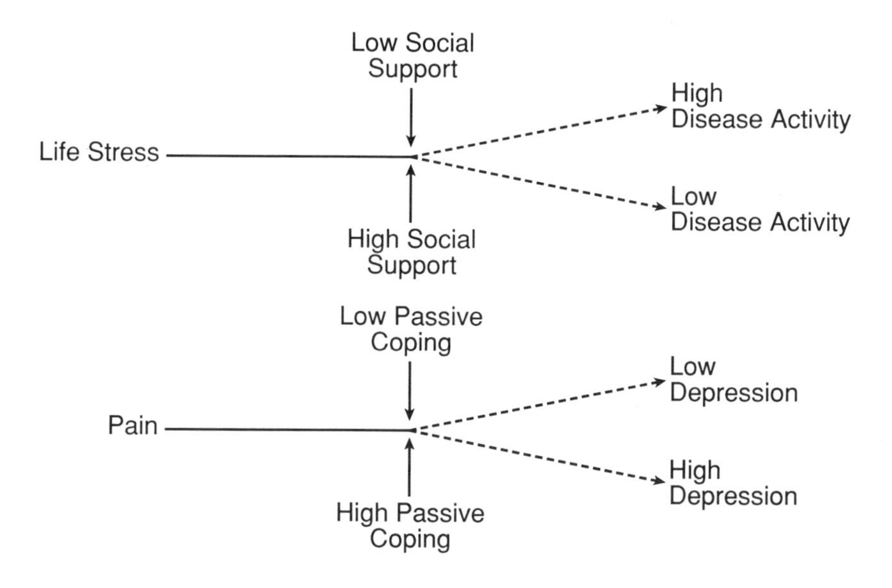

Figure 4. Mechanisms of action: Examples of moderating effects of psychosocial processes on health outcomes.

environmental events and health outcomes. For example, a patient in chronic pain may have more pain at work than at home, or an ulcer patient's gastric discomfort may increase or decrease depending on the presence or absence of interpersonal conflict. Identifying such relationships between psychosocial processes and health outcomes provides the psychologist with a basis for effectively applying the *DSM* code and for rationally developing treatment strategies that take into account important psychosocial and environmental influences.

It is evident that the possible pathways linking psychological processes and physical health are more specific in codes presented in the *DSM-IV* (APA, 1994) than in its predecessors. As a result, these criteria go further in articulating much of the biopsychosocial model for clinical diagnosis. Multiple phases of the disease process may be affected, including onset, exacerbation, and recovery. Many disease outcomes are specified as possibly being influenced by psychological factors, including the pathophysiological process itself, the subjective severity of related symptoms (such as pain), and the behavioral sequelae of the disease (such as impairments in social and vocational roles). The new criteria identify several types of psychological factors as possible influences on the disease and its consequences, including the physiological effects of psychological stress, behavioral factors such as noncompliance or unhealthy habits, and a variety of other psychological factors (e.g., Axis I or II mental disorder, coping styles, and personality traits). Thus, use of the diagnosis of Psychological Factors Affecting Physical Condition acknowledges the inherent complexity and wide range of psychosocial influences on disease and requires the clinician to articulate a working biopsychosocial model in its application.

Somewhat inconsistent with the biopsychosocial model and its foundation in general systems theory is that the connections between psychosocial factors and illness identified in these DSM-III (APA, 1980) and *DSM-IV* (APA, 1994) criteria are largely unidirectional. The criteria do not include the psychological and social effects of physical illness. These diagnostic systems do provide opportunities to identify these reciprocal effects, however, such as by identifying the illness as a likely contributing factor in adjustment disorders or other diagnoses.

Clinical application of the biopsychosocial model certainly can proceed without its inclusion in formal psychiatric diagnostic systems. Indeed, much of the theory and research supporting this model was developed outside of psychiatry and clinical psychology. Nonetheless, inclusion of basic features of the biopsychosocial model in the diagnostic systems is noteworthy as an acknowledgment of its impact within medicine. There are also practical advantages of including the Psychological Factors Affecting Physical Condition diagnosis in the *DSM*. Such formal diagnosis facilitates communication about biopsychosocial processes in clinical care and may be useful in establishing the appropriateness and importance of related health care expenditures and reimbursements. Moreover, the specific elements of the diagnosis may have a heuristic impact on research by serving as sources of hypotheses guiding future research into the biopsychosocial framework.

Outline for Applying the Biopsychosocial Model

Exhibit 3 shows an outline for applying the biopsychosocial model in clinical cases of chronic illness. The outline is not procedural; that is, it does not present a step-by-step guide to clinical assessment and intervention. Such procedures vary considerably according to the specific illness, health care setting, and psychologist's role. Indeed, one might effectively articulate a procedural outline only after considering the remaining chapters in this book. Instead, the outline shown here provides an initial, general organization for conceptualizing cases and gathering relevant information. Once such information is synthesized, one then identifies potential targets for intervention.

It should be recognized at the outset that successfully implementing the biopsychosocial model in large part depends on the validity of information obtained by the psychologist from the patient. It is within this two-person, interactional context that the psychologist gathers information about the patient's physical symptoms, sensory experiences, behavior patterns, and other pertinent data. Because the psychologist–patient relationship is a system in itself, qualities of this system may affect the reporting of data and their subsequent interpretation. Thus, the quality of the interaction between psychologist and patient constitutes the foundation for effectively applying the biopsychosocial framework.

The clinician faced with the task of working with those who are chronically ill will find the basic assumptions of the biopsychosocial model useful in guiding comprehensive assessment and suggesting potential interventions. Implementing this perspective requires that the psychologist have a contextualist orientation, in which interrelated

Exhibit 3

Outline for Assessment and Intervention in the Clinical Application of the Biopsychosocial Model

I. The illness
   A. Pathophysiology
   B. Risk factors
   C. Prognosis
   D. Diagnostic procedures
   E. Treatment procedures
II. The patient
   A. *DSM* Axis I conditions
   B. Disease history
   C. Personality traits and coping styles or mechanisms
   D. Conceptualization of disease and treatment
   E. Educational and vocational status
   F. Impact of illness on subjective distress, social functioning, activity level, self-care, and overall quality of life
III. Social, family, and cultural contexts
   A. Quality of marital and family relationships
   B. Use and efficacy of social support
   C. Patient–physician relationship
   D. Patient's cultural background
IV. The health care system
   A. Medical organization, setting, and culture
   B. Insurance coverage for diagnostic and treatment procedures
   C. Geographical, social, and psychological barriers to accessing health services
   D. Existence of disability benefits for medical condition

biological, psychological, and social conditions are seen as essential in accurate diagnosis and comprehensive care of patients. Many elements to be considered in this contextualist perspective are familiar to mental health professionals; others are unique to medical problems and settings. The patient's psychosocial difficulties are better understood in the context of the nature and likely impact of the disease, the process of its diagnosis and treatment, and the health care system in which these processes are embedded. The elements of the outline articulating these aspects of the context do not operate in isolation. Rather, it is a basic assumption of the biopsychosocial model that these elements overlap and are reciprocally related.

The Illness: Demands of Diagnosis, Treatment, and Prognosis

Psychological services for people who are chronically ill are unlikely to be effective unless psychologists are guided by a thorough understanding of the nature of the disease, of likely procedures involved in diagnosis and treatment, of additional aspects of related medical care, and of the prognosis of the condition. Each of these features of a chronic illness is likely to contain important influences on the patient's emotional, social, and vocational functioning. Clinical health psychologists need not assume the role of independent medical experts, but they should attain a fairly detailed understanding of (a) the medical disorder and health status of the patient, (b) implications and the psychological demands of associated diagnostic tests and treatment procedures, (c) the patient's responsibilities in current and future medical treatment, and (d) the range of potential medical outcomes.

A basic understanding of pathophysiology is an essential element of the biological context of the case. Furthermore, this understanding will identify potential points where psychosocial variables could exert direct, indirect, or moderating effects on the onset and course of the illness. Accurate understanding of the illness also permits the psychologist to track more effectively the outcome of psychosocial interventions designed to influence health status. Although they provide important medical information, many diagnostic tests are experienced by patients as physically painful or emotionally stressful, as are surgical and other procedures. The professional psychologist must have a basic understanding of these procedures to anticipate likely emotional effects of standard medical care. Similarly, some medications used in managing chronic illness have unpleasant side effects and place significant demands on the patient, again requiring that the psychologist appreciate these issues to work effectively with the patient. As noted previously, the patient's compliance with medical regimens is an important psychosocial influence on the disease. Finally, the prognosis of the condition—in terms of life expectancy and likely impact on functioning—is critical in psychological work with patients and their families.

The clinician needing this knowledge can acquire it in many ways, but he or she must not lose sight of the biopsychosocial "forest" for the medical "trees" in acquiring it. This poses an important practical and professional challenge for the clinician (Belar, 1991; see also Belar & Geisser, chap. 2, this book). Becoming familiar with pathophysiology, technically sophisticated diagnostic and treatment procedures, and the nature and consequences of an often bewildering array of medications is a daunting and sometimes consuming challenge in the continuing education of clinical health psychologists. Yet, it is essential that psychologists retain their unique perspective on the psychosocial aspects of medical care, a view that is sometimes at odds with the traditional medical perspective that they must also understand.

The Patient

The discussion above about diagnostic criteria for Psychological Factors Affecting Physical Condition included a partial list of patient characteristics to be considered in applying the biopsychosocial model. Axis I conditions are obviously relevant: Depression is common among patients with chronic physical illnesses (Rodin & Voshart, 1986). It threatens the patient's quality of life and may arise from the stress of the medical illness and its treatment. However, depression in this population is additionally important in that it has been statistically associated with poor medical outcomes for many types of chronic disease (Burton, Kline, Lindsay, & Heidenheim, 1986; Carney, Rich, & Freedland, 1988; Frasure-Smith, Lesperance, & Talajic, 1993). Although precise mechanisms have not been articulated, it is likely that depression exerts indirect effects on the illness through either psychobiological or behavioral mediating mechanisms. It is also important to note that some diseases and medical treatments can produce symptoms of depression. For example, pancreatic cancer and therapeutic corticosteroid medications often cause depressive symptoms.

Other Axis I conditions that are common and clinically quite important include alcohol and other substance abuse disorders, anxiety disorders, organic mental disorders, and adjustment disorders. Each of these conditions can be influenced by chronic illness, can affect the illness directly or indirectly, or can alter the patient's ability to participate effectively in its management.

Personality traits or disorders and coping styles similarly can influence the course of chronic illness and the patient's adjustment to it, through either physiological or behavioral mechanisms. Impulsive patients or those dealing with their illness through denial or minimization may engage in unhealthy behaviors (e.g., continued smoking) or may fail to comply with medication prescriptions (e.g., Levine et al., 1987). Chronic anger and hostility have been implicated in the development of some diseases, presumably through the psychophysiological effects of acute anger and stressful interpersonal conflicts (T. W. Smith, 1992). Hostility may also jeopardize the collaborative relationships between patient and health care team that are necessary to effectively manage the disease.

The patient's understanding and expectations concerning the illness, its prognosis, and the procedures involved in its management significantly influence emotional adjustment, compliance, and the outcome of treatment (Leventhal, Diefenbach, & Leventhal, 1992). Beliefs concerning the nature and cause of an illness and whether important symptoms or the course of an illness can be controlled may affect help-seeking behavior, functional skills, and depressive symptoms (Nicassio, Wallston, Callahan, Herbert, & Pincus, 1985). Evaluating this nexus of illness cognitions is an essential task for the clinical health psychologist, one that requires considerable medical knowledge and communication with other members of the health care team, as we discussed previously (see also Turk & Salovey, chap. 7, this book). Furthermore, any aspects of cognitive or intellectual functioning that might influence the patient's views are important considerations, as are coping styles that might influence his or her willingness or ability to process relevant information. Thus, the patients' phenomenological representation of the illness and its treatment is an important determinant of behaviorally mediated psychosocial effects on health.

Often overlooked in the evaluation of the patient is his or her educational and vocational training and employment history. A person's skills, physical capabilities, and job demands are important features of the biopsychosocial impact of his or her illness. These factors often moderate the impact of stressful aspects of the illness and its treatment on subsequent emotional and social functioning. Many patients face a vocational crisis when chronic illness prevents them from returning to jobs they held before getting sick, especially when their prior training has not prepared them for alternative avenues of employment. The need to change jobs may represent a major threat to the identity and self-esteem of the patient, a problem that may itself become the focus of clinical attention.

The Social, Familial, and Cultural Contexts

Social relationships are important features of a biopsychosocial description of chronic illness. Marital and family relationships are often disrupted by chronic illness, becoming one of the more important psychosocial effects of chronic illness. Changes in role demands within families may result when patients experience various degrees of disability because of their illness. Frequently, such role changes involve having spouses and other family members assume increased responsibility to compensate for various losses, financial and otherwise, caused by the patient's illness. The stressful nature of such changes may have negative emotional consequences for family members and, in some instances, may lead to interpersonal conflict with the patient. It is important for clinicians to assess the preexisting nature of these relationships as well as changes over the course of the illness. Some relationships may be able to withstand the effects of chronic illness more effectively than others. In many chronic illnesses, sexual relationships may be adversely affected—either by physiological features of the disease itself, side effects of medication, psychological sequelae of the illness, or interpersonal conflicts (B. J. Anderson & Wolf, 1986). Sexual difficulties may constitute a hidden source of distress in the marital relationship, because both patients and clinicians may be reluctant to address such issues within the context of the health care setting.

Although chronic illness may significantly affect important social and family relationships, these relationships may have an equally profound influence on the patient. Expressions of symptoms, illness behaviors, or functional limitations are apt to occur in the context of interactions with friends and family members. Indeed, the family itself can be viewed as the primary social context affecting the acquisition of illness beliefs, health behaviors, and the meaning and expression of symptoms (Litman, 1974). Families can exert a range of either positive or negative influences on the health status and psychosocial adjustment of patients (Flor & Turk, 1985; Kerns, chap. 6, this book). Family relationships may constitute an important source of social support for the patient, reducing the stressful impact of illness. In addition, the family may affect the development and use of coping mechanisms by the patient, compliance with medical regimens, recovery from surgical procedures, and performance in vocational roles. Thus, aspects of family and marital relationships can exert a variety of indirect and moderating effects on the disease and its impact.

The relationship of the patient to members of the health care team constitutes a second important social context. Effective communication between physician and patient can influence both the disease and its impact in beneficial ways: For example, it has been shown to contribute to better compliance with prescribed regimens, patient adjustment, and overall medical outcomes (Buller & Buller, 1987; DiMatteo, 1985). This communication is jointly influenced by characteristics of the patient and physician. Physicians sometimes fail to listen to patients sufficiently or to provide enough opportunities for patients to ask questions. They might, for example, use technical language when explaining important features of the illness and its treatment. At times, health care professionals deal with the demands of the work environment by depersonalizing the patient. In turn, the patient's anxiety or adoption of a passive role often undermines the effective exchange of information. These and other barriers to communication can be worsened in cases of chronic illnesses in which many professionals become involved. Fractionated care, differing opinions, and the patient's uncertainty regarding team members' specific functions and responsibilities increase as a function of the complexity of the required medical care.

The cultural background of the patient and health care team members can further complicate these difficulties in communication and effective collaboration. Differences in ethnic, educational, and socioeconomic background often make rapport, trust, and mutual understanding more difficult. Cultural influences on beliefs about health and illness, expression of symptoms, and health care seeking are common and often profound (see Young & Zane, chap. 5, this book).

Problems in patient care arising from the social and cultural aspects of a given case are often the focus of liaison activities for the clinical health psychologist. Rather than typically focusing on the patient in assessment and intervention consultations, the psychologist might more appropriately target the health care team. The clinical health psychologist is often in a unique position to help resolve such difficulties.

The Health Care System

The context of the health care system or organization is also an important consideration. Different types of delivery systems operate under different financial incentives, which, in turn, influence many aspects of patient care. For example, health maintenance organizations and traditional fee-for-service hospitals may provide different types of care for the same condition, within the range of appropriate treatment options. These organizational factors might also influence the number of primary physicians involved in the patient's care and the consistency of patient–physician contacts.

The patient's ability to pay for health care is often an important consideration when one is evaluating the role of psychological factors in chronic illness. For example, insurance coverage can influence a patient's willingness to comply with recommended treatments, and compensation for related disabilities can exert an important effect on emotional adjustment, social functioning, and even recovery rates.

Finally, the health care system can throw up barriers to the effective participation of patients in managing their illness. Transportation can be problematic, as can the fact that the potential cultural or demographic differences between patients and health care professionals may discourage patients from seeking needed treatment and from participating fully in their own care. Assessing and managing health care system concerns often takes the professional psychologist beyond traditional definitions of psychological services. It also underscores the necessity of the psychologist's ability to work collaboratively in interdisciplinary teams with other professionals (e.g., social workers).

Applying the Model to CHD

We now discuss a specific chronic medical illness to illustrate the general features of the biopsychosocial model. CHD provides a useful example for applying the model in clinical practice. Each year, 1.5 million Americans suffer an initial or recurrent myocardial infarction (MI), or heart attack, and over 500,000 die from the disease (American Heart Association, 1989). About 5 million Americans suffer from CHD, and about half of these cases experience some degree of disability or limitation as a result. The associated medical and economic (i.e., lost productivity) costs of this condition are estimated to be between 30 and 40 billion dollars per year. Thus, CHD is a prevalent and expensive chronic disease, and many psychosocial factors are involved in its development, course, management, and impact.

The Illness and Its Usual Management

To understand the illness itself, it is important to note that three distinct clinical events are indicative of CHD—angina pectoris, MI, and sudden cardiac death. *Angina* is the recurrent chest pain associated with insufficient amounts of oxygen reaching the heart muscle (i.e., ischemia). *MI* refers to the actual death of a portion of heart muscle (i.e., myocardium) following prolonged ischemia. *Sudden cardiac death* typically results from a catastrophic disorganization in the rhythm of heart muscle contractions, specifically, ventricular fibrillation. Each of these clinical manifestations of CHD reflects the underlying condition of coronary artery disease—the slow, progressive narrowing of the arteries otherwise supplying blood to the myocardium due to the buildup of fatty deposits on the interior artery walls. Sudden, complete blockage of a partially closed coronary artery can occur if a blood clot lodges in the narrowed passage.

The prognosis of CHD and its impact on psychosocial functioning are influenced by several medical factors. The number, severity, and specific locations of coronary artery disease lesions are important, as is the level of physical exertion required to elicit angina and other indications of myocardial ischemia. For post-MI patients, the location and extent of myocardial damage is a critical consideration, as is the effectiveness of the damaged heart in pumping blood (i.e., ejection fraction). In addition, patients vary considerably in the presence, severity, and potential lethality of their cardiac arrhythmias. These interrelated medical factors are key elements of the biopsychosocial context of CHD.

Acute CHD represents an obvious medical emergency, such as an impending or ongoing MI. The primary objectives of emergency care are to prevent or interrupt MI (e.g., through the use of clot-dissolving medication), to detect and treat arrhythmias, and to maintain adequate pumping function of the heart. Not surprisingly, this medical emergency is typically experienced by patients as an emotional crisis, because the prospect of death or serious disability is frightening.

Nonemergency care also raises many psychosocial issues that are typical of other chronic diseases. Clinically evaluating the extent and precise location of coronary artery disease lesions requires an invasive procedure: cardiac catheterization with coronary arteriography. In this radiographic procedure, a special dye is repeatedly administered through a catheter into the coronary arteries, producing an x-ray image of their interior. Patients are awake during this approximately 1- to 2-hour procedure and understandably describe it as emotionally stressful and uncomfortable. Brief psychological preparations for this procedure, such as coping skills training or modeling, have been effective in reducing its stressfulness (K. Anderson & Masur, 1989; Kendall et al., 1979). Results of this test and others are used in deciding among the various treatment approaches to the illness.

Medical management of CHD typically involves prescribing a program of progressive aerobic exercise training and one or more of three general classes of medications (i.e., nitrates, beta-blockers, and calcium channel blockers). CHD patients often have problems maintaining exercise programs, with most dropping out during their first 3 months (Carmody, Senner, Malinow, & Matarazzo, 1980; Dubbert, Rappaport, & Martin, 1987). Similarly, patients often do not follow their medication regimens, such as when side effects of beta-blockers (e.g., fatigue or decreased sexual activity) discourage appropriate use (see Dunbar-Jacob, Burke, & Puczynski, chap. 9, this book).

Doctors typically prescribe a variety of lifestyle changes for CHD patients because of the association of specific risk factors with future cardiac morbidity and mortality (Blumenthal & Emery, 1988). Smoking cessation is strongly encouraged, although only about one third to one half of smokers with CHD do quit smoking (Perkins, 1988). A low-fat diet is typically prescribed, given the atherogenic effects of high cholesterol. Overweight individuals are encouraged to lose weight through exercise and caloric restrictions. Finally, a combination of dietary restrictions, exercise, weight loss, and medication is often prescribed for CHD patients with high blood pressure. Despite the fact that such lifestyle interventions can be quite effective in managing CHD (e.g., Ornish et al., 1990), many patients do not comply with doctors' recommendations. The fact that patients' behavior figures so prominently in the routine medical management of CHD underscores the importance of the biopsychosocial, as opposed to the simple biomedical, perspective.

Psychological stress and related personality and social factors have been implicated as risk factors for the initial development of CHD (for reviews, see Krantz, Contrada, Hill & Friedler, 1988; T. W. Smith, 1992; Syme, 1987). Among patients with established CHD, high levels of stress have been associated with recurrent cardiac events and cardiac arrhythmias (Follick et al., 1988; Ruberman, Weinbla, Goldberg, & Chadhary, 1984). Emotionally stressful events or situations have also elicited temporary myocardial ischemia in many CHD patients (Barry et al., 1988; Rozanski et al., 1988). Such ischemic changes would in turn increase the likelihood of angina, MI, and potentially life-threatening arrhythmias. Thus, psychological stress can exert psychobiologically mediated indirect effects on underlying CAD and acute CHD events.

Researchers have found that interventions designed to reduce psychological stress and alter related personality characteristics can reduce recurrent cardiac events among CHD patients (Frasure-Smith & Prince, 1989; Powell & Thoresen, 1988). However, the traditional biomedical approach to the course and treatment of CHD does not involve considering psychological and social risk factors and interventions, which again, demonstrates the usefulness of the biopsychosocial approach for patient management.

Surgical treatment of CHD is typically accomplished through a coronary artery bypass graft. In the case of less severe coronary artery disease, balloon angioplasty can be used as a less invasive and stressful treatment; procedurally, this is similar to coronary artery angiography. In addition to the extensive physical trauma inherent to the graft procedure and the related physical discomfort, this surgery is usually experienced by patients and their families as highly stressful. As in the case of cardiac catheterization, brief psychological preoperative interventions have been shown to effectively facilitate patients' emotional adjustment before and after surgery, to reduce postoperative pain and complications, and even to reduce the likelihood of the postoperative delirium that sometimes accompanies this procedure (E. A. Anderson, 1987; Leserman, Stuart, Mamish, & Benson, 1989; Pimm & Feist, 1984; L. W. Smith & Dimsdale, 1989).

The Patient

CHD is often associated with pronounced disruption in patients' emotional, social, vocational, and sexual functioning. Although most patients return to relatively normal functioning following the acute crises posed by MI or coronary artery bypass graft surgery, a substantial minority continues to have clinically significant difficulties in one or more of these areas (Croog & Levine, 1982).

Most MI and bypass patients who were working previously return to work within a few months; this convalescence is medically appropriate. However, some take longer to return to work than is medically necessary, and some fail to resume employment altogether (Langeluddecke, Fulcher, Baird, Hughes, & Tennant, 1989). More severe disease, increasing age, less education, and employment in blue-collar occupations are all factors contributing to decreased likelihood of a patient returning to work (Dimsdale, Hackett, Hutter, & Block, 1982; Hlatky, Haney, & Barefoot, 1986). Anxiety, depression, and hypochondriasis are also associated with a decreased likelihood of returning to work (Dimsdale et al., 1982; Hlatky et al., 1986), as is the patient's belief that job stress contributed to his or her CHD (Bar-on & Cristal, 1987). Patients' expectations of returning to work are excellent predictors of later vocational functioning, and patients' confidence in their capabilities is a better predictor of later physical activity levels than are medical indicators of such capabilities (Ewart, Taylor, Reese, & DeBusk, 1983; Maeland & Havik, 1987). Thus, it is obvious that psychological factors are influential in one of the more personally and economically important outcomes of CHD.

Many CHD patients cope with the acute stress of MI or bypass graft surgery by denying or minimizing the seriousness of their condition (Blumenthal, 1982). Some evidence has suggested that such a coping style might be adaptive, at least initially. Denial in MI victims, for example, has been found to predict more rapid medical stabilization in the initial hours and days following a heart attack (Leserman et al., 1989; Levine et al., 1987). However, denial has also been associated with a decline in psychosocial functioning and compliance following discharge from the hospital (Havik & Maeland, 1988; Levine et al., 1987).

Depressed mood is a normal response in the days and weeks following MI or bypass graft surgery. However, some CHD patients develop more severe and lasting depressive conditions (Carney, Rich, & Tevelde, 1987; Croog & Levine, 1982). The clinical significance of this in the CHD population is underscored by findings indicating that major depression is associated with an increased risk of recurrent cardiac events, even when the severity of disease and other coronary risk factors are controlled for (Carney et al., 1988; Frasure-Smith et al., 1993).

CHD patients often report levels of sexual activity well below their premorbid levels (Papadopoulos, Shelley, Piccolo, Beaumont, & Barnett, 1986). Temporarily reduced sexual functioning is an appropriate reaction to MI or graft surgery and may even reflect the adaptive responses of well-functioning couples (Michela, 1987). However, prolonged difficulties do suggest a cause for concern. For example, decreased sexual interest and activity in cardiac patients sometimes reflect current or impending depressive episodes (Folks, Blake, Freeman, Sokol, & Baker, 1988). Erectile dysfunction and decreased desire are commonly reported side-effects of beta-blocking cardiac medications. Furthermore, some patients may curtail sexual activity because they fear that another cardiac event will be triggered through physical exertion (Papadopoulos et al., 1986).

The emotional, vocational, and social difficulties displayed by some CHD patients are quite amenable to treatment. Brief counseling interventions during hospitalization have been found to reduce distress and increase social and vocational activity levels in the months following MI and coronary artery bypass graft patients' discharge (e.g., Gruen, 1975; Langosch et al., 1982). Here again, the biopsychosocial perspective provides more comprehensive care of the patient with chronic illness, with the beneficial result of better psychosocial functioning.

Social Context

Marital and family relationships are also potentially important factors in the course, impact, and management of CHD. Among MI victims, the availability of marital and family support has been shown to reduce the likelihood of recurrent coronary events (Berkman, Leo-Summers, & Horowitz, 1992; Case, Moss, Case, McDermott, & Eberly, 1992; Chandra, Szklo, Goldberg, & Tonascia, 1983). Social support from spouses has also been associated with more rapid recovery following bypass graft surgery (Kulik & Mahler, 1989). Spouses of MI patients and other family members often report feeling insufficiently informed about prognosis, treatment, and rehabilitation (Bramwell, 1986). Directly involving the spouse when evaluating the patient's functional capability is useful in helping the spouse to develop a more thorough and accurate understanding of any physical limitations imposed by the disease (Taylor, Bandura, Ewart, Miller, & DeBusk, 1985). Furthermore, positive involvement of the spouse can help to maximize both the psychological and physical benefits of cardiac rehabilitation following MI or bypass surgery (Davidson, 1987).

We now return to the outline for clinical application of the biopsychosocial model, presented in Exhibit 3. It is clear how a variety of interacting aspects of illness and its treatment, patients' emotional status, personality, and vocational status, and surrounding family and other social contexts are essential features of health care problems posed by CHD. This illness has behavioral, emotional, and social causes and consequences, and its effective management involves biological, psychological, and even social interventions. A complete application of the model would also involve consideration of the availability and accessibility of, and insurance coverage for, acute cardiac care and subsequent rehabilitation.

This brief overview of the psychosocial aspects of CHD illustrates the potential value of the biopsychosocial model in the clinical management of chronic illness. This is not intended to underestimate the invaluable contributions from the traditional biomedical approach to the condition in diagnosis, treatment, and rehabilitation of patients with CHD. Rather, this review demonstrates the additional improvements in medical, emotional, social, and economic outcomes that can follow from adoption of this broader, interactional perspective.

Conclusion

The biopsychosocial model does not offer a specific blueprint for working with chronically ill patients because its application will justifiably vary from patient to patient, depending on the health outcomes of concern and factors identified as contributing to the outcomes of a particular case. Instead, adopting this framework allows the clinician to contextualize the patient's health problems by considering the full gamut of factors within different systems that may require specific evaluation and management. Health care interventions will differ in scope, complexity, the systems targeted, and specific techniques or treatments used to bring about change. The major strengths of this framework lie in its adaptability and accommodation to the needs of the individual patient, its flexibility of application, and the creative approaches to health care that follow from its implementation.

Chronic physical illness does indeed provide professional psychologists with important opportunities in the rapidly changing health care environment. Their clinical assessment and intervention skills can be of great use to many different patient populations and medical services. Yet, to successfully apply these skills, clinicians must transpose them to accommodate the unique circumstances of medical disorders and medical care environments. The biopsychosocial model is an invaluable guide for professional psychologists seeking to meet this challenge.

REFERENCES

American Heart Association. (1989). *Heart facts*. Dallas, TX: Author.

American Psychiatric Association. (1968). *Diagnostic and statistical manual of mental disorders* (2nd ed.). Washington, DC: Author.

American Psychiatric Association. (1980). *Diagnostic and statistical manual of mental disorders* (3rd ed.). Washington, DC: Author.

American Psychiatric Association. (1987). *Diagnostic and statistical manual of mental disorders* (3rd ed., revised). Washington, DC: Author.

American Psychiatric Association. (1994). *Diagnostic and statistical manual of mental disorders* (4th ed.). Washington, DC: Author.

Anderson, B. J., & Wolf, F. M. (1986). Chronic physical illness and sexual behavior: Psychological issues. *Journal of Consulting and Clinical Psychology, 54,* 168–175.

Anderson, E. A. (1987). Preoperative preparation for cardiac surgery facilitates recovery, reduces psychological distress, and reduces incidence of acute preoperative hypertension. *Journal of Consulting and Clinical Psychology, 55,* 513–520.

Anderson, K. O., & Masur, F. T. (1989). Psychologic preparation for cardiac catheterization. *Heart and Lung, 18,* 154–163.

Bar-on, D., & Cristal, N. (1987). Causal attributions of patients, their spouses and physicians, and the rehabilitation of the patients after their first myocardial infarction. *Journal of Cardiopulmonary Rehabilitation, 7,* 285–298.

Baron, R. M., & Kenny, D. A. (1986). The moderator–mediator variable distinction in social psychological research: Conceptual, strategic, and statistical considerations. *Journal of Personality and Social Psychology, 51,* 1173–1182.

Barry, J., Selwyn, A. P., Nabel, E. G., Rocco, M. B., Mead, K., Campbell, S., & Rebecca, G. (1988). Frequency of ST-depression produced by mental stress in stable angina pectoris from coronary artery disease. *American Journal of Cardiology, 61,* 989–993.

Belar, C. D. (1991). Professionalism in medical settings. In J. J. Sweet, R. H. Rozensky, & S. M. Tovian (Eds.), *Handbook of clinical psychology in medical settings* (pp. 81–92). New York: Plenum Press.

Berkman, L. F., Leo-Summers, L., & Horowitz, R. I. (1992). Emotional support and survival after myocardial infarction. *Annals of Internal Medicine, 117,* 1003–1009.

Bloom, B. R., & Murray, C. J. L. (1992). Tuberculosis: Commentary on a re-emergent killer. *Science, 257,* 1055–1061.

Blumenthal, J. A. (1982). Assessment of patients with coronary heart disease. In F. J. Keefe & J. A. Blumenthal (Eds.), *Assessment strategies in behavioral medicine* (pp. 37–97). New York: Grune & Stratton.

Blumenthal, J. A., & Emery, C. F. (1988). Rehabilitation of patients following myocardial infarction. *Journal of Consulting and Clinical Psychology, 56,* 374–381.

Bramwell, L. (1986). Wives' experiences in the support role after husbands' first myocardial infarction. *Heart and Lung, 15,* 578–584.

Brown, G. K., Nicassio, P. M., & Wallston, K. W. (1989). Pain coping strategies and depression in rheumatoid arthritis. *Journal of Consulting and Clinical Psychology, 57,* 652–657.

Buller, M. K., & Buller, D. B. (1987). Physicians' communication style and patient satisfaction. *Journal of Health and Social Behavior, 28,* 375–388.

Burton, H. J., Kline, S. A., Lindsay, R. M., & Heidenheim, A. P. (1986). The relationship of depression to survival in chronic renal failure. *Psychosomatic Medicine, 48,* 261–269.

Carmody, T. P., Senner, J. W., Malinow, M. R., & Matarazzo, J. D. (1980). Physical exercise rehabilitation: Long-term dropout rate in cardiac patients. *Journal of Behavioral Medicine, 3,* 163–168.

Carney, R. M., Rich, M. W., & Freedland, K. E. (1988). Major depressive disorder predicts cardiac events in patients with coronary-artery disease. *Psychosomatic Medicine, 50,* 627–633.

Carney, R. M., Rich, M. W., & Tevelde, A. (1987). Major depressive disorder in coronary artery disease. *American Journal of Cardiology, 60,* 1273–1275.

Case, R. B., Moss, A. J., Case, N., McDermott, M., & Eberly, S. (1992). Living alone after myocardial infarction: Impact on prognosis. *Journal of the American Medical Association, 267,* 515–519.

Catania, J. A., Kegeles, S. M., & Coates, T. J. (1990). Towards an understanding of risk behavior: An AIDS risk reduction model (ARRM). *Health Education Quarterly, 17,* 53–72.

Chandra, V., Szklo, M., Goldberg, R., & Tonascia, J. (1983). The impact of marital status on survival after an acute myocardial infarction: A population-based study. *American Journal of Epidemiology, 117,* 320–325.

Cohen, S. (1988). Psychosocial models of the role of social support in the etiology of physical disease. *Health Psychology, 7,* 269–297.

Cohen, S., & Wills, T. H. (1985). Stress, social support, and the buffering hypothesis. *Psychological Bulletin, 98,* 310–357.

Croog, S. H., & Levine, S. (1982). *Life after a heart attack: Social and psychological factors eight years later.* New York: Human Sciences Press.

Davidson, D. M. (1987). Social support and cardiac rehabilitation: A review. *Journal of Cardiopulmonary Rehabilitation, 7,* 196–200.

DiMatteo, M. R. (1985). Physician–patient communication: Promoting a positive health care setting. In J. C. Rosen & L. J. Solomon (Eds.), *Prevention in health psychology* (pp. 328–365). Hanover, NH: University Press of New England.

Dimsdale, J. E., Hackett, T. P., Hutter, A. M., & Block, P. C. (1982). The association of clinical, psychosocial, and angiographic variables with work status in patients with coronary artery disease. *Journal of Psychosomatic Research, 26,* 215–221.

Dubbert, P. M., Rappaport, N. B., & Martin, J. E. (1987). Exercise in cardiovascular disease. *Behavior Modification, 11,* 329–347.

Engel, G. L. (1977). The need for a new medical model: A challenge to biomedicine. *Science, 196,* 129–136.

Engel, G. L. (1980). The clinical application of the biopsychosocial model. *American Journal of Psychiatry, 137,* 535–544.

Ewart, C. K., Taylor, C. B., Reese, L. B., & DeBusk, R. F. (1983). Effects of early postmyocardial infarction exercise testing of self-perception and subsequent physical activity. *American Journal of Cardiology, 51,* 1076–1080.

Flor, H., & Turk, D. C. (1985). Chronic illness in an adult family member: Pain as a prototype. In D. C. Turk & R. D. Kerns (Eds.), *Health, illness, and families: A life-span perspective* (pp. 255–278). New York: Wiley.

Folks, D. G., Blake, D. J., Freeman, A. M., Sokol, R. S., & Baker, D. M. (1988). Persistent depression in coronary bypass patients reporting sexual maladjustment. *Psychosomatics, 29,* 387–391.

Follick, M. J., Gorkin, L., Capone, R. J., Smith, T. W., Ahern, D. K., Stabein, D., Niaura, R., & Visco, J. (1988). Psychological distress as a predictor of ventricular arrhythmias in a post-myocardial infarction population. *American Heart Journal, 116,* 32–36.

Frasure-Smith, N., Lesperance, F., & Talajic, M. (1993). Depression following myocardial infarction: Impact on 6-month survival. *Journal of the American Medical Association, 270,* 1819–1825.

Frasure-Smith, N., & Prince, R. (1989). Long-term follow-up of the Ischemic Heart Disease Life Stress Monitoring Program. *Psychosomatic Medicine, 51,* 485–513.

Gruen, W. (1975). Effects of brief psychotherapy during the hospitalization period on the recovery process in heart attacks. *Journal of Consulting and Clinical Psychology, 43,* 223–232.

Havik, O. E., & Maeland, J. G. (1988). Verbal denial and outcome in myocardial infarction patients. *Journal of Psychosomatic Research, 32,* 145–157.

Haynes, S. N., & O'Brien, W. H. (1990). Functional analysis in behavior therapy. *Clinical Psychology Review, 10,* 649–668.

Hlatky, M. A., Haney, T., & Barefoot, J. C. (1986). Medical, psychological, and social correlates of work disability among men with coronary artery disease. *American Journal of Cardiology, 58,* 911–915.

Kendall, P. C., Williams, L., Pechacek, T. F., Graham, L. E., Shisslak, C., & Herzoll, N. (1979). Cognitive–behavioral and patient education interventions in cardiac catheterization procedures: The Palo Alto Medical Psychology Project. *Journal of Consulting and Clinical Psychology, 47,* 49–58.

Krantz, D. S., Contrada, R. J., Hill, R. O., & Friedler, E. (1988). Environmental stress and biobehavioral antecedents of coronary heart disease. *Journal of Consulting and Clinical Psychology, 56,* 333–341.

Kulik, J. A., & Mahler, H. I. M. (1989). Social support and recovery from surgery. *Health Psychology, 8,* 221–238.

Langeluddecke, P., Fulcher, G., Baird, D., Hughes, C., & Tennant, C. (1989). A prospective evaluation of the psychosocial effects of coronary artery bypass surgery. *Journal of Psychosomatic Research, 26,* 475–484.

Langosch, W., Seer, P., Brodner, G., Kallinke, D., Kulick, B., & Heim, F. (1982). Behavior therapy with coronary heart disease patients: Results of a comparative study. *Journal of Psychosomatic Research, 26,* 475–484.

Leserman, J., Stuart, E. M., Mamish, M. E., & Benson, H. (1989). Denial and medical outcome in unstable angina. *Psychosomatic Medicine, 51,* 27–35.

Leventhal, H. S., Diefenbach, M., & Leventhal, E. A. (1992). Illness cognition: Using common sense to understand treatment adherence and affect cognition interactions. *Cognitive Therapy and Research, 16,* 143–163.

Levine, J., Warrenburg, S., Kerns, R., Schwartz, G., Delaney, R., Fontana, A., Gradman, A., Smith, S., Allen, S., & Cascione, R. (1987). The role of denial in recovery from coronary heart disease. *Psychosomatic Medicine, 49,* 109–117.

Litman, T. J. (1974). The family as a basic unit in health and medical care: A behavioral overview. *Social Science and Medicine, 8,* 495–519.

Maeland, J. G., & Havik, O. E. (1987). Psychological predictors for return to work after a myocardial infarction. *Journal of Psychosomatic Research, 31,* 471–481.

Michela, J. L. (1987). Interpersonal and individual impacts of a husband's heart attack. In A. Baum & J. E. Singer (Eds.), *Handbook of psychology and health: Vol. 5.* Stress (pp. 255–301). Hillsdale, NJ: Erlbaum.

National Center for Health Statistics. (1992). *Vital statistics of the United States, 1992.* Washington, DC: U.S. Government Printing Office.

Nicassio, P. M., Wallston, K. A., Callahan, L. F., Herbert, M., & Pincus, T. (1985). The measurement of helplessness in rheumatoid arthritis: The development of the Arthritis Helplessness Index. *Journal of Rheumatology, 12,* 462–467.

Ornish, D., Brown, S. E., Scherwitz, L. W., Billings, J. H., Armstrong, W. T., Ports, T. A., McLanahan, S. M., Kirkeeide, R. L., & Gould, K. L. (1990). Can lifestyle changes reverse coronary heart disease? *Lancet, 336,* 129–133.

Papadopoulus, C., Shelley, S. I., Piccolo, M., Beaumont, C., & Barnett, L. (1986). Sexual activity after coronary bypass surgery. *Chest, 90,* 681–685.

Perkins, K. A. (1988). Maintaining smoking abstinence after myocardial infarction. *Journal of Substance Abuse, 1,* 91–107.

Pimm, J. B., & Feist, J. R. (1984). *Psychological risks of coronary bypass surgery.* New York: Plenum.

Powell, L. H., & Thoresen, C. E. (1988). Effects of Type A behavioral counseling and severity of prior acute myocardial infarction on survival. *American Journal of Cardiology, 62,* 1159–1163.

Rodin, G., & Voshart, K. (1986). Depression in the medically ill: An overview. *American Journal of Psychiatry, 143,* 696–705.

Rozanski, A., Bairey, C. S., Krantz, D. S., Friedman, J., Resser, K. J., Morrell, M., Hilton-Chalfen, S., Hestrin, L., Bietendorf, J., & Berman, D. S. (1988).

Mental stress and the induction of silent myocardial infarction. *New England Journal of Medicine, 311,* 552–559.

Ruberman, W., Weinbla, H. E., Goldberg, J. D., & Chadhary, B. S. (1984). Psychosocial influences on mortality after myocardial infarction. *New England Journal of Medicine, 311,* 552–559.

Schwartz, G. E. (1982). Testing the biopsychosocial model: The ultimate challenge facing behavioral medicine? *Journal of Consulting and Clinical Psychology, 50,* 1040–1053.

Smith, L. W., & Dimsdale, J. E. (1989). Postcardiotomy delirium: Conclusions after 25 years? *American Journal of Psychiatry, 146,* 452–458.

Smith, T. W. (1992). Hostility and health: Current status of a psychosomatic hypothesis. *Health Psychology, 11,* 139–150.

Syme, S. L. (1987). Coronary artery disease: A sociocultural perspective. *Circulation, 76*(Suppl. 1), 112–116.

Taylor, C. B., Bandura, A., Ewart, C. K., Miller, N. H., & DeBusk, R. F. (1985). Exercise testing to enhance wives' confidence in their husbands' cardiac capability soon after clinically uncomplicated acute myocardial infarction. *American Journal of Cardiology, 55,* 635–638.

von Bertalanffy, L. (1968). *General systems theory.* New York: Braziller.

Chapter

2

Roles of the Clinical Health Psychologist in the Management of Chronic Illness

Cynthia D. Belar and Michael E. Geisser

Until the mid-1960s, the major role for psychologists in treating chronic illness was to assess psychopathology in patients. With the growth of knowledge regarding the importance of psychosocial factors in the etiology and maintenance of chronic illness, psychologists have become more expert in brain–behavior relationships; issues of compliance and coping; and measurement of behavioral, affective, cognitive, and psychophysiological aspects of illness. Psychological interventions aimed at modifying etiologic factors, concomitant symptoms, and disease sequelae have been developed, and over the past several decades, clinical health psychologists have come to occupy multiple roles in the management of chronic illness—consultant, teacher, researcher, administrator, and health care service provider. In this chapter, we describe the roles of the clinical health psychologist in the management of chronic illness. Although the roles presented above are not mutually exclusive and, in fact, do more often overlap, they are discussed separately below for organizational purposes.

Psychologist as Health Care Service Provider

Patient services related to managing chronic illness include psychological assessment, intervention, and consultation activities. Although there are no data on psychologists who work solely with chronic illness problems, as a group, clinical health psychologists do spend from 35% to 60% of their professional time in direct service activities (Morrow & Clayman, 1982).

Assessment

The assessment services of clinical health psychologists can be used to perform many different functions associated with diagnosis and treatment of people who are chronically ill.

Differential diagnosis. In some cases, psychological assessment methods are an integral part of the medical diagnostic process itself. For example, an assessment may be directed toward making a differential diagnosis of dementia versus depression or of malingering versus chronic pain syndrome. Clinical health psychologists are also frequently asked to distinguish various medical conditions from either somatoform disorders (such as conversion disorder) or a factitious disorder (e.g., Munchausen syndrome). Given that psychological assessment methods in general have not been shown to have good sensitivity or specificity for making these diagnoses, decisions regarding these diagnoses are often made on the basis of clinical judgment and the lack of an organic basis for the patient's symptoms. Thus, it is important for the psychologist assessing a chronically ill patient to work in close consultation with the physician who is responsible for the medical diagnostic procedures.

Although some medical diagnostic procedures are highly accurate, the clinical health psychologist should not assume that lack of medical evidence for a patient's symptoms rules out an underlying pathophysiological process. In some cases an underlying physical cause is too early to detect medically. Moreover, some physical causes of chronic illnesses (e.g., myofascial pain) are difficult to substantiate through medical diagnostic testing.

In cases where the cause of the patient's symptoms is not clear, the psychologist should consider the impact that labeling a patient with a psychological diagnosis may have on his or her subsequent medical care, particularly in cases where the patient has a history of medical difficulties that produced the same or similar symptoms. For example, one of us was referred a chronic pain patient who had been previously diagnosed as having hysterical features and drug dependence. The referring physician believed that her current pain complaints reflected her desire to obtain narcotic medications. The patient had a history of spinal tumor, but the physician indicated that current examinations were normal, and he referred her for therapy for substance abuse. However, the patient's pain continued to increase, and she subsequently went to another physician, who conducted further diagnostic testing; this time she was found to have another spinal tumor. The original physician's opinion that the patient's pain complaints were psychologically based had influenced decisions regarding diagnostic studies and follow-up.

More consistent with a biopsychosocial approach to illness and with the fact that most diseases are influenced by both physical and psychosocial factors to varying degrees, clinical health psychologists are also frequently asked to assess whether there is a significant psychosocial contribution to a person's illness. This type of approach to "diagnosing" a person's illness fosters a collaborative and comprehensive approach to addressing the patient's medical and psychosocial needs.

Provision of treatment. Other assessments are oriented toward decision making regarding various treatments after the diagnosis of chronic illness is already established. The following types of questions are frequently addressed by clinical health psychologists: Is this patient a good candidate for cardiac transplant? Could this patient comply with, for example, a home dialysis regimen? Is this patient competent to make a decision regarding termination of life support systems? Is this patient likely to benefit from, for example, bariatric surgery? What are the chances of good functional recovery after surgery for this patient? Psychologists are either integral members of multidisciplinary teams that make these decisions or consultants to the physician responsible for final decision making. Their input can therefore vary: from providing definitive opinions about a patient's psychological readiness to undergo a procedure, to recommending that a patient (a) be treated for a particular problem and reevaluated for readiness for the procedure once treatment is completed or (b) receive concurrent treatment to facilitate the likelihood of a favorable outcome. For example, in the case of a cardiac transplant candidate who is a smoker, the psychologist can recommend that he or she undergo smoking cessation treatment and be reevaluated for transplantation if he or she can remain abstinent for a specific period of time. The psychologist can also recommend that the patient continue to undergo relapse prevention therapy if cardiac transplantation takes place.

Treatment planning. Other assessments serve to provide an understanding of the concomitants of a chronic disease, the sequelae of a particular event, and issues of individual differences and reaction to illness so as to facilitate either medical or psychological treatment planning. For example, the clinical health psychologist may need to delineate the cognitive deficits in an AIDS patient to plan for appropriate support services. In other cases, medical and nursing staff need to be alerted to issues that are likely to affect adherence to medical regimens—a major area of concern in chronic illness. Anxiety and depression components in chronic pain patients must be identified and treated if medical treatment is to be maximally effective, or effective at all. Individual and family coping strategies need to be understood to foster adaptation among cancer patients. Muscle tension components of muscle contraction headache and myofascial pain syndromes must be delineated to design biofeedback treatment. And individual psychopathology must be understood before these services are provided to any patient. The role of the psychologist in these activities may be as either a consultant providing information to other providers of treatment or the primary clinician who gathers assessment data to be used for planning the psychological treatment to be provided.

Intervention

Intervention services of clinical health psychologists can be directed toward the patient, the family, the health care system, or sociocultural features of the environment of patients with chronic illness. In many cases, the intervention is carried out by others with whom the psychologist consults.

Patient. The psychologist may serve as an individual therapist to the patient and, in that role, may provide interventions to accomplish one or more of the following goals: (a) relieving symptoms (e.g., using hypnosis for cancer pain or managing anxiety for terminally ill patients); (b) controlling behavior related to specific physical problems (e.g., using biofeedback to control fecal incontinence or desensitization techniques for anticipatory nausea associated with chemotherapy); (c) achieving adherence to medical regimens (e.g., monitoring glucose in people with diabetes or medication compliance in people with hypertension); (d) preparing for stressful medical procedures (e.g., stress inoculation training before open heart surgery; (e) coping with the chronic illness itself (e.g., stress management for patients with multiple sclerosis or sexual counseling for disease-related impotence problems), and (f) dealing with emotional and behavioral problems that may exacerbate the disease itself or interfere with rehabilitation (e.g., alcohol abuse among those with chronic liver disease, poor self-esteem among obese patients, body image problems among those with arthritis, and anger management among cardiac patients).

Family. The psychologist's role may also involve family interventions, either to facilitate one of the goals described above or as a primary focus of intervention itself. For example, marital therapy may be required to help patients deal successfully with a chronic headache problem because marital stress and conflict may precipitate many of the headache episodes, and family counseling is often needed when chronic disease results in major role reversals. Family members must also learn when their behavior inhibits rehabilitation (e.g., unwitting reinforcement of pain behavior, such as assisting the patient too much with the activities of daily living) and should be taught how to respond to the patient to help facilitate recovery (e.g., praise for completing exercises and increasing independence). In some cases, intervention designed to modify a family's maladaptive response to the threatened loss (e.g., increased blaming of other family members for the patient's condition) of a loved one may be the sole intervention provided by a clinical health psychologist.

Health care system. More often than not, the role of the psychologist is to intervene at the level of the health care system. Among other activities, psychologists counsel nursing, physical therapy, and occupational therapy staff to help them develop more effective relations with patients; for example, by teaching assertiveness skills to help them deal with and decrease demanding patient behavior. Psychologists also help health care providers deal with the stressors of particular health care environments (such as intensive care units) by teaching stress management skills that may help decrease the affective impact of their jobs and, it is hoped, increase job satisfaction. Otherwise, nurses who work in high-stress units and frequently experience death may develop feelings of hopelessness and helplessness that can lead to withdrawal from patients. Finally, a clinical health psychologist may provide information to a physician about the psychosocial aspects of a particular patient (e.g., their health beliefs or personality style) that may decrease a physician's frustration with a particular patient, facilitate good patient–doctor relations, and lead to increased patient compliance and satisfaction.

Sociocultural context. Clinical health psychologists also intervene in the sociocultural context of chronic disease. For example, the psychologist may counsel employers on such issues as activity pacing or job modification to facilitate the return to work of patients with chronic pain or may consult with community service organizations to design a self-help group for, say, patients with systemic lupus erythematosus. Although interventions at this level are sometimes neglected by clinicians, they often play a critical role in rehabilitation attempts.

Psychologist as Teacher

To provide the direct services described above, the psychologist must assume the role of teacher, because it is well accepted that education is a major component of all treatment. Thus, psychologists are teachers of their patients, as well as patients' families, their health care providers and their relevant social–occupational contacts regarding individual patients' needs and concerns.

Patient education can serve several purposes. First, educating the patient regarding the role of psychosocial factors in the etiology and maintenance of disease helps to increase understanding of the psychologist's role in health care and helps promote patient acceptance that psychological interventions can affect health and health behavior. In addition, education regarding psychosocial influences on health may help patients develop better self-care and self-management skills, which in turn may decrease the impact of disease and prevent future health complications. Second, patient education is also believed to importantly affect increasing patient compliance. Research has demonstrated that increasing patients' knowledge of their treatment regimen and instructing them on how to implement treatment regimens are important factors in increasing adherence (Meichenbaum & Turk,

1987). Third, education regarding the development and implementation of self-management skills, such as relaxation training and cognitive and behavioral coping skills, has been found to be beneficial to patients by helping them cope with their illness and other stressors.

In addition to services related to a specific patient, clinical health psychologists serve in a variety of other teaching roles in the management of chronic illness. For example, they provide continuing education programs for many health care disciplines, including physicians, nurses, dentists, physical therapists, and pharmacists. This role, although not related to a specific patient, is nevertheless a very important one in the management of chronic illness. Other disciplines often have more continuing contact with patients, and many psychological interventions are actually delivered by these members of the health care team.

Clinical health psychologists also participate in educating and training future and practicing professional psychologists through lecturing and scholarly endeavors. Teaching at the community level may involve participating in health education programs and health advisory councils, as more communities concern themselves not only with the prevention and management of known chronic illnesses but also with the impact of such problems as noise level, environmental threats, victimization, and crowding on community health. Psychologists teaching in industry might provide knowledge of work-site health promotion, disease prevention, and such illness-management programs as stress management, weight control, and "behavior and your health" type programs. These programs often reach more people if implemented in the workplace than if offered in a hospital or outpatient care setting.

Finally, it is not uncommon for the psychologist to assume a teaching role by preparing briefs or testimony for government groups considering policies or legislation likely to significantly affect the management of chronic illness. For example, in the early 1980s, Belar engaged in an informal educational process with the worker's compensation board of the state of Florida during its development of policies for authorizing treatment in chronic pain programs.

Psychologist as Researcher

The clinical health psychologist as researcher has a very important role in chronic illness, in that psychologists create new knowledge in the areas of prevention, etiology, treatment, and rehabilitation that is crucial to successful management. For example, the most successful management strategy for AIDS at present is to adopt behaviors that prevent the spread of HIV infection. The body of knowledge related to behavior change and health promotion is, of course, fundamental. With regard to etiology, psychologists conducting research in psychoneuroimmunology are making major contributions to the basic understanding of chronic disease—its precursors, onset, and mechanisms. Psychologists have also substantially contributed to the body of knowledge regarding treatment of chronic disease (e.g., psychophysiological self-regulation, psychological management of pain, adherence to medical regimens, preparation for stressful medical procedures, coping with illness, and the impact of treatment environments).

Additional roles for psychologists include program developer and program evaluator—roles for which good research skills are also required. The measurement, design, and data-analysis skills obtained during research training are fundamental to (a) assessment of quality of care, (b) analysis of cost-effectiveness, (c) documentation of service needs, (d) systematic clinical management, and (e) measurement of quality of life—all of which are being increasingly demanded by society and the health care industry.

Although professionals in a number of other disciplines are independently licensed to provide the direct patient services described above, roles involving clinical research are ones for which psychologists are uniquely trained. In our opinion, the scientist–practitioner clinical health psychologist has the brightest future for contributing to the management of chronic illness, because it is the integration of scientific and practice skills that fosters the development of new treatments and methods of service delivery. It is the empirical approach that will ensure the survival of psychology through the health care revolution.

Psychologist as Administrator

Many clinical health psychologists occupy positions involving a significant amount of administrative activity that can affect the management of chronic illness. For example, as chief psychologist in a major health maintenance organization, Belar (1991a) advocated services for preventing and managing chronic disease. She has designed and implemented programs across administrative units for chronic headache sufferers. She also established the Behavioral Medicine Team and a Behavioral Health Service that provided diagnostic, treatment, and behavioral health promotion programs for a wide variety of problems associated with chronic illness. Although not responsible for the design itself, she administratively encouraged and supported team psychologists to establish Alzheimer's caretakers' groups, a behavioral cardiac rehabilitation program, and HIV-positive support groups. Other psychologists have developed and administered the psychological and behavioral components of rehabilitation programs in the areas of chronic obstructive pulmonary disease, spinal cord injury, diabetes self-management, and coping with arthritis, to name only a few. Prevention programs have focused on HIV infection, periodontal disease, lung disease, cancer, cardiovascular disease, and presurgical counseling. Psychologists also take on multidisciplinary-team leadership roles that have administrative components—leading psychosocial rounds, coordinating team activities, and infusing interdisciplinary teams with psychological sophistication that directly facilitates treatment appropriate to patient needs.

Psychologists in administrative roles also have a significant impact on the management of chronic illness through their support of good quality assurance programs. As Jospe, Shueman, and Troy (1991) noted, such support is critical to the survival of a good quality assurance program, which in turn ensures that quality care is being delivered to those who are chronically ill.

In general, it is our opinion that clinical health psychologists in administrative roles have more potential than do psychologists who function solely as individual service providers to affect the provision and maintenance of quality care to people who are chronically ill. Those who work at legislative levels have perhaps the most impact, in that they can promote smoke-free environments, accessibility to health care, and environmental design friendly to those with disabilities, among other efforts that are fundamental to the management of chronic illness.

Practice Issues in Managing Chronic Illness

In carrying out the roles described above, clinical health psychologists are likely to encounter a variety of issues that require careful attention to practice ethically and to maximize their effectiveness in the management of chronic illness. An extensive review of practice issues is outside the scope of this chapter and can be found elsewhere (Belar, 1991b; Belar & Deardorff, 1995), but a brief overview is provided below.

Competence to Practice

In performing the functions required by their many roles, clinical health psychologists need to possess the knowledge, skills, and attitudes fundamental to professional practice in this area. Recognizing these needs, leaders in the field gathered in May 1983 for the National Working Conference on Education and Training in Health Psychology, sponsored by the Division of Health Psychology (Stone, 1983). Three of the conference recommendations regarding service provision in health psychology are particularly noteworthy here.

First, the scientist–practitioner model was endorsed at every level of training. The integration of science and practice, and the ability to conduct both consistent with the highest standards in psychology were considered fundamental to the role of the clinical health psychologist.

Second, in addition to advocating core education and training in psychology and professional psychology within an APA-accredited program, conference delegates agreed that service providers in health psychology should be broadly trained in the following areas:

1. Biological bases of health and disease
2. Social bases of health and disease
3. Psychological bases of health and disease
4. Health assessment, consultation, and intervention
5. Health policy and organization
6. Interdisciplinary collaboration
7. Ethical, legal, and professional issues
8. Statistics and experimental design in health research.

Third, supervised training in a health care setting by experienced professional health psychology mentors was considered crucial. Skills in interdisciplinary collaboration and knowledge of the sociopolitical aspects of health care settings (e.g., hospitals, managed care systems, rehabilitation centers, and nursing homes) were considered fundamental to successful practice. Professional behavior can spell the difference between success and disuse of psychological services, because consultees can often better judge quality of service than quality of care.

For health service providers, conference delegates asserted the need for a 2-year postdoctoral training program, the parameters of which have been more fully developed by Sheridan et al. (1988). These authors noted that to be

> properly prepared for the role of health service provider, the health psychologist must be (a) familiar with and comfortable with today's medical settings. . . , (b) skilled in a broad range of diagnostic techniques and capable of rendering treatment for a wide variety of conditions. . . , (c) familiar with and experienced in disease prevention/health promotion strategies, (d) competent in consultation and related writing skills, and (e) an individual who appreciates the value of interdisciplinary collaboration. (p. 8)

Although these standards are useful in providing the underpinnings for practice related to chronic illness, the particular health problems dealt with by a clinical health psychologist require additional knowledge specific to the pathophysiology, illness course, medical management, and treatment settings involved. For example, the knowledge base of the psychologist counseling patients with diabetes will differ from that of the psychologist providing services to patients recovering from stroke. The former requires more understanding of immunology, measurement of blood glucose, nutrition, peripheral neuropathies, relationships between behavior and insulin levels, and outpatient ambulatory care services. The latter requires more expertise in human brain functioning, the impact of trauma, prosthetic environments, cognitive skills training, relationships between brain damage and affect, and rehabilitation settings. However, both psychologists require knowledge and skills related to psychological coping, management of pain, adherence to treatment regimens, and working with other health care disciplines in addition to the training described above.

With respect to specific skills, Sheridan et al. (1988) indicated that health psychologists should be competent in at least six of the following 14 areas:

1. Relaxation therapies
2. Short-term psychotherapy
3. Group therapy
4. Family therapy

5. Consultation skills
6. Liaison skills
7. Assessment of specific patient populations (e.g., pain patients or spinal-cord-injury patients)
8. Neuropsychological assessment
9. Behavior modification techniques
10. Biofeedback
11. Hypnosis
12. Health promotion and public education skills
13. Major treatment programs (e.g., chemical dependence or pain management)
14. Compliance motivation.

Managing chronic illness demands all of these skills from the profession of clinical health psychology, even if individual psychologists do not possess each and every one. However, it is hard to imagine how any health care provider of services to people who are chronically ill could manage without expertise in at least consultation, relaxation, short-term treatment, family therapy, and compliance.

The professional practice of health psychology has been formally recognized as a specialty by the American Board of Professional Psychology since 1991. Diplomates in Health Psychology from this board are granted through the American Board of Health Psychology to psychologists who have demonstrated an advanced level of competency in practice. After credentials review, candidates submit work samples and participate in an examination process to demonstrate professional and scientific knowledge, skills, and attitudes in their area of practice.

We believe that all psychologists involved in managing chronic illness should meet these education, training, and practice standards before considering themselves qualified as experts in this area.

Settings for Health Psychology Practice

The increased importance of psychosocial factors in chronic illness has expanded the roles of clinical health psychologists and the settings in which they practice. For example, whereas many psychologists employed in academic medical settings have been affiliated with departments of psychology, psychiatry, or behavioral sciences, more departments of medicine—such as anesthesiology, oncology, orthopaedics, physical medicine and rehabilitation, and cardiology—have begun hiring clinical health psychologists for their expertise in particular areas of specialization. According to a survey of Division 38 members of the American Psychological Association presented in 1982 (Morrow & Clayman, 1982), the principal work settings reported by members of the Division of Health Psychology were colleges and universities (28%), medical centers (25%), and private practice (20%). Below, we discuss the principal work settings of clinical health psychologists briefly along with the various skills that are relevant to these settings. We wish to acknowledge that all of the issues below are generally of concern to all clinical health psychologists no matter what the setting; however, they are presented where they may be most relevant for the sake of brevity.

Private practice. Clinical health psychologists in private practice may see a wide variety of chronically medically ill patients depending on the practitioner's area or areas of expertise and referral sources. Because clinical health psychologists in private practice may be isolated from other health care providers, significant efforts to contact other health care providers may be required to coordinate patient care. Some patients may actually view private-practice settings favorably because they are removed from potentially aversive and unpleasant hospital settings, and this may aid the clinical health psychologist in not being labeled as "part of the health care system" when such a label would be a barrier to care for the patient. However, private-practice settings may contribute to fragmented patient care among patients with chronic medical illness who have several, ongoing therapies at different locations. Continuity of care with a frequently hospitalized patient may be difficult for the clinical health psychologist in private practice if he or she does not have practice privileges at the admitting facility. In addition, psychologists in private practice may have fewer opportunities to interact with peers and other health care providers. Because of this, psychologists in private practice may need to make greater efforts to gain visibility among colleagues and other health care professionals.

Medical and surgical hospital. Clinical health psychologists working within hospitals may have a wide range of responsibilities, including working with both patients and staff. Working within a hospital setting requires good knowledge of the health care system and effective interaction with other health care providers. Clinical health psychologists may work in a specific area (e.g., chronic pain or cardiovascular disorders) or may be part of a consultation–liaison service that offers psychological services to a number of different medical or surgical departments. In a particular area, the psychologist may work as part of a program or multidisciplinary team (e.g., cardiac transplantation or spinal cord injury) that often requires the psychologist to coordinate his or her efforts with the other team members and participate in team staff meetings. Performing consultation and liaison tasks requires the clinical health psychologist to have a broad range of knowledge and experience with a wide range of medical problems. The clinical health psychologist may also provide services to medical and support staff on such issues as dealing with job stress and patient care. In addition, he or she may also serve as a hospital administrator or be involved in the planning and evaluation of health service delivery (Altman & Cahn, 1987).

When working in a medical or surgical hospital setting, the clinical health psychologist must become accustomed to the social environment and organization of the hospital. Psychologists in hospital settings may have less autonomy in comparison with colleagues in other settings because hospital-based psychologists often act only as consultants to attending physicians, whereas the attending often makes the final decisions regarding a patient's care. This can be frustrating for the psychologist, because physicians may not adopt some or all of the recommendations made. In addition, it is often difficult to coordinate times to see a patient with the physicians and other hospital staff and services; interruptions while consulting with patients are common. The psychologist in this setting must be able to both tolerate functioning in a secondary role and to work in settings that may not be optimal for conducting therapy.

Academic settings. According to Altman and Cahn (1987), academic jobs in health psychology with a clinical emphasis are relatively common. Many clinical health psychologists hold appointments in departments traditionally involved with mental health (e.g., psychology or psychiatry); however, a larger number of positions are emerging in many other departments of medicine, as noted above. Also, health psychologists are employed in other colleges, such as dentistry and nursing. With increased recognition of psychosocial factors in illness, many chronic and acute illnesses are believed to be best treated from a multidisciplinary or "team" approach. For example, many chronic pain programs rely on the expertise of different health professionals to provide a total treatment package to the patient (e.g., an orthopedic surgeon, neurosurgeon, psychologist, physical therapist, occupational therapist, vocational rehabilitation counselor, pharmacist, and dietitian). The multidisciplinary approach requires the clinical health psychologist to have a good working knowledge of the individual roles played by various team members, both to interact effectively with other health professionals and to assist in coordinating various aspects of patient care.

Health psychology research is also a core activity in academic settings. There are special challenges for clinical health psychologists hired in departments in which they have few or no other colleagues in psychology to maintain their professional identity.

Government-related organizations. According to Altman and Cahn (1987), clinical health psychologists are ideally suited to become involved in the development of health policy and regulation of health services, yet few psychologists are presently employed in this area. Activities include becoming involved with national and state governmental agencies that reimburse health care, regulate and evaluate health service delivery, enact laws to regulate health behaviors, regulate environmental policies that may affect disease, and organize programs designed to affect health and health behavior. This setting confronts the clinical health psychologist with the challenges of working and communicating effectively with various public officials and of translating behavioral research findings and other information into a form that can be easily understood by such individuals. Several fellowship programs have now been established to provide trainees the opportunity to gain relevant experience.

Private industry. With the escalating costs of health care, many insurance companies and private industries hire behavioral researchers to investigate patterns of health care utilization and behavior and how these patterns may be altered to reduce health care costs. Examples of this are the incentives that insurance companies provide for nonsmokers and demonstrated cost-effective treatments, such as outpatient versus inpatient detoxification. Private businesses may also hire clinical health psychologists to conduct programs to alter the environment or increase "well" behaviors to reduce illness among employees, which may translate into lower insurance premiums and savings for the company, as well as higher productivity. The psychologist may also work in private industrial settings to help screen employees for illness risk factors (e.g., obesity) and to design risk management programs. Finally, private consulting firms may find clinical health psychologists desirable because of their expertise in health issues and their research skills. For example, Geisser was employed by a private consulting firm to develop medical reimbursement systems and to analyze how changes in health policy affected health care use.

Clinical health psychologists in these settings should know about organizational dynamics, consulting, assessment of risk factors, program evaluation, health education, and cost–benefit analyses (Altman & Cahn, 1987).

Interdisciplinary Issues

As noted above, psychologists working with patients who have chronic illnesses must be skilled in interdisciplinary collaboration. Communicating with professionals from other disciplines requires an understanding of their perspective and the ability to be concrete, practical, and succinct in verbal and written communications. However, Elfant (1985) has cautioned against inappropriate "medical socialization" and the dangers of overidentifying with the traditional medical model, with its authoritarian stance that portrays the patient as sick and dependent. The health care system contains strong pressures to arrive at quick decisions and to "fix people"—a role that is not necessarily appropriate for the psychologist to assume.

Bleiberg, Ciulla, and Katz (1991) have described different ways in which psychologists can function when working with multidisciplinary teams. First, the psychologist may be a fully integrated member of the team. In this model, the psychologist usually evaluates all patients treated by the team, provides intervention services as needed, and offers behavioral expertise to all team members on a continuing basis. This model facilitates the team understanding of all patients, thus maximizing the individualization of treatment and minimizing opportunities for misperceptions of the patient that can raise barriers to successful treatment. It also facilitates the use of the team in the actual delivery of psychological interventions.

A second role is for the psychologist to act as consultant to the team. In this role, the psychologist sees only those patients referred for evaluation or treatment—which can sometimes be after an impasse has already developed between a patient and a treatment team or after a problem has unnecessarily worsened. For example, a University of Florida service received a midmorning request for an urgent afternoon recommendation as to whether a young girl was a good candidate for a heart transplant. Although the girl had been hospitalized and had shown gradually increasing behavior problems (voluntary bed-wetting and withdrawal) over the prior 2 weeks, the request was triggered primarily by the timing of a medical review meeting. Had a psychologist been involved earlier, what turned out to be a major problem with anxiety could have been treated, and perhaps some of the presenting problems (as well as physician impatience with the time needed to complete psychological evaluations) could have been prevented. This consultant model also results in a team focus on psychopathology: Patients with subtle disturbances or others who may benefit from psychological interventions may not receive any help at all.

Sometimes the psychologist finds herself or himself in a mediating role between the patient and the physician or the health care system. This requires sensitivity, tact, and good conflict-resolution skills. To the extent that patient autonomy in obtaining services is limited (e.g., in some managed care systems), psychologists are likely to become more involved in advocacy related to patient welfare, a role that clinicians may not always be comfortable with.

Ethical Issues

Practice in the management of chronic illness can bring with it unique ethical issues because of the special settings and patient populations encountered, only a few of which have been mentioned here. First, given that the clinical health psychologist is in part working to help improve a patient's physical health, increased responsibility is placed on the clinical practitioner for coordinating and managing physical health problems. Goals of treatment might be to reduce the amount of hypertension medication needed, to decrease attacks of spastic colitis or migraine headaches, or to increase compliance with an exercise program for a cardiac patient. Clinical health psychologists must ensure that adequate medical evaluation and monitoring are integrated with such interventions.

Second, given the fact that other health care providers are involved in providing treatments simultaneously, there is the risk of diffusion of responsibility or referring to a collective entity (e.g., the team) as responsible for some aspect of care, such as record keeping, follow-up, communicating with other professionals, and obtaining informed consent. The clinical health psychologist must ensure that psychological care has been responsibly delivered in keeping with the General Guidelines for Providers of Psychological Services (American Psychological Association [APA], 1987).

Third, Weiss (1982) has noted the importance of the psychologist as a role model to patients and other professionals. Principle C of the Ethical Principles of Psychologists and Code of Conduct (APA, 1992) addresses the ethical issues involved when personal behavior reduces the "public trust" or compromises the fulfillment of professional responsibilities. Should a psychologist lead a relaxation group for emphysema patients with a pack of cigarettes in his or her pocket? Should an extremely overweight psychologist be a service provider in a cardiac rehabilitation program? Although behavior should not be rigidly defined for the field, the "clinical health psychologist must be aware of personal health habits and make decisions about acceptable, ethical public behavior" (Belar & Deardorff, 1995, p. 161).

Fourth, issues related to confidentiality abound in the management of chronic illness. How much information should be shared with other health care providers? What information should be documented in the more widely accessible medical chart? How confidential is an interview in a multiple-bed hospital room? Patients must be informed about the limits of confidentiality, and the psychologist must use his or her judgment about what kind of information should be shared with the treatment team. Every effort must be made to maximize confidentiality.

Fifth, informed-consent issues often arise when patients are sent by their physicians for consultation. Although inpatients sign a consent to evaluation and treatment on admission, this does not necessarily mean that they are informed about psychological consultation. Outpatients often do not know why they have been referred, to whom information will be provided, or how it might be used. Consider the case of the patient hoping for cardiac transplantation who is seen for presurgical psychological evaluation. If the team uses such information in making decisions about suitability for transplantation, then the patient should be made aware of this before he or she reveals information to the psychologist. Another important aspect of informed consent is presenting the patient with accurate information about the function or purpose of psychological intervention along with its potential benefits. For example, many individuals have misconceptions regarding their ability to be hypnotized and the effectiveness of hypnosis that may lead to unrealistically high expectations regarding the effectiveness of this intervention for such problems as pain and modifying habit disorders.

Sixth, in providing professional services in health care settings, the psychologist might well have to deal with conflicts of interest and cope with competing agendas regarding a specific patient. The health care team may want compliance from a patient whose values are at variance with the treatment protocol. For example, a surgeon might want a "clean bill of health" for a potential kidney donor or documentation of malingering in a pain patient. Standard 1.21 of the APA's Ethical Principles states that when conflicts of interest arise psychologists clarify the nature and direction of their loyalties and responsibilities and keep all parties informed of their commitments (APA, 1992). Psychologists who depend on physicians for consultations are especially sensitive to these issues, and they must develop adequate skills in providing sometimes unwelcome feedback to consultees.

Seventh, continuing to provide services that do not benefit the patient is also an ethical problem. Patients are sometimes referred to psychologists as a last resort when all previous treatments have failed. For instance, a tinnitus patient may be seeking symptom relief and be willing to undergo relaxation sessions over an extended period of time. But when has an adequate trial of treatment been provided? Many patients with chronic illness present clinical challenges for the application of scientific knowledge. Psychologists must "gauge carefully, in realistic negotiation with the patient, when an adequate trial of treatment has been accomplished without significant benefit" (Belar & Deardorff, 1995, p. 169).

Malpractice Issues

As Knapp and Vandecreek (1981) have noted, psychologists working in the area of clinical health psychology have additional malpractice liability risks to be aware of. For example, patients with chronic illness provide more opportunities for inadvertently practicing medicine without a license (e.g., independently diagnosing "tension headache" or advising a decrease in medication). Wording of recommendations to patients and recording of information in charts should thus always reflect the scope of one's licensed practice. It is prudent to record the source of the Axis III diagnosis (per patient, per medical record, or per Dr. X) and to base medication usage recommendations on decisions made in consultation with the primary physician.

Another issue is that physical harm is easier to document and prove in court than emotional harm. And physical harm is perhaps more likely to occur as a result of psychological treatments or diagnostic decisions in patients who are chronically ill and worsen, do not improve, or are not recommended for complex—yet desired—medical treatments. Although data on this are not available, Knapp and Vandecreek (1981) have asserted that patients being seen by clinical health psychologists might be more likely to bring legal suits because they often do not have an ongoing psychotherapy relationship with the psychologist—a relationship that has been thought to protect the traditional mental health service provider in the past.

Wright (1981) suggested that the area of practice most likely to result in malpractice litigation is that of psychological evaluation. Indeed, there have been many consultation reports in which classic psychiatric interpretations (made on the basis of standardization samples of psychiatric patients) have been inappropriately applied to medical–surgical patients. Grounds for a legitimate malpractice suit might also involve the use of psychometric techniques to conclude that physical symptoms are "functional" in nature. Neither of these practices is in keeping with sound clinical practice.

Personal Issues

In fulfilling their roles in the management of chronic illness, psychologists will also need to deal with a variety of personal issues that can affect their performance or satisfaction with the field. Chronic illness confronts the psychologist with threats to body image; it highlights human physical vulnerability and triggers concerns over death and dying. Thus, the psychologist who is repulsed by the thought of sexual activity after mastectomy can exacerbate a mastectomy patient's basic fears. Likewise, the psychologist who cannot accept death can prevent a patient from adequately preparing for his or her own passing. Clearly the psychologist's role requires self-examination and efforts to address many significant life issues that might not be encountered in other areas of psychological practice.

Another personal issue related to psychologists' roles is the fact that although psychology is an independent profession, practice with chronically ill patients requires some dependency on medicine. Such forced dependency can be difficult for some practitioners, especially when it involves depending on a professional of greater social status and income. However, the close association of clinical health psychology with medicine also permits insight into the tensions among medical specialties, which can alleviate defensiveness by psychologists, as well as increased awareness of the unknowns in medical practice. This awareness can sometimes facilitate confidence in psychology's science base for practice.

Working with people who are chronically ill also requires perseverance and a high frustration tolerance to weather the fluctuating interest of patients, providers, and the health care system. Many patients are reluctant to see psychologists, themselves believing in the functional versus organic myth. To establish a good working relationship, the clinician needs to help the patient shift from a biomedical to a biopsychosocial orientation and to provide a rationale for psychological services in an atmosphere of open negotiation. Additionally, much work must be done to dispel the mind–body dualism that pervades both the health belief models of patients and professionals and the reimbursement policies of the health insurance industry.

Future Issues

We have identified a number of important roles for clinical health psychologists in the management of chronic illness and addressed some of the practice issues that psychologists will be likely to encounter in fulfilling these roles. In closing, we would like to make some comments about the future, because certain trends are occurring that have significant implications for psychologists' future roles. First, the field is becoming increasingly technologically oriented. Computerized assessment methods are becoming more available to nonpsychologist users, and so the potential for abuse or misapplication of psychometric instruments is increasing. There is the risk of a backlash similar to that which occurred in the school system over intelligence testing. Psychologists will thus need to take a stronger advocacy role with respect to the appropriate use of psychological measurements.

Increased knowledge will also bring increased opportunities for coercive control of patients—for example, in terms of having them comply with the values of health care providers. Psychologists will need to address more intensively the ethical issues involved in providing services to those who are chronically ill, giving special attention to issues associated with diversity and working with patients from different backgrounds (see Ethical Principle D, APA, 1992).

Although the future is bright with respect to the development of new knowledge and programs related to managing chronic illness, there is also the risk of overselling psychological approaches in this endeavor. Already we have heard from patients who feel inadequate that they cannot cure their own illnesses (e.g., thwart tumor growth or enhance their immune systems). In addition, many people confuse causal and correlational models or believe that because a psychological treatment can help an illness, it might have been caused psychologically. These patients are at more risk for self-blame and guilt in the face of an illness, which can then aggravate their physical condition. Above all, psychologists working with chronically ill people must not contribute to this process.

Within professional psychology, considerably more attention has been paid to issues of specialization and proficiency in the last few years. Standards and credentials for psychologists with expertise in such areas as pain management, cognitive rehabilitation, neuropsychological assessment, organ transplant evaluations, and pediatric psychology (to name only a few) are likely to be developed, and subspecialization within the Diploma in Health Psychology will probably occur. These new credentials will affect who gets reimbursed for certain services by third-party carriers and the government, which will continue to play the major role in determining health care policy in the United States. And, as the profession of medicine loses its total grip on the health care system, there will be opportunities for more policy-making and administrative roles for psychologists.

The marketplace for psychologists offering specialized services in clinical health psychology (and targeted treatment programs) will do well until service providers from other disciplines (e.g., health educators, social workers, and nurse practitioners) offer these services more economically. At that time, psychologists will need to use their research skills to develop new products or to act as program developers and evaluators as well as service providers if they are to remain valuable to the health care system.

Finally, clinical health psychologists must also learn to deal with changing philosophies in the delivery of and in reimbursement for health care. There are risks that psychological services could be unaffordable for some people and that there will be inadequate coverage for individuals requiring long-term care. In addition, there might be coverage for "mental health cases" but not for psychological services for physical health care. We hope that clinical health psychologists can become more actively involved in educating policy makers as well as the public about the role of psychologists in health care, the effectiveness of psychological interventions on health, and health behavior and quality of life, so that they can provide input regarding adequate coverage for psychological services in any health care plan.

Psychologists must also cope with the increasing numbers of people participating in managed care plans. Under many managed care plans, primary care physicians act as gatekeepers to other services offered; thus, the physician's attitude about the utility of psychological services can affect referrals and the number of visits allowed. Some plans place caps on the number of visits, and services are typically reimbursed at a negotiated fee that is often lower than the charged fee, or the provider is offered a flat fee to treat a negotiated number of patients under the plan, or the psychologist must obtain authorization to treat a patient from the managed care organization or a peer reviewer. These policies are attempts to encourage psychologists and other health care providers to become more effective and cost-efficient, further emphasizing the need to develop practice standards for health psychology. Despite this, many health care providers, including psychologists, believe that managed care policies decrease provider control over care and attempt to decrease costs by lowering reimbursement for and restricting access to care. People with chronic illness may suffer the most under these types of plans because they are typically in need of more intensive and long-term treatment. As with health care reform, clinical health psychologists should work with other health care providers to educate the public and policy makers about the contributions of psychologists to health care and the impact of managed care policies on quality of health care. They should work with third-party payors and policy makers to develop adequate coverage and reimbursement policies.

In conclusion, if roles for psychologists in the management of chronic illness continue to expand at the rate they have over the past few decades, we believe that the future will be rich with opportunities and challenges for the health psychologist. This growth should be ongoing, as long as the field's commitments to cost-effective, scientifically sound practice and to the creation of new knowledge for practice are maintained.

REFERENCES

Altman, D. G., & Cahn, J. (1987). Employment options for health psychologists. In G. C. Stone, S. M. Weiss, J. D. Matarazzo, N. E. Miller, J. Rodin, C. D. Belar, M. J. Follick, & J. E. Singer (Eds.), *Health psychology: A discipline and profession* (pp. 231–244). Chicago: University of Chicago Press.

American Psychological Association. (1987). *General guidelines for providers of psychological services.* Washington, DC: Author.

American Psychological Association. (1992). Ethical principles of psychologists and code of conduct. *American Psychologist, 47,* 1597–1611.

Belar, C. D. (1991a). Behavioral medicine. In C. S. Austad & W. H. Berman (Eds.), *Psychotherapy in managed health care* (pp. 65–79). Washington, DC: American Psychological Association.

Belar, C. D. (1991b). Professionalism in medical settings. In J. J. Sweet, R. H. Rozensky, & S. M. Tovian (Eds.), *Handbook of clinical psychology in medical settings* (pp. 81–92). New York: Plenum Press.

Belar, C. D., & Deardorff, W. W. (1995). *Clinical health psychology in medical settings.* Washington, DC: American Psychological Association.

Bleiberg, J., Ciulla, R., & Katz, B. L. (1991). Psychological components of rehabilitation programs for brain-injured and spinal-cord-injured patients. In J. J. Sweet, R. H. Rozensky, & S. M. Tovian (Eds.), *Handbook of clinical psychology in medical settings* (pp. 375–400). New York: Plenum Press.

Elfant, A. B. (1985). Psychotherapy and assessment in hospital settings: Ideological and professional conflicts. *Professional Psychology: Research and Practice, 16,* 55–63.

Jospe, J., Shueman, S. A., & Troy, W. G. (1991). Quality assurance and the clinical health psychologist: A programmatic approach. In J. J. Sweet, R. H. Rozensky, & S. M. Tovian (Eds.), *Handbook of clinical psychology in medical settings* (pp. 95–112). New York: Plenum Press.

Knapp, S., & Vandecreek, L. (1981). Behavioral medicine: Its malpractice risks for psychologists. *Professional Psychology, 12,* 677–683.

Meichenbaum, D., & Turk, D. C. (1987). Patient education: Organizing and structuring. In D. Meichenbaum & D. C. Turk (Eds.), *Facilitating treatment adherence: A practitioner's guidebook* (pp. 111–148). New York: Plenum Press.

Morrow, G., & Clayman, D. (1982). *A membership survey of the Division of Health Psychology, American Psychological Association.* Unpublished manuscript.

Sheridan, E. P., Matarazzo, J. D., Boll, T. J., Perry, N. W., Weiss, S. M., & Belar, C. D. (1988). Postdoctoral education and training for clinical service providers in health psychology. *Health Psychology, 7,* 1–17.

Stone, G. C. (1983). Proceedings of the National Working Conference on Education and Training in Health Psychology. *Health Psychology,* 2(Suppl.), 1–153.

Weiss, S. M. (1982). Health psychology: The time is now. *Health Psychology, 1,* 91.

Wright, R. H. (1981). Psychologists and professional liability (malpractice) insurance. *American Psychologist, 36,* 1484–1493.

Chapter

3

Psychological Assessment

Leonard R. Derogatis, Megan P. Fleming, Nanette C. Sudler, and Lynn DellaPietra

Chronicity relative to a medical condition typically comes about when medical science is unable to definitively treat or resolve the pathophysiology underlying the disorder. In such instances, medical science is often capable of offering patients therapeutic interventions that slow or impede the progress of the disease, ameliorate its symptoms, and maintain health and functional status at levels notably higher than would be found in an untreated course of the disease. Variability in the levels of disability associated with chronic illnesses, even within the same disease state, is great, however, and chronic medical conditions often have pervasively degrading effects on people's well-being and quality of life.

Because definitive medical resolution of these conditions is impossible, if they are sufficiently distressing and debilitating chronic medical illnesses can overwhelm coping styles oriented toward more acute stress situations. Their unremitting and unsalutary character can frequently bring on reactive psychological disorders, resulting in comorbid conditions that magnify the pernicious impact of the patient's primary medical condition. These circumstances, coupled with the well-established fact that primary care physicians have a poor record of identifying psychiatric disorders in their patients (Anderson & Harthorn, 1989; Seltzer, 1989), emphasize the need for efficient psychological assessment approaches to treating patients with chronic medical illnesses. Such systems should be designed to accurately apprise health care professionals of patient status and alert them to emerging dysfunctional states.

Currently, systematic protocols for psychologically assessing chronically ill patients are rare. Most clinical health psychologists develop local assessment batteries, which tend to be dissimilar and lack standardization. This practice results in a hodgepodge of information being communicated in psychological reports that is rarely consistent from one treatment center to the next. Modern assessment paradigms with chronic medical patients must involve more case-relevant, standardized assessment that recognizes the persistent nature of such conditions as medicine and health care move toward more protocol-driven treatment standards.

The realities of modern health care systems suggest that the proportion of chronically ill patients who will be exposed to formal psychological assessment is likely to increase sharply in the future, because of the documented capacity of psychological screening measures both to detect cost-multiplying, comorbid (co-occurring) psychological disorders (Derogatis & DellaPietra, 1994) and to serve as valid outcome measures for effective health care delivery (Derogatis & Lazarus, 1994). For such systems of assessment to function efficiently with those who are chronically medically ill, their design must be distinct from that of traditional systems of psychological assessment focused on psychiatric patients. Multiple prospective assessment windows must be designed for the chronic patient so that, from the outset, psychological evaluation is appreciated as a prospective and integral aspect of both treatment planning and outcome assessment. Because many chronic illnesses are progressive and debilitating, assessment time must be carefully monitored. The traditional battery of psychological tests, requiring hours to administer, must be replaced with brief, specifically targeted assessments. Because the time allotted for assessing medical patients' psychosocial status tends to be limited, the clinical health psychologist must efficiently determine which functions are central to successful adjustment and integrate valid measures of those functions into the psychological evaluation paradigm.

Major Issues

Time of Assessment

An important variable when working with patients who have chronic medical illnesses is the specific time of assessment, because the natural history of many conditions contains specific medical epochs (e.g., discovery of metastases in cancer or vascular degeneration of the retina in diabetes) at which stress on patients' coping resources is increased. Therapeutic interventions may also carry noxious effects that can generate psychosocial liabilities (e.g., sexual dysfunction associated with antihypertensive drugs or nausea, vomiting, and alopecia associated with cancer chemotherapy). Baseline assessment prior to the introduction of any significant treatment or intervention should serve as a benchmark in any assessment paradigm with chronically ill patients. By establishing baseline psychosocial status when patients enter the health care system or institution, psychologists can monitor and evaluate the cumulative effects of the disease, the impact of acute medical crises, and the effectiveness of coping strategies by contrasting subsequent assessments with these baseline values throughout the course of the illness. Ideally, psychological assessments should systematically coincide with substantive medical evaluations, so that information on the patient's psychological status can be integrated with the overall clinical picture and play a significant role in helping to guide treatment planning.

Chronic anxiety or panic disorder, emerging depressive illness, marital discord, and cognitive dysfunction are all examples of significant psychological comorbidities that require accurate identification and effective treatment to circumvent their potential exacerbating influences on primary medical problems. At a minimum, one comprehensive psychological evaluation should be completed annually with chronically ill patients, and more circumscribed psychological assessments—focusing on well-being, coping efficacy, and psychological distress—should be accomplished during scheduled treatment or evaluation visits. Such a model establishes a sound assessment baseline and enables the clinician to link psychological status to medical status and treatment response.

Modality of Measurement

An issue that is a frequent source of confusion, particularly among nonpsychologist health care professionals, is optimum measurement modality. Arguments about the advantages and disadvantages associated with self-report versus clinical observer-based assessment have led to the reification of one or the other approach in some circles. In reality, however, both modalities of measurement represent reliable, valid approaches to evaluating patients' psychological status. As has been pointed out repeatedly (Derogatis & DellaPietra, 1994), each of the two techniques carries its own intrinsic strengths and weaknesses. Thus, each measurement situation must be evaluated uniquely to determine which is the most effective method to use in achieving valid assessment. For example, self-report approaches are advantageous when external observers cannot achieve sufficient access to the phenomena being measured (e.g., affects or attitudes), cost is a critical variable, staff time is at a premium, or psychologically trained clinicians are unavailable. Clinical observer rating scales and interviews are usually preferred in situations where clinical judgment is essential (e.g., diagnosis), debilitation or disease has robbed the patient of the ability to report accurately (e.g., delirium or dementia), or sophisticated clinical decisions are required (e.g., neuropsychological testing). Prevailing wisdom holds that certain constructs (e.g., quality of life) are best measured through self-report (Ferrans, 1990); other measurement tasks have been determined to exclusively require judgments from clinical observers (e.g., diagnostic assignment for the *Diagnostic and Statistical Manual of Mental Disorders,* 4th ed. [American Psychiatric Association, 1994]); and still other foci of psychological assessment (e.g., psychological distress) may be approached effectively through either modality.

Identity of the Respondent

Another important issue in psychological assessment of chronically ill patients concerns the identity of the respondent. In most assessment contexts there is an implicit assumption that the respondent will be the "patient" or "client." However, in many instances of chronic illness, the impact of the illness is felt by the entire family (e.g., see chap. 6 of this book; Rabins, Fitting, Eastham, & Fetting, 1990). Thus, it is often desirable to assess the effects of the illness on the spouse or parents of the patient as well as on the patient per se. In addition, it may be useful in certain instances to enlist a family member to provide an independent assessment of the patient's status from a well-informed, external perspective. In such situations, a slightly modified (spousal or parental) version of the same measuring instrument used with the patient may be used with the family member. Although such external evaluations should not be viewed as a "gold standard" against which the validity of patient responses should be judged, these assessments can usefully highlight areas of the patient's life experience that may be subject to illness- or need-induced distortions.

Selection of Norms

A related topic that is central to the effective psychological assessment of chronically ill patients involves selecting the most appropriate norms to use as referents. This issue usually centers around the question of whether general (usually community-based) norms of the test or specialized, illness-specific norms should be used to evaluate patient status. Determining norms really comes down to examining the nature of the comparison that the evaluator wishes to make and the specific question that he or she is addressing. For example, is it more meaningful to compare a cancer patient's psychological distress score with norms derived from a healthy community population or with norms developed from a sample of like cancer patients? The answer to this question lies in one's particular query of interest.

If the fundamental question is whether or not the patient's psychological distress has reached "clinical" proportions, then the community norm should probably be used because it is much more likely to have well-established "caseness" criteria associated with it. Although there are notable exceptions (e.g., illness-induced somatic symptoms), psychiatric disorders (e.g., anxiety disorders and depressions) tend to be relatively invariant in their symptomatic presentations. Comparison with a general norm thus addresses the question "Does this patient have a psychological disorder of sufficient (i.e., clinical) magnitude to initiate a therapeutic intervention?" Alternatively, if the primary question concerns the quality of a patient's adjustment to the illness at a particular stage or milestone in comparison with the typical patient, then an illness-specific norm, if available, will probably provide the most meaningful comparison.

The question of general versus illness-specific norms is also colored by the nature of the construct being assessed. In the example given above, psychological distress and psychiatric disorder are constructs that are sufficiently robust to generalize across specific groups of individuals. Criteria for assessing these constructs are sufficiently consistent, such that a general norm will usually provide a clinically meaningful interpretation of symptomatic distress levels. Alternatively, adjustment to illness is a construct that is much more illness specific. Diabetes typically results in a very different illness from breast cancer, and both of these are in turn quite distinct from renal failure resulting in the need for chronic kidney dialysis. The measurement of a construct such as adjustment to illness, then, should be accomplished with a "library" of norms (Derogatis, 1986) that enable the evaluator to interpret adjustment profiles in terms of a specific illness referent.

Still other constructs, such as quality of life, are best approached in a "modular" manner that combines normative data from both general and illness-specific populations. Ideally, a general quality-of-life measure will generate a very broad score continuum—from a status reflecting optimum health, social functioning, and so on at one pole, to one revealing serious degradation of well-being at the other. In addition, specific medical disorders carry with them specific symptoms, problems, and disabilities that require detailed determination if an accurate picture of a patient's status is to be gained. Investigators in the field (Bullinger, 1991; Derogatis & DellaPietra, 1994; Mayou, 1990) are increasingly embracing a modular strategy, combining general instruments with modules developed from illness-specific samples. In this paradigm, the illness-specific module may then be treated as an additional domain of the general test instrument or as a distinct, stand-alone measure.

Central Constructs in the Psychosocial Assessment of Chronic Illness

Clearly, the most essential question to be answered in the psychosocial assessment of the patient with chronic illness is, Which attributes should be measured? Given the multitude of overlapping psychological constructs that have predictive value concerning health status, it is difficult to definitively determine those that possess both substantive relevance and the potential for satisfactory operational definition. In this chapter, we identify and examine a set of constructs that possess both high relevance for psychological assessment in chronic illness and valid operational definition. In doing so, we review a number of instruments designed around specific constructs that have demonstrated validity and prior utility with chronically ill patients. We have not attempted to definitively evaluate either the constructs discussed or the instruments designed to measure them. Instead, the commentaries provided here represent capsule reviews and recommendations intended to familiarize readers with the application of these measures in assessing the chronically ill patient. We examine the following five sets of constructs: (a) well-being (affect balance), (b) psychological distress, (c) cognitive functioning, (d) psychosocial adjustment to illness, and (e) personality (health-related constructs).

Well-Being

Historically, well-being has been conceived as a construct defined by a unitary bipolar continuum extending from extreme positive affect (e.g., joy or happiness) at one pole to extreme negative affect (e.g., depression or sadness) at the other. According to this model, an individual's well-being is defined by his or her point location on this single affective continuum. Positive and negative affectivity are assumed to have an inverse linear relationship, so that the relative ascendance of one affective state necessarily results in the diminution of the other. More recently, however, this historical model of well-being has been impressively challenged by a conceptualization that has come to be known as *two-factor theory.*

Consistent with the World Health Organization's (1960) definition of health as being "more than merely the absence of disease" (p. 4), researchers broadened their previously narrow focus on negative affects and began to more vigorously investigate the bases of positive affectivity as well as the nature of the relationship between the two. Similarly, the realization that well-being is defined by more than the mere absence of psychological distress became more clearly appreciated. What has emerged is an impressive collection of empirical research that argues persuasively for a definition of well-being encompassing two distinct dimensions of positive and negative affectivity that vary independently.

One of the earliest investigators to formally define well-being in terms of independent dimensions of positive and negative affects, Bradburn (1969) developed his posture as a further refinement of motivation-hygiene theory (Herzberg, Mathapo, Wiener, & Wiesen, 1974). Bradburn operationalized affect balance through the use of a 10-item checklist that he called the *Affect Balance Scale.* Although the scale was found to be somewhat lacking in terms of psychometric refinement (Watson, Clark, & Tellegen, 1988), a great deal of productive research has been done with it over the past 20 years—much of it lending support to a two-factor theory of affectivity. Recently, L. A. Baker, Cesa, Gatz, and Mellins (1992) published an interesting study with the Affect Balance Scale suggesting that the independence of positive and negative affectivity arises from distinct origins: Positive affect has its foundation in the environment, whereas negative affect appears to be heritable to some degree.

Derogatis (1975) has also defined emotional experience in terms of independent positive and negative affective coordinates, using a distinct test instrument similarly termed the *Affects Balance Scale.* His psychometric model postulates four positive and four negative primary affective dimensions—a paradigm that has been confirmed in large measure through a factor analytic study of a large sample of psychiatric outpatients (Derogatis, 1982; Derogatis & Rutigliano, in press). Further analysis of the primary factor correlation matrix from this sample identified two higher order factors: positive affectivity and negative affectivity.

More recently, Watson (1988) has convincingly shown positive and negative affectivity to function as independent dimensions of emotional experience—across time, scale of measurement, and response mode. He and his colleagues posited positive and negative affectivity as two essentially orthogonal constructs that make up the cardinal components of subjective well-being. They went on to discriminate state versus trait versions of these attributes, which, at the trait level, they likened to extraversion and neuroticism, respectively (Watson & Tellegen, 1985). Watson and associates (Watson, Clark, & Tellegen, 1988) also developed a test instrument, the Positive and Negative Affect Schedule, on the basis of their theoretical position.

The various two-factor measures of well-being have been increasingly used in recent years in a comprehensive range of health applications and have proven to be extremely sensitive to differences or changes in health status. For example, Derogatis and his colleagues have shown the Affects Balance Scale (Derogatis, 1975) to be sensitive to the attenuation of well-being associated with sexual dysfunctions in both men and women (Derogatis & Meyer, 1979). They also have demonstrated distinct affect balance profiles between male and female gender-dysphoric patients, with the former revealing very high levels of negative affectivity (Derogatis, Meyer, & Vasquez, 1978) and the latter showing profiles essentially in the "normal" range (Derogatis, Meyer, & Boland, 1981). In seriously ill cancer patients, Derogatis, Abeloff, and Melisaratos (1979) as well as Levy, Lee, Bagley, and Lippman (1988) showed the Affects Balance Scale scores to be sensitive to differences in survival time. Likewise, Irvine, Brown, Crooks, Roberts, and Browne (1991) used this scale to document the subjective well-being and adjustment of breast cancer patients. Concerning spousal adjustment to chronic illness, Northhouse (1988) disclosed that Derogatis's Affects Balance Scale was attuned to husbands' as well as patients' affective postures regarding breast cancers, and Rabins et al. (1990) used the test effectively in documenting the status of well-being and its determinants in groups of cancer and Alzheimer's caregivers. Both Hoehn-Saric (1983) and Holland and her colleagues (Holland et al., 1990) have provided substantial evidence of the instrument's ability to detect drug-induced therapeutic changes in anxious and depressed patient groups. Wolf and associates (T. H. Wolf, Elston, & Kissling, 1989; T. M. Wolf, Von Almen, Faucet, Randall, & Franklin, 1991) have used the scale to document the well-being of medical students and relate their affective status to daily hassles and life events.

Watson and his collaborators have published a systematic series of studies with the Positive and Negative Affect Schedule, both supporting the validity of the two-factor theory of well-being and demonstrating a number of relationships between health attributes and affectivity. Watson and Tellegen (1985) defined *Trait PA* as a persistent inclination to respond to the environment with an active, enabling posture, reflecting a general sense of competence and mastery. They described *Trait NA* as a broadly based tendency to experience life events in the context of dysphoric emotional coloring, which ultimately extends to pervasively influence one's cognitive style and self-concept. L. A. Clark & Watson (1988) also observed that high levels of positive affects were strongly related to levels of social interaction and physical activity and were inversely related to health complaints among young adults. In a more clinical context, Watson, Clark, and Carey (1988) have demonstrated affect levels to effectively discriminate psychiatric outpatients diagnosed with anxiety disorders from those with a primary diagnosis of depression. Although both groups revealed high levels of negative affectivity, only those with depression showed a significant reduction in positive affect. D. A. Clark, Beck, and Stewart (1990) have elaborated on this phenomenon, which has also found support in recent research by Garamoni et al. (1991), using Derogatis's Affects Balance Scale.

Affects balance has been shown to be a characteristic highly reflective of individuals' subjective sense of well-being and to be correlated with a broad spectrum of health-related variables. Measures of affectivity are also highly sensitive to changes in health status that have clinical implications. Frequently in our experience, affective measures have revealed the effects of therapeutic interventions substantially earlier than symptom-based scales; conversely, such measures also tend to reveal any decline in well-being more readily. The measures discussed here are extremely brief (less than 5 minutes), cost-efficient, and nonintrusive self-report inventories that conform well to the stated requisite of providing an ongoing, prospective depiction of chronic patients' psychosocial adjustment. These qualities lead us to recommend that one of these instruments should be a component of every psychological assessment of chronically medically ill patients.

Psychological Distress

Recent results from the Epidemiologic Catchment Area study, sponsored by the National Institute of Mental Health and assessing almost 20,000 individuals, confirmed the widely held belief that community rates of psychiatric disorder are substantial (e.g., the 1-month prevalence rate for any psychiatric disorder was 15.4%; Regier et al., 1988). In medical populations, prevalence rates have been consistently found to be even higher. Derogatis and Wise (1989), in reviewing a representative series of medical conditions, observed prevalence rates ranging from 22% to 33%. Similarly, Barrett, Barrett, Oxman, and Gerber (1988) observed rates from 25% to 30%.

When focus is restricted to chronic medical illnesses, rates of psychiatric comorbidity rise even higher. In a dramatic demonstration of the increased liability for psychiatric disorder associated with chronic illnesses, K. B. Wells, Golding, and Burnham (1988) published data comparing prevalence rates across 2,550 patients from eight chronic illness groups with rates from an illness-free control group. Evaluating both 6-month and lifetime prevalence estimates, these investigators found significantly higher rates of psychiatric disorder in the majority of chronic illness cohorts (exceptions being those with hypertension, etc.) in comparison with those in the control group. Lifetime prevalence rates ranged from 38.5% to 63.8%. These data clearly illustrate that psychiatric comorbidity is a very common problem among those who are chronically ill—a problem that is not only a substantial burden in its own right, but one that often seriously complicates treatment of the primary medical condition.

In light of these considerations, the accurate and timely assessment of psychological distress in chronically ill patients assumes enhanced importance. The evaluation not only serves as a means of descriptively documenting an individual's level of psychological integration at a given stage of illness but also provides a mechanism for identifying the emergence of comorbid psychiatric disorders. Effective treatment planning and efficient management of the chronic patient can only be accomplished with an accurate appreciation of his or her cognitive and emotional status, and currently, psychological assessment is the most valid and cost-efficient means of gaining this perspective.

Although there are many well-established psychological tests designed to measure psychological distress, some of these are long and time-consuming. Others measure various interrelated aspects of psychopathology and personality, but do not deliver results in terms of pure measures of symptomatic distress. Our approach involves the use of brief self-report symptom inventories in conjunction with the methodology of formal screening models. This enables us to immediately address the question, "What is the probability that this patient currently has a psychiatric disorder?" If the patient screens negative, then further evaluation of psychological distress is not necessary. If the patient screens positive, then a more specific series of diagnostic assessments are initiated.

Screening has been traditionally defined as follows:

> the presumptive identification of unrecognized disease or defect by the application of tests, examinations or other procedures which can be applied rapidly to sort out apparently well persons who probably

> have a disease from those who probably do not. (Commission on Chronic Illness, 1957, p. 45)

Screening is an operation conducted in an ostensibly well population (relative to the index disorder) to identify occult instances of the disease or disorder in question.

As clinical assessments go, the screening process represents a relatively unrefined sieve that is designed to partition any sample under assessment into *positives*, who presumptively have the condition in question, and *negatives*, who are apparently free of the disorder. Screening is not a diagnostic procedure per se; rather, it represents a preliminary filtering technique for identifying individuals with the highest probability of having the disorder in question for subsequent specific diagnostic evaluation. Individuals found negative by the screening process are typically not further evaluated.

The conceptual foundation for screening rests on the premise that early detection of unrecognized disease carries a measurable advantage in achieving effective treatment or cure of the condition. Although logical, however, this assumption is not always valid. In certain conditions, early detection does not measurably improve the capacity to alter morbidity or mortality, either because diagnostic procedures are unreliable or because effective treatments for the condition are not yet available. In the case of psychiatric disorders occurring with chronic medical illnesses, validity of this assumption is not a problem. Psychologists currently possess any number of valid and reliable screening tests, and, in general, most psychological conditions can be treated effectively. In addition, reductions in health care facility use, unnecessary diagnostic tests, substance abuse secondary to psychiatric disorders, and health care costs (not to mention improved treatment response to the primary medical condition) are explicit benefits associated with screening and early detection.

Because many psychologists are not familiar with formal screening paradigms, we briefly review the basic epidemiologic screening model here. Basically, a cohort of individuals who are apparently well, or have a condition distinct from the index disorder (e.g., a chronic medical illness), are evaluated through tests to determine if they are at high risk for a particular (index) disorder or disease. The disorder should have sufficient incidence or consequence to be considered a serious health problem and should be characterized by a distinct early or asymptomatic phase during which detection will substantially improve the results of treatment.

The screening test itself (e.g., pap smear or Western blot) should be both reliable (i.e., consistent in its performance from one administration to the next) and valid (i.e., capable of identifying those with the index disorder and of eliminating individuals who do not). In psychometric terms, this form of validity has been traditionally referred to as *predictive validity.* In epidemiologic models, the predictive validity of the test is divided into two distinct parts: (a) the degree to which the test correctly identifies those individuals who actually have the disorder, termed its *sensitivity,* and (b) the extent to which those free of the condition are correctly identified as such, or its *specificity.* Correctly identified individuals who have the index disorder are referred to as *true positives,* whereas those accurately identified as free of the disorder are *true negatives.* Misidentifications of healthy individuals as affected are labeled *false positives,* and affected individuals missed by the test are referred to as *false negatives.* It is not appropriate to further detail these screening paradigms in the present chapter, but readers may consult recent reviews of screening for psychiatric disorders (e.g., Derogatis & DellaPietra, 1994; Derogatis, DellaPietra, & Kilroy, 1992). The basic fourfold epidemiological table, as well as the algebraic definitions of each of the validity indexes are given in Table 1.

In our review of screening inventories, we chose to document five tests. Administration time for all of the instruments is brief (7–15 minutes), and all are self-report inventories. Three instruments are multidimensional in nature, whereas the remaining two measure only depression. Our assessment is not intended to be comprehensive but, rather, to touch on the nature of each measure and provide some information about its psychometric characteristics and background. For the commercially available tests, detailed discussions and comprehensive psychometric data are available from their published administration manuals. Scholarly reviews provide similar information for others. Table 2 shows a brief summary of the relevant characteristics of each test.

SCL-90-R. The SCL-90-R (Derogatis, 1977, 1983, 1994) is a 90-item, multidimensional, self-report symptom inventory derived from the Hopkins Symptom Checklist (Derogatis, Lipman, Rickels, Uhlenhuth, & Covi, 1974) and first published in 1975. The inventory measures symptomatic distress in terms of nine primary dimensions and three

Table 1

Epidemiological Screening Model

	Actual	
Screening test	Cases	Noncases
Test positive	a	b
Test negative	c	d

Note. Algebraic definitions of the validity indexes are as follows:

Sensitivity (Se) = a/(a + c)
False negative rate = (1 − Se) = c/(a + c)
Specificity (Sp) = d/(b + d)
False positive rate = (1 − Sp) = b/(b + d)
Positive predictive value (PPV) = a/(a + b)
Negative predictive value (NPV) = d/(c + d)

From *The Use of Psychological Testing for Treatment Planning and Outcome Assessment* (p. 25), edited by M. Maruish, 1994, Hillsdale, NJ: Erlbaum. Copyright 1994 by Erlbaum. Adapted with permission.

global indexes of distress. The dimensions include somatization, obsessive–compulsive, interpersonal sensitivity, depression, anxiety, hostility, phobic anxiety, paranoid ideation, and psychoticism. SCL-90-R norms have been developed for adult community nonpatients, psychiatric outpatients, psychiatric inpatients, and adolescent nonpatients. Geriatric and other specialized norms for the test are currently under development. The SCL-90-R takes from 12 to 15 minutes to complete.

Brief Symptom Inventory. The Brief Symptom Inventory (Derogatis, 1993; Derogatis & Melisaratos, 1983; Derogatis & Spencer, 1982) is the abbreviated form of the SCL-90-R. It measures the same nine symptom dimensions and three global indexes using only 53 items. Dimension scores on this inventory correlate highly with comparable SCL-90-R scores (Derogatis & Spencer, 1982), and it shares most psy-

Table 2

Psychological Screening Tests for Use With Chronic Medical Populations

Instrument	Author & date	Mode	Description	Completion time	Application	Sensitivity	Specificity
SCL-90-R	Derogatis (1975)	Self	90 items, multi	15–20 months	1, 2, 3	.73	0.91
Brief Symptom Inventory	Derogatis (1975)	Self	53 items, multi	10–15 min	1, 2, 3	0.72	0.90
General Health Questionnaire	Goldberg (1972)	Self	60, 30, & 12 items, multi	5–15 min	1, 2, 3, 4, 5	0.60–1.0	0.75–0.92
Center for Epidemiological Studies Depression Scale	Radloff (1977)	Self	20 items, uni	10 min	1, 2, 3, 4	0.83–0.97	0.61–0.90
Beck Depression Inventory	Beck et al. (1961)	Self	21 items, uni	5–10 min	2, 3, 4	0.76–0.92	0.64–0.80

Note. 1 = community adults, 2 = community adolescents, 3 = inpatient–outpatient, 4 = medical patients, 5 = elderly, 6 = children, 7 = college students. Multi = multidimensional; uni = unidimensional.

From *The Use of Psychological Testing for Treatment Planning and Outcome Assessment* (p. 29), edited by M. Maruish, 1994, Hillsdale, NJ: Erlbaum. Copyright 1994 by Erlbaum. Adapted with permission.

chometric characteristics of the longer scale. Approximately 10–12 minutes are required to complete the 53-item inventory.

Both the SCL-90-R and the Brief Symptom Inventory have been used as outcome measures in an extensive array of research studies, among them a number of investigations focusing specifically on screening (Derogatis et al., 1983; Zabora, Smith-Wilson, Fetting, & Enterline, 1990). A recent review of the two tests (Derogatis & Lazarus, 1994) examined several hundred research reports in which they have been used to measure symptomatic distress. Additionally, both versions have been translated into 26 languages.

General Health Questionnaire. The General Health Questionnaire was originally developed as a 60-item, multidimensional self-report symptom inventory by Goldberg (1972). Subsequently (Goldberg & Hillier, 1979), four subscales were derived through factor analysis: somatic symptoms, anxiety and insomnia, social dysfunction, and severe depression. The General Health Questionnaire has been widely used internationally as a measure of psychiatric disorder, its popularity arising in part from the fact that several brief forms of the test are available. The General Health Questionnaire–30 and General Health Questionnaire–12 represent brief forms of the original inventory and also follow the basic four-subscale format of the longer parent scale. These brief versions of the questionnaire do not include physical symptoms as indicators of distress (Malt, 1989), a methodological innovation that is very helpful in reducing error variance in populations with chronic medical illnesses. The General Health Questionnaire has been validated for use in screening and outcome assessment in numerous populations, including traumatically injured patients, cancer patients, geriatric patients, and many community samples (Goldberg & Williams, 1988). It takes from 5 to 15 minutes to complete.

Center for Epidemiological Studies Depression Scale. Developed by Radloff (1977), this brief, unidimensional self-report depression scale comprises 20 items to assess the respondent's perceived mood and level of functioning within the past 7 days. Four fundamental dimensions—depressed affect, positive affect, somatic problems, and interpersonal problems—have been identified as basic to the scale. Scores of 16 or greater suggest depressive disorders in nonmedical populations.

This depression scale has been used effectively to screen a number of community samples (Comstock & Helsing, 1976; Frerichs, Aneshensel, & Clark, 1981; Radloff & Locke, 1985) as well as samples of medical cohorts (Parikh, Eden, Price, & Robinson, 1988) and clinical populations (Roberts, Rhoades, & Vernon, 1990). Investigators have adopted the scale in research on the predictors of depressed mood in patients with such chronic illnesses as rheumatoid arthritis (Nicassio & Wallston, 1992) and fibromyalgia (Nicassio & Radojevic, 1993). Turk and Okifuji (1994) recommended a cutoff score of 19 for detecting depressive disorder in chronic pain populations. Recently, Shrout and Yager (1989) demonstrated that the CES-D could be shortened to five items and still maintain adequate sensitivity and specificity, as long as prediction was limited to traditional two-class categorizations. Typically, the Depression Scale can be completed in less than 10 minutes.

Beck Depression Inventory. The Beck Depression Inventory is a unidimensional self-report depression measure that uses 21 items to measure depression. It was developed by Beck and his colleagues (Beck, Ward, Mendelson, Mock, & Erbaugh) in 1961. Each of the items represents a characteristic symptom of depression (e.g., pessimism or self-contempt) on which the respondent is instructed to rate himself or herself on a 4-point scale. These scores are then summed to yield a total depression score. Beck's justification for this system was based on the notion that the frequency of depressive symptoms is distributed along a continuum, from "nondepressed" to "severely depressed." In addition, number of symptoms is viewed as correlating with intensity of distress and severity of depression. A short (13-item) version of the inventory was introduced in 1972 (Beck & Beck, 1972), and additional psychometric evaluation was subsequently accomplished (Reynolds & Gould, 1981).

The Beck Depression Inventory has been used to screen renal dialysis patients as well as medical inpatients and outpatients (Craven, Rodin, & Littlefield, 1988). Recently, Whitaker et al. (1990) used the inventory with a group of 5,108 community adolescents and noted its moderate validity for screening for major depression in this previously undiagnosed population. The inventory usually requires only 5–10 minutes for completion.

All of the instruments mentioned above have performed effectively in screening studies designed to establish the presence of either psychiatric disorder (in the case of the multidimensional tests) or clinical depression (with the Depression Scale and the Beck Depression Inventory). The sensitivities and specificities provided in Table 2 are typical of the performances by each test in medical populations. It should be noted, however, that these validity coefficients are specific to the populations from which they were generated. New validity coefficients should be developed for each new population (i.e., disorder or disease) in which the tests are applied.

Cognitive Functioning

Screening for cognitive impairment, particularly in geriatric populations, takes on a special significance in light of estimates that place the proportion of undetected organic mental disorder at close to 70% in some samples (Strain et al., 1988). Because some organic mental disorders are reversible if detected early enough, screening programs for cognitive impairment in high-risk populations can be very useful. Even in irreversible conditions, early detection and diagnosis can facilitate treatment planning and aid in the education of the family. In chronically medically ill populations, the sheer numbers of patients involved and the extensive time required for assessment preclude formal neuropsychological testing of all patients. The most meaningful alternative is to select patients for detailed cognitive evaluation on the basis of cognitive screening.

There are a number of cognitive instruments available that provide rapid and efficient screening of distinct cerebral dysfunction. Most of these have been used primarily with elderly people and address the general categories of cognitive functioning covered in the standard Mental Status Examination (McDougall, 1990): attention, concentration, intelligence, judgment, learning ability, memory, orientation, perception, problem solving, psychomotor ability, reaction time, and social intactness. However, not all instruments include items from all of the categories above. These general instruments can be contrasted with another class of cognitive-screening measures characterized by a more specific focus. For example, the Stroke Unit Mental Status Examination was designed specifically to identify cognitive deficits and plan rehabilitation programs for stroke patients (Hajek, Rutman, & Scher, 1989), whereas the Dementia of Alzheimer's Type Inventory was designed to distinguish Alzheimer's disease from other dementias (Cummings & Benson, 1986). These more specific types of measures tend to be less common, primarily because of their limited range of applicability.

Unlike other screening tests, which tend to be based on self-reports, the majority of cognitive impairment scales are administered by an examiner. Of the instruments that we review here, none are self-report measures. Instead, these tests are designed to be administered by a professional and require a combination of oral and written responses. Most of the tests are highly transportable, however, and can be administered by a wide variety of properly trained health care workers.

In the section that follows we provide a brief summary of five popular measures of cognitive impairment screening. Again, this exposition was intended as a brief review, to provide some data on the nature of each measure and its psychometric profile (see Table 3 for a comparative list of various attributes).

Mini-Mental State Examination (MMSE). The MMSE was developed by Folstein, Folstein, and McHugh (1975) to determine the level of a person's cognitive impairment. This 11-item scale measures six aspects of cognitive functioning: orientation, registration, attention and calculation, recall, language, and praxis. Scores can range from 0 to 30, with lower scores indicating greater impairment.

The MMSE has proved successful at assessing levels of cognitive impairment in many populations, including community residents (Kramer, German, Anthony, Von Korff, & Skinner, 1985), hospital patients (Teri, Larson, & Reifler, 1988), residents of long-term care facilities (Lesher & Whelihan, 1986), and neurological patients (Dick et al., 1984). However, Escobar et al. (1986) have recommended using an alternative instrument with Spanish-speaking individuals, because the MMSE appears to overestimate dementia in this population. Similarly, Roca et al. (1984) have also recommended other instruments for use with patients who have less than 8 years of schooling. In contrast, there is some evidence that the MMSE may underestimate cognitive impairment in psychiatric populations (Faustman, Moses, & Csernansky, 1990). Finally, the MMSE has shown lower sensitivity with mildly impaired individuals who are more likely to be labeled as demented (Doyle, Dunn, Thadani, & Lenihan, 1986). As such, the MMSE is most useful for patients who have moderate to moderately severe dementia.

Cognitive Capacity Screening Examination (CCSE). The CCSE is a 30-item scale designed to detect diffuse organic disorders, especially delirium, in medical populations. The instrument was developed by Jacobs, Berhard, Delgado, & Strain (1977). Items include questions of orientation, digit recall, serial 7s, verbal short-term memory, abstractions, and arithmetic—all of which facilitate the detection of delirium (F. Baker, 1989).

The CCSE has been used with geriatric patients (McCartney & Palmateer, 1985) as well as with hospitalized medical–surgical patients

Table 3

Screening Instruments for Cognitive Impairment

Instrument	Author & date	Description & purpose	Application	Sensitivity	Specificity
Mini-Mental State Examination	Folstein, Folstein, & McHugh (1975)	11 items; to determine level of cognitive impairment	1, 3, 4	0.83	0.99
Cognitive Capacity Screening Examination	Jacobs, Berhard, Delgado & Strain (1977)	30 items; to detect presence of organic mental disorder	2, 3, 4, 5	0.73	0.90
Short Portable Mental Status Questionnaire	E. Pfeiffer (1975)	10 items; to detect presence of cognitive impairment	1	0.55–0.88	0.72–0.96
High Sensitivity Cognitive Screen	Faust & Fogel (1989)	15 items; to estimate presence, scope, and severity of cognitive impairment	2	0.94	0.92
Mental Status Questionnaire	Kahn, Goldfarb, Pollack, & Peck (1960)	10 items; to quantify dementia	1, 4, 5, 6	0.550–.96	NA

Note. 1 = community populations, 2 = cognitively intact, 3 = hospital inpatients, 4 = medical patients, 5 = geriatric, 6 = long-term-care patients. NA = not applicable.

From *The Use of Psychological Testing for Treatment Planning and Outcome Assessment* (p. 39), edited by M. Maruish, 1994, Hillsdale, NJ: Erlbaum. Copyright 1994 by Erlbaum. Adapted with permission.

(Foreman, 1987). In a comparison study of several similar brief screening instruments, the CCSE was shown to be the most reliable and valid (Foreman, 1987). Like the MMSE, the CCSE is also influenced by the educational level of the subject. However, unlike the MMSE, the CCSE cannot differentiate levels of cognitive impairment or types of dementias, and it is felt to be most appropriate for patients who are essentially cognitively intact (Judd et al., 1986).

Short Portable Mental Status Questionnaire. This 10-item scale (E. Pfeiffer, 1975) is for use with community or institutional residents. It is unique in having been used with rural and less educated populations (F. Baker, 1989). The items assess orientation as well as recent and remote memory; however, visuospatial skills are not tested. The questionnaire is a reliable detector of organicity (Haglund & Schuckit, 1976), but it should not be used longitudinally to predict the progression or course of the disorder (Berg, Edwards, Danzinger, & Berg, 1987).

High Sensitivity Cognitive Screen. This scale was designed to be as sensitive and comprehensive as lengthier instruments while still being clinically convenient. It was developed by Faust & Fogel (1989) for use with 16-year-old to 65-year-old native-English–speaking subjects with at least an 8th-grade education who are free from gross cognitive dysfunction. The 15 items of this screen include reading, writing, immediate and delayed recall, and sentence construction, among others. It has shown adequate reliability and validity and appears to be best used to estimate the presence, scope, and severity of cognitive impairment (Faust & Fogel, 1989). The High Sensitivity Cognitive Screen is not designed to identify specific areas of the central nervous system involved; and as is true for most screening tests, it should represent a first step toward cognitive evaluation, not an end in and of itself.

Mental Status Questionnaire. The Mental Status Questionnaire is a 10-item scale developed by Kahn, Goldfarb, Pollack, and Peck (1960). It has been used successfully with medical geriatric patients (LaRue, D'Elia, Clark, Spar, & Jarvik, 1986), community residents (Shore, Overman, & Wyatt, 1983), and long-term-care patients (Fishback, 1977). Disadvantages of this measure include its sensitivity to the education and ethnicity of the subject, its reduced sensitivity with individuals suffering less dramatic impairment, and its omission of tests of retention, registration, and cognitive processing (F. Baker, 1989).

The five screening instruments reviewed above have been validated either principally or exclusively in individuals with primary central nervous system disease and, with the exception of the High Sensitivity Cognitive Screen, in individuals who are elderly. Thus, readers should be cautioned that none of these instruments has yet been specifically validated in populations with chronic systemic disease. In another chapter in this book, on neuropsychological assessment, Kelly & Doty discuss other approaches to screening aimed at detecting more subtle impairment in young and middle-aged adults.

Additional instruments. We deem three additional measures to be appropriate for testing cognitive impairment in chronically medically ill populations because their primary function is to simply rule out or detect the presence of dementia. The FROMAJE (Libow, 1981) classifies individuals into normal, mild, moderate, and severe dementia groups and has been used successfully with long-term-care patients (Rameizl, 1984). The Blessed Dementia Scale (Blessed, Tomlinson, & Roth, 1968) measures changes in activities and habits, personality, interests, and drives and has shown utility in determining the presence of dementia—although not in measuring its progression. Finally, the Global Deterioration Scale (Reisberg, Ferris, deLeon, & Crook, 1982) has shown utility in distinguishing between normal aging, age-associated memory impairment, and primary degenerative disorders (such as Alzheimer's disease). This scale is useful for assessing the magnitude and progression of cognitive decline (Reisberg, 1984).

A special challenge in screening for cognitive impairment involves evaluation of the geriatric patient. Elderly patients often present with sensory, perceptual, and motor problems that seriously limit the use of many standardized tests. Problems with vision, diminished hearing, and numerous other physical disabilities can subvert the suitability of tests that depend on these skills. Similarly, required medications can cause drowsiness, inalertness, or unwanted pharmacological effects that interfere with optimal cognitive functioning. Illnesses such as cardiovascular disorders and hypertension, which are highly prevalent among elderly people, have also been shown to affect cognitive functioning (Libow, 1977). These limitations demand that screening instruments be both flexible enough for adaptation to the patient with disabilities and sufficiently standardized to enable normative comparisons.

Another problem in assessing geriatric populations involves distinguishing cognitive impairment from memory loss associated with aging and from characteristics of normal aging. This distinction demands a sensitive screening instrument, because the differences between these conditions are often quite subtle. Normal aging and dementia can be distinguished through their differential effects on such functions as language, memory, perception, attention, information-processing speed, and intelligence (Bayles & Kaszniak, 1987). The Global Deterioration Scale (discussed above) was designed for this specific purpose; it has been demonstrated to successfully describe magnitude of cognitive decline as well as to predict functional ability (Reisberg, Ferris, deLeon, & Crook, 1988).

An additional problem encountered in screening for cognitive impairment in geriatric populations is the comorbidity of depression. Depression is highly prevalent among the elderly and is one of several disorders that may imitate dementia. The resulting condition is a syndrome known as *pseudodementia.* Patients with this syndrome have no currently discernible organic impairment, and the symptoms of dementia will usually remit when the underlying affective disorder is treated. Variability of task performance can help to distinguish these patients from truly demented patients, who are more likely to have a generally lowered performance level on all tasks (C. Wells, 1979). If the patient has a history of depression or there are other reasons to suspect depression, a more detailed diagnostic workup should be initiated.

Screening for cognitive impairment in medical inpatients by its nature involves a number of the problems discussed above with regard to elderly patients. Medical patients are often limited by their illness and may not be capable of responding legitimately to tests. In addition, these patients are often bedridden, necessitating the use of a portable, bedside assessment. Often, the most demanding task when evaluating this population is discriminating between the dementing patient and the patient who is in an acute confusional state, or delirious. This distinction is particularly important, not only because of the increased occurrence of delirium in medical patients but also because if left untreated it can progress to an irreversible status. Delirium can arise from multiple etiologies, such as drug intoxication, metabolic disorders, fever, cardiovascular disorders, or effects of anesthesia. Geriatric and medical patients are both susceptible to misuse or overuse of prescription drugs as well as to metabolic or nutritional imbalances. Hypothyroidism, hyperparathyroidism, and diabetes are a few of the medical conditions that are often mistaken for dementia (Albert, 1981).

In addition, cognitive impairment can also be caused by a variety of infections, such as pneumonia.

Fortunately, three cardinal characteristics facilitate the distinction between dementia and delirium. The first of these is the rate of onset of symptoms. Delirium is marked by acute or abrupt onset of symptoms, whereas dementia is characterized by a more gradual progression. Second is the impairment of attention. Delirious patients reveal a particular difficulty in sustaining attention on such tasks as serial 7s, and digit span. The third distinguishing feature is nocturnal worsening, which is characteristic of delirium but not of dementia (Mesulam & Geschwind, 1976).

In general, the majority of patients with chronic medical illnesses do not present with questions of cognitive impairment, and so from a strict "current functioning" perspective, they probably do not require a cognitive screening assessment. A broader, more prospective view of the assessment process, however—particularly in the case of the chronic patient—suggests that it is an excellent idea to include a screen for cognitive impairment at baseline. In general, most chronic illnesses show increasing morbidity with time. It is not uncommon for dramatic medical events to transpire, either as direct or indirect results of the disease process or its treatment. On the occasion of such an event, it is very useful for the psychologist to conduct an assessment of the event's possible impact on central nervous system functioning; at this time, a record of pre-event functioning, even a relatively gross one, can be of enormous value. In addition, implementing a routine cognitive screen enables the psychologist to identify unsuspected cognitive dysfunction arising from the primary medical illness or a second, unanticipated source.

Psychosocial Adjustment to Illness

The construct of psychosocial adjustment to illness had its formal beginnings in the 1950s in the context of attempts to systematically document the quality of adjustment achieved by psychiatric patients returning to the community. More recently, an increased focus on reintegrating and rehabilitating such patients in the community has heightened interest in this issue (Weissman, 1975). During the 1960s and 1970s, as enormous technological strides were made in medicine over a broad spectrum of diseases, increasing numbers of chronic medical disorders emerged in which protracted morbidity replaced mortality. The enhanced demands on people's coping and adjustment skills initiated by prolonged illnesses with little possibility of definitive resolution have highlighted the importance of being able to systematically quantify psychosocial adjustment to illness.

The very nature of the term *psychosocial adjustment* implies that the construct has to do with more than just intrapsychic processes. The concept also includes interactions between the individual (respondent) and other individuals and institutions in the environment. These associations are usually mediated through somewhat vaguely prescribed behavioral patterns called roles. How efficiently an individual performs his or her role functions (e.g., as spouse, parent, or worker) has been shown to be consistently correlated with judgments concerning his or her level of psychosocial adjustment. Furthermore, it has been demonstrated in the context of numerous chronic diseases (De-Nour, 1982; Murawski, Penman, & Schmitt, 1978; Zyzanski, Stanton, Jenkins, & Klein, 1981) that the quality of a patient's psychosocial adjustment can function on par with the status of his or her physical disease as a determinant in the outcome of an illness experience.

Some have been tempted to represent psychosocial adjustment as simply the converse of psychological distress—thus, to construe the degree of absence of the latter as a measure of the quality of the former. These models fail to recognize the inherently multidimensional nature of the adjustment construct, with its principal dimensions deriving from strong associations with salient role functions. Psychological distress, alternatively, represents an inverse indicator of quality of adjustment, which often signals a failure of the adjustment process. The vocational role, domestic role, and social-leisure roles, for example, are intrinsic to almost all definitions of psychosocial adjustment. Which additional attributes are included in any given operational definition of psychosocial adjustment (i.e., test or interview instrument) are determined by judgments of relevance, measurability, time, and cost-efficiency. Such attributes should be highly relevant to the superordinate construct of adjustment, should be measurable in brief operational terms, and should have unique predictive value relative to the effort taken to measure them. As is evidenced below, different authors have arrived at somewhat comparable, but distinct, operational definitions.

Although numerous instruments have been developed over the years to assess the psychosocial adjustment of psychiatric patients to their illnesses (Weissman, 1975; Weissman, Sholomskas, & John, 1981), fewer measures have been generated to evaluate the quality of adjustment of medical patients. Of those that have been published, we briefly highlight and review three scales. Each instrument discussed approaches the definition of adjustment in a somewhat distinct fashion, but each has demonstrated sound psychometric design, high outcome sensitivity, and predictive validities across a spectrum of chronic medical disorders.

Psychosocial Adjustment to Illness Scale (PAIS/PAIS-SR). The Psychosocial Adjustment to Illness Scale (PAIS; Derogatis, 1986) is a 46-item semistructured interview designed to evaluate and quantify the level of adjustment of a chronically ill medical patient to his or her disease or disorder. Seven principal domains of adjustment—health care orientation, vocational environment, domestic environment, sexual relationships, extended family relationships, social environment, and psychological distress—are reflected in the profile, as well as a total adjustment score. The PAIS interview takes approximately 20–30 minutes to complete. In addition, a matching self-report version of the instrument, the PAIS-SR, is also available. Self-report items were designed to be as similar as possible to PAIS interview items, to ensure the comparability of the PAIS-SR and the PAIS. The original administration manual for the PAIS and PAIS-SR (Derogatis & Lopez, 1983) has been superseded by a second edition (Derogatis & Derogatis, 1990). The latter provides formal norms for seven distinct illness groups: lung cancer, renal dialysis, burns, hypertension, cardiovascular disorder, mixed cancer, and diabetes. Several additional norms (e.g., for breast cancer and gynecological cancers) are currently under development.

The dimensional structure of the PAIS has been substantiated in a confirmatory factor analysis based on a sample ($N = 120$) of lung cancer patients (Derogatis, 1986). The independence of the primary dimensions in contributing to the measurement variance of the overall construct of psychosocial adjustment has also been well-established. Interdimensional correlations in three distinct illness samples—under treatment for lung cancer, kidney dialysis, and Hodgkin's disease—averaged .33, .29, and .10, respectively, whereas average correlations of dimension scores with total score were much higher in each instance (Derogatis, 1986).

De-Nour (1982) has reported significant convergent relationships between the PAIS-SR total score and the Multiple Affects Adjective Checklist and between physicians' ratings for psychological impairment and the psychological distress score on the PAIS-SR. In a study with 70 cardiac transplantation patients, Freeman, Fahs, Kolks, & Sokol (1988) demonstrated high correlations between appropriate PAIS scores and both the Zung Depression Scale and the State–Trait Anxiety Inventory across a postoperative period of 2 years. Similarly, Hochberg and Sutton (1988) showed substantial correlations between the dimensions of the PAIS-SR and the disability index, pain score, and global assessment rating of the Stanford Health Assessment Questionnaire in a sample of patients with systemic lupus erythematosus. Moguilner, Bauman, and De-Nour (1988) investigated the adjustment of children and their parents to the latter's chronic hemodialysis and found consistently high correlations between the parents' PAIS scores and a variety of measures of child adjustment, including the Tennessee Self-Concept Scale and the Thematic Apperception Test. Conrady, Wish, Agre, Rodriguez, and Sperling (1989) investigated the psychological status of polio survivors and correlated PAIS domain scores with the global scores of the SCL-90-R. Findings revealed that the global severity index of the SCL-90-R correlated .72 with the PAIS psychological distress scale.

Numerous studies have contributed substantially to the predictive and construct validity of the PAIS. De-Nour (1982) contrasted the PAIS-SR scores of dialysis patients rated as "good" and "bad" adjusters by their treating physicians and observed statistically significant differences between the groups on PAIS-SR total and domain scores. S. P. Murphy (1982) observed consistent predictive relationships between PAIS domain scores and external measures of adjustment with a similar cohort. Lamping (1981), who also worked with dialysis patients, demonstrated significant correlations between the PAIS and appropriate scales from the Profile of Mood States, Minnesota Multiphasic Personality Inventory, and medical compliance measures. In addition, she observed PAIS scores to discriminate patients in terms of life events, stress, work status, severity of illness and coping styles. Oldenburg, MacDonald, and Perkins (1988) also used the PAIS and the SCL-90-R with a sample of end-stage renal disease patients, observing that the PAIS was instrumental in predicting adjustment to disease. Similarly, Moguilner, Bauman, and De-Nour (1988) demonstrated high correlations between patients and spouses on the PAIS in a chronic hemodialysis sample and, furthermore, showed that adult PAIS scores correlated well with independent measures of their children's adjustment.

The PAIS and PAIS-SR have also been used frequently in cancer populations. Evans et al. (1988) used the PAIS to definitively demonstrate differences in adjustment between cancer patients suffering from clinical depression who were appropriately treated and similar patients who did not receive appropriate treatment. Gilbar and De-Nour (1988) used both the PAIS and the Brief Symptom Inventory to demonstrate marked differences between 53 patients who dropped out of chemotherapy and a matched control group who did not. In a study focused on family dynamics in breast cancer, L. C. Friedman and her colleagues (1988) related PAIS dimension scores to measures of family type, cohesion, and satisfaction in a sample of 57 women with breast cancer. PAIS scores significantly discriminated between family types and levels of cohesion, and showed substantial correlations with measures of family satisfaction and adjustment. Similarly, Wolberg, Tanner, Malec, and Romsaas (1989) contrasted three groups of women with breast disease (benign, unconfirmed malignancy, and confirmed malignancy) at time of initial evaluation and found that the PAIS successfully discriminated the benign sample from the two cohorts with cancer. Those with neoplasia were then offered either mastectomy or surgery with breast conservation procedures. PAIS measures continued to discriminate the benign biopsy sample from the two with cancer for up to 16 months after surgery.

Perhaps the widest use of the PAIS and PAIS-SR has been in studies of psychosocial adjustment among cardiac patients. In an innovative study with 410 coronary-bypass patients, Folks, Baker, Blake, Freeman, and Sokol (1988) demonstrated high predictive validity for the PAIS sexual functioning score in predicting postsurgical levels of clinical depression. Using both the Zung Scale and the Center for Epidemiological Studies Depression Scale as measures of depression, these investigators demonstrated average correlations of .30, .45, .53, and .57 between preoperative PAIS sexual functioning scores and depression scores at prebypass and at 3, 6, and 12 months postbypass, respectively. These investigators concluded that they were able to predict with "80% accuracy who will be at risk for a 'poor' outcome as defined by a PAIS score of >55 preoperatively" (1988, p. 390). Freeman et al. used the PAIS to predict adjustment in 19 patients who underwent cardiac transplants. In this study, the PAIS was able to document significant improvements in psychosocial adjustment at both 6- and 12-month posttransplant periods ($p < .001$).

In an Australian study, Langeluddecke, Baird, Hughes, Tennant, and Fulcher (1989) also used the PAIS to evaluate adjustment in coronary-artery-bypass surgery. Eighty-nine patients were prospectively followed for 1 year after surgery. All seven PAIS domain scores and the PAIS total score showed significant improvements in psychosocial adjustment at both 6 and 12 months postsurgery, with reductions in distress carrying patients from the clinical range into normative levels of adjustment. In a companion study, Langeluddecke and her colleagues (Langeluddecke, Tennant, Fulcher, Baird, & Hughes, 1989) used the PAIS-SR along with other psychological measures to evaluate the adjustment of spouses of coronary-artery-bypass patients to the index patient's illness. Preoperative evaluations revealed high levels of psychological distress and disturbances in social environment, with slightly smaller but significant elevations in constructs of vocational and domestic environments and sexual functioning. At 12 months after surgery, almost all scores were significantly reduced, as were scores on independent measures of anxiety and depression.

Shifting from cardiac patients per se, we can cite other examples of PAIS use. Powers and Jalowec (1987) used the PAIS and a number of other measures to predict blood pressure control in a sample of 450 persons with hypertension. The PAIS was also used as a dependent measure of adjustment to illness. The investigators used discriminant-function analysis to distinguish people with controlled hypertension from people with uncontrolled hypertension and found the PAIS health care orientation score to have the highest standardized coefficient in making the discrimination. Approximately 80% of hypertensive patients were correctly classified by using the determined set of predicator variables. Also, in a unique study of the long-term psychosocial adjustment of polio survivors, Conrady, Wish, Agre, Rodriguez, and Sperling (1989) used the PAIS-SR and SCL-90-R to evaluate levels of psychological distress and psychosocial adjustment status. Psychological morbidity on the somatization, depression, and anxiety measures of the SCL-90-R characterized the group, as did high levels of maladjustment on PAIS measures of health care orientation, social environment, and extended family relations. For those interested, a detailed review of PAIS and PAIS-SR research has recently become available (Derogatis & Fleming, in press).

Sickness Impact Profile. The Sickness Impact Profile is a self-report inventory comprising 136 items presented in a dichotomous format (e.g., "true of me" vs. "not true of me") that are organized into 12 categories of "health-related behavioral dysfunctions": sleep and rest, eating, work, home management, recreation and pastimes, ambulation, mobility, body care and movement, social interaction, alertness behavior, emotional behavior and communication. In addition, factor and cluster analytic studies of the primary categories (M. Bergner, 1993) have repeatedly demonstrated that seven of these categories consistently converge into two higher order dimensions: physical dysfunction and psychological dysfunction. M. Bergner, Bobbitt, Carter, and Gilson (1981)—in summarizing the 6 years of research leading to the final version of the instrument—characterized the inventory as "designed to be broadly applicable across types and severities of illness and across demographic and cultural subgroups" (p. 787). As opposed to the PAIS and PAIS-SR, the Sickness Impact Profile may also be viewed as a measure of functional status (Brook, Jordan, Divine, Smith, & Neelon, 1990), because many of its items are designed to reflect physical and cognitive functional status.

The Sickness Impact Profile is based on a specific model of sickness-related behavior that represents such behavior as independent of conceptualizations of health, health systems, or care-seeking activities (M. Bergner, 1993). In operationalizing the model in terms of a health-adjustment outcome measure, M. Bergner et al. (1981) treated sickness impacts as dysfunctional alterations in daily life activities that essentially reflected impairments in major role performances. They viewed these dysfunctions as potentially arising from self-report or from clinical judgments or as determined through objective testing and evaluation.

Scoring of this inventory is somewhat unique in that each item has a "severity of illness" weight associated with it. M. Bergner et al. (1981) determined relative severity weights by using a cohort of 133 "judges" composed of patients and health care professionals. An overall score for the profile is developed by summing the scale weights for each of the items endorsed by the respondent and dividing that sum by the total of all item scale weights. One then converts this ratio to a centile score by multiplying by 100. Similar scores may be computed for each profile category and the two higher order dimensions, with higher scores being equated with greater dysfunction.

M. Bergner (1993) reported very good test–retest reliabilities for the Sickness Impact Profile score categories (*r*s = .75–.92), with evidence of moderate (*r*s = .45–.60) item-endorsement consistency across time. Internal consistency reliability was reported to be very high (*r*s =

.94–.97) for the profile categories. Greenwald (1987) evaluated the convergent-discriminant validity of the profile in a multitrait–multimethod matrix design along with several other psychological measures. In a sample comprising 536 individuals who had recently been diagnosed with cancer, Greenwald found that the pattern of correlations supported the validity of the profile. Additional factor analyses of all instruments in which the entire patient sample was used produced a factor structure in which the large majority of the profile's categories loaded on the primary (physical disorder) dimension.

In clinical trials, the Sickness Impact Profile has been demonstrated to be a sensitive measure of adjustment to illness across an extensive array of disorders. For example, M. Bergner and her colleagues (M. Bergner, Bobbitt, Pollard, Martin, & Gilson, 1976) used the profile to demonstrate the therapeutic efficacy of a home-care regimen in the treatment of patients with chronic obstructive pulmonary disease. Later, Bergner used the instrument to effectively register the health status of cardiac-arrest patients after a specialized emergency medical service program had been implemented (L. Bergner, Hallstrom, Bergner, Eisenberg, & Cobb, 1985). Likewise, with the sample from the National Study of End Stage Renal Disease, Hart and Evans (1987) used the profile to demonstrate significant differences across the study's four major treatment groups. Transplantation showed decided advantages on a majority of the measures in comparison with home dialysis, medical-center-based dialysis, and continuous-peritoneal dialysis. In a different venue, Deyo, Diehl, and Rosenthal (1986) used the Sickness Impact Profile to evaluate patients who had distinct periods of bed rest following acute back pain. Deyo et al. found few, if any, differences between patients who had 2 versus 7 days of bed rest.

In a study aimed at establishing construct validity for the two superordinate dimensions of physical and psychological dysfunction on the Sickness Impact Profile, Brook et al. (1990) correlated profile scores with scores on the Minnesota Multiphasic Personality Inventory and the Carol Depression Rating Scale using a sample of 332 patients who had medical and comorbid psychiatric disorders. Total score and psychological dimension scores correlated significantly with the other psychological measures, whereas the physical dimension score correlated moderately. Multiple regression analysis revealed that psychological variables accounted for 40% of the total score variance, 62% of psychological dimension variance, and 19% of physical dimension variance. Brook et al. concluded that the profile was capable of discriminating psychological from physical dysfunction, even in a medical population with prominent psychological comorbidity, and that the measure of psychological dysfunction on the profile is strongly correlated with clinical depression.

In research highly pertinent from the perspective of outcome measurement, MacKenzie, Charlson, DiGioia, and Kelley (1986) evaluated the Sickness Impact Profile for its ability to reliably document intrapatient change across time. An instrument's capacity as an outcome measure is directly related to its ability to sense change within individuals. Therefore, MacKenzie et al. compared profile scores to an independent index that estimated maximum physical and emotional functioning by patients across time. Findings indicated that the profile was reasonably effective in documenting patients who were characterized as "becoming worse" but that it did not possess the sensitivity to detect either improvement or an unchanged status. Receiver Operating Characteristic analysis confirmed this result, suggesting that the profile has at least some difficulty discriminating improved adjustment. In another outcome-relevant study, Rothman, Hedrick, Bulcroft, Hickam, and Rubenstein (1991) investigated the validity of the profile for proxy scoring in comparison with standard self-report scoring. Approximately 275 patient–proxy pairs from a national adult day health care program completed the profile on the basis of the patients' perceived health status. Correlations between the two sets of assessments were generally high; however, proxy ratings of patients' psychosocial adjustment were not sufficiently convergent to suggest that they could be used as valid estimates of patient status.

Millon Behavioral Health Inventory (MBHI). The MBHI is a self-report inventory designed to evaluate the principal dimensions of health-related psychological coping among adult medical patients (Millon, Green, & Meagher, 1979, 1982a, 1982b). The MBHI is based on 150 true–false items, which generate a profile of 20 distinct dimensions. The dimensions are subsumed under four higher order categories: basic coping styles, psychogenic attitudes, psychosomatic correlates, and prognostic indicators. Norms for the MBHI were developed by using clinical groups from diverse medical populations and nonpatient "normals" recruited from a variety of settings. The MBHI also contains several validity scales designed to help identify patients who have uncooperative attitudes, those for whom comprehension is a problem, and patients who are not sufficiently competent to respond validly.

Since its introduction more than a decade ago (Millon, Green, & Meagher, 1979) the MBHI has been used with medical cohorts suffering from a broad variety of disorders. Green, Millon, and Meagher (1983) have described the use of the MBHI in assessing and managing patients who are undergoing coronary-artery-bypass surgery, whereas Gatchel, Mayer, Capra, Barnet, and Diamond (1986) have elucidated its effectiveness in predicting the functional status of patients suffering from low back pain. Murphy, Sperr, and Sperr (1986) have also conducted studies of the MBHI with chronic pain patients, in which results contrasted with those from the Minnesota Multiphasic Personality Inventory. They found that prognosis and sensitivity favored the MBHI; however, at a 1-year follow-up neither scale could successfully predict patients' functional status, medication use, or need for hospitalization. Wilcoxon, Zook, and Zarski (1988) also used the MBHI and the Minnesota Multiphasic Personality Inventory to predict criteria of functional status for patients attending a 20-day pain rehabilitation program. Using a discriminant-function model, these researchers found that both scales effectively discriminated functional from dysfunctional patients. Labbe, Myron, Fishbain, Rosomoff, and Rosomoff-Steele (1989) developed a norm for the MBHI based on chronic pain patients and, somewhat surprisingly, reported few differences between pain patients and normal control distributions. Those differences that did exist were observed on measures of anxiety and depression.

In addition to what researchers have done with chronic pain patients, Weisberg and Page (1988) have used the MBHI to contrast home- and hospital-based dialysis in the treatment of renal disease. Findings indicated that coping styles, psychogenic attitudes, and prognostic scale categories were highly predictive of patient adjustment and satisfaction, and a number of basic MBHI dimensions successfully discriminated between home dialysis and hospital-based treatments. Focusing specifically on repressive coping styles, Goldstein and Antoni (1989) compared a sample of 44 breast cancer patients undergoing multimodal treatment with a group of 34 women who were free of cancer. As they hypothesized, the women suffering from breast cancer demonstrated significantly higher levels of repressive coping styles than did healthy women.

In a cohort of duodenal ulcer patients, Tosi, Judah, and Murphy (1989) focused their attention on differential treatment efficacy across four distinct psychological treatments. These investigators subsequently contrasted the MBHI scores of the four treatment groups in whom frequency of gastrointestinal distress was also monitored. Results demonstrated that the MBHI measure of coping styles successfully discriminated cognitive experiential therapy as being more effective in reducing frequency of gastrointestinal distress. Also concerned with documenting treatment efficacy, Clifford, Tan, and Gorsuch (1991) used the MBHI to compare three treatment groups of overweight adults who differed in the nature of social support that was provided to them. The course of treatment was scheduled over a 12-month period, and although certain MBHI scores correlated with healthy changes over this period, there were no significant differences across treatment groups. Dickson et al. (1992) studied the psychological characteristics of patients who were referred to a special clinic for somatizers. In addition to revealing a higher prevalence of psychiatric disorder and substance abuse, somatizing patients showed elevated scores on anxiety and mood measures of the MBHI, a finding confirmed by elevated scores on the SCL-90-R for this group.

Middelboe, Birket-Smith, Andersen, and Friis (1992) used the MBHI and the General Health Questionnaire to study how the personality traits of 51 patients affected their adjustment to postconcussional sequelae. Patients were partitioned into two groups on the basis of their psychiatric caseness status as measured by the General Health Questionnaire. Numerous personality and coping style dimensions discriminated the two groups at 1 week postinjury and remained observable in patients with postconcussional sequelae at both 3- and 12-month follow-ups. The relative etiologic roles of premorbid personality factors and the traumatic events were discussed by Middleboe et al. in some detail.

Health-Related Personality Constructs

Personality typically refers to an enduring collection of attributes and traits that characterize an individual and are consistently reflected in his or her patterns of cognition, affectivity, and behavior. The notion that personality has relevance for health and disease can be traced back at least 2,000 years to Hippocrates' humoral theory of temperament and, even later, to the physician Galen's conviction that these same humoral elements are etiologic in disease (Goldfarb, Driesen, & Cole, 1967). Although there are diverse theoretical postures concerning personality (e.g., trait vs. process or interactional theories), it is ultimately the behavioral consistencies associated with personality attributes that make it a compelling area for psychological assessment.

Before turning to the specifics of personality assessment in chronic medical illness, researchers need to distinguish between health-related and general personality constructs. A second issue requiring clarification concerns distinguishing among the different avenues of influence through which personality attributes can act to affect health and illness status. The former question relates to the nature and breadth of personality constructs that are likely to have predictive value in chronic medical illness; the latter addresses the scientific necessity of maintaining viable personality–health linkages as conceptually distinct.

Concerning general versus health-related constructs, Mischel (1968) has argued that—although they are valid in a broad, descriptive sense—the enduring general traits measured by traditional personality tests lack predictive specificity. He contended that they have failed to predict behaviors and other specific outcomes of interest both because they tend to be extremely general and because they are person-oriented, nonsituational constructs. Health psychologists (e.g., Lamping, 1985) have further argued that such constructs are relatively insensitive to the context-specific changes (e.g., alteration in residence or modifications of coping requirements) associated with the exacerbations and remissions that characterize chronic medical illness. Although committed proponents of traditional trait theory remain (e.g., Eysenck, 1967) and advocates are clearly present in the health care arena (Costa & McCrae, 1987), many recent personality theorists have adopted a more interactional, process-oriented posture (Bandura, 1977; Contrada, Leventhal, & O'Leary, 1991).

Turning to the putative mechanisms through which personality may affect health, one must appreciate that multiple paths exist through which personality can potentially influence health and illness. Personality can conceivably function in an etiologic role relative to health status; that is, it can serve as a proximal causal agent (e.g., Type A personality and hypertension) or distal causal agent (e.g., unhealthy habits). Personality attributes can also plausibly operate as mediating factors—that is, as intervening variables that either facilitate or impede good health habits and positive adjustment to illness (Drory &

Florian, 1991; Suls & Rittenhouse, 1987). As an example, personality characteristics such as extraversion and agreeableness could act to promote a patient's cooperation with a demanding treatment regimen, ultimately promoting better health and well-being, whereas traits such as neuroticism and antagonism could initiate counterproductive health behaviors. Personality attributes can also serve as concomitants or marker variables for health status, the result of a common underlying biogenic agent which also causes a disease. In the latter situation, the personality attribute is a concomitant and a signal of disease risk, but has no causal bearing on the disease process. Regardless of which of the above schemes represents the most accurate depiction of the relationship between a personality pattern and a specific disease, it is essential to recognize that the majority of diseases have multifactorial etiologies. Even if personality does have a causal relationship in disease, the most likely scenario is that it is only one of a number of causal agents (H. S. Friedman & Booth-Kewley, 1987).

Because of the exciting recent findings suggesting that neuropeptide and cytokine networks may provide mechanisms through which thoughts and emotions directly influence physiologic functions of the body, including those of the immune system (Daruna & Morgan, 1990; Pert, 1986; Vingerhoets & Assies, 1991), it is tempting to focus our review on those personality attributes that have been suggested to have a direct causal relationship to disease. At the very least, one might be tempted to address the persistent question of the fact or fiction of the disease-prone personality. Because our commission was to review psychological assessment in chronic medical illnesses and not the etiologic role of psychological factors in disease, we have refrained from addressing either of these fascinating areas here (see reviews by Blalock, 1989, and Vingerhoets & Assies, 1991, on the former, and by Contrada et al., 1991, and H. S. Friedman & Booth-Kewley, 1987, on the latter topic). Instead, we have selected for discussion several personality attributes that share sound psychometric definition, a demonstrable predictive relationship to health status, and substantive utility in the health environment.

Type A Personality/Cynical Hostility. The Type A personality construct originated from the observations of two cardiologists regarding a consistent behavior pattern manifested by many of their patients who presented with coronary heart disease (M. Friedman & Rosenman, 1959). They identified this behavior pattern as *Type A Personality* and defined such individuals as those who characteristically exhibit high ambition, driven competitiveness, compulsive preoccupation with deadlines, time urgency and impatience, hostility, and a certain pronounced style of speech and posture. Individuals who matched this behavioral profile were identified as coronary prone. By exclusion, individuals who did not match the profile were designated *Type B*. After repeated small studies showed support for this hypothesis, a large prospective investigation—the Western Collaborative Group Study (Rosenman et al., 1975)—was launched to definitively evaluate the relationship between Type A behavior and coronary heart disease. Follow-up of approximately 3,500 men who were apparently free of disease at baseline revealed a rate of heart disease that was twice as high among the Type A men in comparison with Type B men. Subsequently, Drory and Florian (1991) proposed that Type A behavior patterns are associated not only with increased risk for coronary heart disease but also with increased risk for recurrent coronary events.

Essentially, two instruments have been developed that appear to validly measure Type A behavior pattern: the Structured Interview for Assessing Type A Behavior (Rosenman, 1978) and the Jenkins Activity Survey (Jenkins, Zyzanski, & Rosenman, 1979), a self-report inventory. The first instrument is a structured interview of 25 items addressing exemplary Type A behaviors, whereas the second uses statistical procedures (discriminant function and factor analysis) to identify 21 of its 50 items as optimum predictors of Type A behavior. Although the two measures do converge, Matthews, Krantz, Dembroski, and MacDougall (1982) reported a correlation between them of only .30. This finding and similar empirical evidence strongly suggest that the construct of Type A personality is not a unitary construct but, rather, that it comprises a number of specific but related behavioral patterns (Matthews, 1982).

An impressive array of evidence supports the hypothesis that the "lethal" component in the global Type A construct is an element labeled *cynical hostility* (Barefoot, Dahlstrom, & Redford, 1983; Matthews, 1988; Williams et al., 1980). Although various authors have defined cynical hostility somewhat distinctly, the core of this behavior pattern revolves around a tendency to quickly experience anger and resentment, accompanied by a pervasive distrustful view of the world. A cynical, negative perception of other people that characterizes them as unreliable and untrustworthy promotes a vigilant, aggressive posture and social and emotional alienation in individuals who score high on this trait. Contrada et al. (1991) thoroughly reviewed research linking cynical hostility to coronary heart disease, and H. S. Friedman and Booth-Kewley (1987) reported the results of their meta-analytic study, showing linkages of more broadly defined hostility constructs with five chronic medical illnesses (i.e., chronic heart disease, asthma, peptic ulcer, rheumatoid arthritis, and headache). More recently, Houston and Vavak (1991) published an interesting report exploring some of the developmental factors that may lead to the cynical hostility pattern.

In addressing the measurement of cynical hostility, the Cook–Medley Hostility Scale (Cook & Medley, 1954)—derived from the Minnesota Multiphasic Personality Inventory—has been far and away the most consistently predictive instrument relative to coronary heart disease. Dozens of other measures of hostility, anger, and aggression, manifested in overt or covert forms, have shown predictive value for the health status of patients with chronic medical illnesses; however, the similarity or convergence of these operational definitions is unclear.

Extraversion and Neuroticism. Extraversion and neuroticism are two higher order personality constructs defined initially through the work of Eysenck (1960, 1967) and subsequently adopted by many other personality theorists and investigators as major dimensions in their personality paradigms. In most representations, extraversion and neuroticism are posited as orthogonal dimensions—the former associated with positive affect states, effective coping, and enabling behavior patterns (Miller, 1991) and the latter observed as fundamental to negative affectivity, devalued self-concept, reduced self-esteem, and general life dissatisfaction (McCrae, 1991).

Although both personality constructs have repeatedly been shown to have substantial predictive effects for a broad spectrum of behaviors (Eysenck, 1967), neuroticism has been much more thoroughly investigated relative to health and illness. In their meta-analytic review, H. S. Friedman and Booth-Kewley (1987) cited only 32 reports in which extraversion was studied as a factor in adjusting to chronic medical illnesses, but they cited hundreds of reports in which neuroticism (in terms of its more specific components, e.g., anxiety or depression) was evaluated. The relatively disproportionate interest in neuroticism as a health influence has shifted in recent years, as Watson and his colleagues (Watson & Tellegen, 1985) have equated positive affectivity with extraversion at the trait level and have shown it to have substantial relevance for health-related behavior (Clark & Watson, 1988). As positive affectivity and general well-being increasingly become the focus of health-related research, the role of extraversion in patients' adjustments to chronic medical illnesses will almost certainly become much better defined and elaborated.

In terms of specific measuring instruments for extraversion and neuroticism, numerous tasks and inventories are available. The Eysenck Personality Inventory (Eysenck & Eysenck, 1968) and the Maudsley Personality Inventory (Eysenck, 1959) measure both of these constructs, as does the more recent NEO Personality Inventory (Costa & McCrae, 1985). The 16 Personality Factor Inventory (Cattell, Eber, & Tatsuoka, 1970) also contains dimensions that are the equivalents of these broad personality constructs.

Hardiness. The personality construct of hardiness was introduced by Kobasa (1979). Hardiness is a positive personality characteristic in that it is associated with successful coping patterns, optimism, an enabling style, and an orientation toward mastery. It is represented as a composite construct, comprising the three related dimensions of commitment, control, and challenge. *Commitment* refers to a tendency to appreciate self and the environment as engaging entities and to be constantly involved in activities that are viewed as interesting and worthwhile. *Control* alludes to the belief that an individual can determine his or her own destiny, through personal effort and actions that affect other individuals and the environment. *Challenge* represents a belief in which self-actualization and growth are linked to new learning and successful confrontation with new challenges.

Hardy individuals appear more resistant to the effects of stress, in some measure because their appraisal of potentially threatening events is more positive (i.e., they are not overwhelmed) and their coping strategies are more effective (Kobasa, 1982). The decisive and enabling coping style emblematic of hardy individuals is characterized as "transformational coping," being distinguished by a persistent tendency to take decisive actions that permanently recast the stressful event into a less stressful form. In contrast, Kobasa has referred to a less effective form of coping called *regressive coping*; people with this style of coping perceive stressful events as potentially catastrophic, calling forth primitive, regressive coping mechanisms, such as repression and denial (Kobasa, 1982). For the short term, regressive coping enables the individual to feel better by avoiding and escaping the stressor; however, in the long run, coping by evasion is not effective because the initial threatening circumstance goes unresolved.

Hardiness is a personality construct with high relevance for individuals suffering from chronic mental illnesses in that it has been proposed as an effective moderator and a resistance resource in stress-illness relationships. Those researchers centrally involved in developing the hardiness construct (e.g., Kobasa, 1982; Kobasa, Maddi, & Covington, 1981; Maddi, 1990) have maintained that hardiness acts to decrease illness through both direct effects and secondary effects of buffering. In terms of empirical findings, Maddi (1990) has reported significant negative correlations between levels of hardiness and annual blood pressure measures in a sample of executives over a course of 6 years; alternatively, Okun, Zautra, and Robinson (1988) have demonstrated a positive relationship between hardiness and measures of immune system efficiency in patients with rheumatoid arthritis. In a revealing study, Kobasa, Maddi, Pucetti, and Zola (1985) have constrasted and evaluated the buffering effects of hardiness, exercise, and social supports for a sample of executives whose stressful life events scores placed them in the upper half of the distribution. Results revealed that the buffering effect of hardiness relative to serious illness during the ensuing year was approximately twice as strong as either of the other two resistance resources. Drory and Florian (1991) also included hardiness in their examination of variables influencing the quality of adjustment by patients diagnosed with coronary heart disease; they found hardiness to be the most salient correlate of positive adjustment.

There have been some methodologic (Funk & Houston, 1987; Hull, Van Treuren, & Virnelli, 1987) as well as conceptual (Rhodewalt & Zone, 1989) criticisms of hardiness research, specifically relating to item construction in the second-generation test and to the idea that hardiness may simply be an inverse reflection of neuroticism and negative affectivity. A third-generation version of the test, addressing most of the psychometric issues, has recently been completed (Maddi, 1990), and there appears to be sufficient uniqueness preserved in the hardiness construct that it should continue to be a useful construct in health psychology. Additionally, Pollock and Duffy (1990) have developed the Health-Related Hardiness Scale specifically to measure hardiness among the medically ill. This more specific focus may improve the predictive specificity of hardiness in chronic illness populations.

Health-related locus of control. The locus of control construct originated from the social learning theory of Rotter (1954, 1982), where it was formally referred to as "internal versus external control of reinforcement" (1982, p. 489). Essentially, the locus of control construct describes a belief system focused on the expectancies that one has concerning the deterministic sources responsible for the events or outcomes of his or her life. Individuals who believe that outcomes depend on their personal behaviors or attributes (i.e., those who believe they have substantial control over their own destinies), are referred to as possessing an internal locus of control. Those who believe that outcomes or events are randomly or chance determined, or are determined by powerful entities beyond their governance, are characterized as having an external locus of control. Excellent reviews on locus of control have been published by Lefcourt (1981) and by Strickland (1989). In addition, Rotter (1990) has recently published a stimulating commentary on the heuristic value of the construct and why he believes it has continued to generate substantial interest and research for over 30 years.

An operational definition of locus of control was provided by the Internal–External Locus of Control Scale (Rotter, 1966), which dichotomizes individuals across the locus of control gradient into internals and externals. Lumpkin (1988) also provided a review of the validities and other psychometric qualities of a series of brief locus of control scales.

The Wallstons and their colleagues (B. S. Wallston, Wallston, Kaplan, & Maides, 1976)—deriving their motivation from the recognized importance of the area of health and well-being and from the fact that health-related locus of control research showed a number of significant inconsistencies—developed a health-specific version of Rotter's (1966) internal–external scale that they called the *Health Locus of Control Scale*. In a summary of health-related research applications of locus of control somewhat later, B. S. Wallston and Wallston (1978) reviewed a number of examples of locus of control in prevention research (e.g., smoking or birth control use) and sick-role behaviors (i.e., postdiagnosis responses involving adherence to regimen and compliance with appointments). They concluded that substantial evidence exists confirming the predictive validity of the locus of control construct in the area of health-related behaviors.

More recently, as Rotter (1990) indicated, there have been numerous studies using the locus of control construct in the broad area of physical health and illness. As examples, C. A. Pfeiffer and Wetstone (1988) compared health locus of control and affectivity among (a) patients with systemic lupus erythematosus, (b) a large sample of individuals with a variety of other chronic illnesses, and (c) a sizable sample of control subjects. They found that, in general, patients with lupus had substantially higher levels of affectivity than did control patients and a more external health locus of control. However, among those lupus patients who had significantly more experience with the disease and could predict their exacerbations, internal health beliefs were higher. Christensen, Turner, Smith, Holman, and Gregory (1991) evaluated the health locus of control construct and depression in a cohort of patients suffering from end-stage renal disease. Results indicated that, among patients who had not previously experienced a failed transplant, high internal locus was associated with lower levels of depression. Internals who had previously experienced a failed transplant, however, experienced significantly higher depression. A further interactive effect was that the interaction between health locus of control, depression, and previous transplant was only observed among patients who were severely ill.

In the area of chronic pain and its management, Crisson and Keefe (1988) evaluated the relationship between health locus of control, coping strategies, and psychological distress as measured by the SCL-90-R. They observed that chronic pain patients with an external locus of control revealed poorer pain-coping strategies and reported higher levels of psychological distress, particularly anxiety and depression. Also in the area of chronic pain, Harkapaa, Jarvikoski, Mellin, & Hurri (1991) evaluated the relationship of health locus of control, psychological distress, and short-term outcome in a low-back-pain rehabilitation program. They found that patients with higher internal locus of control gained significantly more from treatment. McLean and Pietroni (1990) recently showed the relevance of health locus of control to a self-care approach to treating stress conditions. They used an intervention combining behavioral techniques with active health promotion for a sample of 111 patients. A significant improvement in stress-related symptoms was observed at both 6 months and the 1-year follow-up and was found to be significantly related to an internal health locus of control.

Evidence that the original Health Locus of Control Scale is not a unidimensional measure led to the development of the Multidimensional Health Locus of Control (MHLC) scale (K. A. Wallston, Wallston, & DeVellis, 1978). The MHLC scale has three subscales, each assessing a separate dimension of the LOC construct: (a) Internal Health Locus of Control (IHLC)—the belief that one can directly influence health outcomes; (b) Chance Health Locus of Control (CHLC)—the belief that health outcomes result from fate and chance factors; and (c) Powerful Others Health Locus of Control (PHLC)—the belief that health professionals (doctors or nurses) or other people (family or friends) determine one's health status. There are two equivalent forms (A and B) of the MHLC.

Although the original HLOC Scale continues to receive research attention, the multidimensional scale is the preferred measure because its different components provide greater flexibility of application and have proven to be associated with varying health behaviors and outcomes. For example, in a review of the construct of control and its relationship to health, K. A. Wallston, Wallston, Smith, & Dobbins (1987) pointed out that CHLC and IHLC are better predicators of preventive health behaviors in healthy people than PHLC. In contrast, the PHLC Scale has shown evidence of predicting medical adherence responses in people with such chronic illnesses as rheumatoid arthritis more effectively than either the CHLC or IHLC scales (Roskam, 1986). High PHLC scores tend to be associated with higher adherence. K. A. Wallston et al. also made the important point that the three scales may yield better results in predicting health behaviors and outcomes when other pertinent variables are taken into account. Situation variables and other factors—such as the value placed on health, other behavioral and outcome expectancies, or the severity of one's illness—in people with chronic illnesses, may interact with the MHLC dimensions to predict specific health behaviors.

Recently, K. A. Wallston (1993) reported on the development of a condition-specific version of the MHLC scales (Form C)—one that can easily be modified to assess locus of control beliefs pertinent to any existing health condition (e.g., arthritis, cancer, pain, or diabetes). Use of Form C allows both the respondent and the investigator to be clear about which aspect of the respondent's health is being assessed.

As Rotter (1990) has pointed out, it is apparent that the locus of control construct remains a viable and productive scientific concept in the area of clinical health psychology. It has predictive validity for health-related behaviors in a broad variety of chronic illnesses and retains considerable heuristic value.

Conclusion

In this chapter, we have pointed out the major issues and methods central to the psychological assessment of individuals suffering from chronic medical illnesses. In doing so, we have tried to emphasize that illness is a broader concept than disease—one that inherently involves intrapsychic, interpersonal, and psychosocial facets, which interact with the primary pathophysiology of disease. By the nature of chronic illnesses, behavior—and its affects, attitudes, and cognitions—plays a significant role in the ultimate determination of a patient's morbidity and his or her response to therapeutic intervention. For this reason, it is vital that those responsible for treating chronic medical conditions possess a valid appraisal of the patient's psychological functioning, in terms of not only current status but also historical capacity and potential for future functioning.

Change is intrinsic to chronic illnesses (e.g., biological, functional, and residential), necessitating continual alterations in coping and adjustment by the patient. The psychologist's ability to document patients' responses to disease- and treatment-induced alterations in status accurately is critical to achieving an optimal therapeutic plan. Psychological assessment, if designed as a dynamic, prospective enterprise that is an integral aspect of the chronic patient's care system, will contribute unique and highly relevant information to the patient's treatment regimen. Carefully planned, programmatic assessments of the patient's psychological coping and adjustment can identify problematic patients as well as those generally well-adjusted patients who are entering problematic periods. Indications that coping resources are taxed or faltering can signal the need for specific intervention efforts designed to avert serious adjustment problems and restore patient well-being.

Future developments in this area will almost certainly evolve around two concepts: specificity and standardization. Assessments will be targeted to address specific outcome questions rather than general psychological status and will increasingly become standardized within and across large health care organizations and systems. The increased predictive power derived from large databases with standardized assessments of constructs such as those discussed here will make the adoption of such standardized approaches increasingly more compelling. Psychological assessment data will increasingly become incorporated in cost-utility analyses, as outcomes involving patients' adjustment and well-being become a more central and quantifiable aspect of the economic dimensions of treatment (Howard, Kopta, Krause, & Orlinsky, 1986; Kopta, Howard, Lowry, & Beutler, 1994). Brevity, cost-efficiency, minimal intrusiveness, and broad applicability will be dominant concepts in the design of future assessment systems.

REFERENCES

Albert, M. (1981). Geriatric neuropsychology. *Journal of Consulting and Clinical Psychology, 49,* 835–850.

American Psychiatric Association. (1994). *Diagnostic and statistical manual of mental disorders* (4th ed.). Washington, DC: Author.

Anderson, S. M., & Harthorn, B. H. (1989). The recognition, diagnosis and treatment of psychiatric disorders by primary care physicians. *Medical Care, 27,* 869–886.

Baker, F. (1989). Screening tests for cognitive impairment. *Hospital and Community Psychiatry, 40,* 339–340.

Baker, L. A., Cesa, I. L., Gatz, M., & Mellins, C. (1992). Genetic and environmental influences on positive and negative affect: Support for a two-factor theory. *Psychological Aging, 7,* 158–163.

Bandura, A. (1977). *Social learning theory.* Englewood Cliffs, NJ: Prentice Hall.

Barefoot, J. C., Dahlstrom, W. G., & Redford, B. W. (1983). Hostility, child incidence, and mortality: A 25-year follow-up study of 255 physicians. *Psychosomatic Medicine, 45,* 59–63.

Barrett, J. E., Barrett, J. A., Oxman, T. E., & Gerber, P. D. (1988). The prevalence of psychiatric disorders in a primary care practice. *Archives of General Psychiatry, 45,* 1100–1106.

Bayles, K., & Kaszniak, A. (1987). *Communication and cognition in normal aging and dementia.* Boston: Little, Brown.

Beck, A. T., & Beck, R. W. (1972). Screening depressed patients in family practice: A rapid technique. *Postgraduate Medicine, 52,* 81–85.

Beck, A. T., Ward, C., Mendelson, M., Mock, J. E., & Erbaugh, J. K. (1961). An inventory for measuring depression. *Archives of General Psychiatry, 4,* 53–63.

Berg, G., Edwards, D., Danzinger, W., & Berg, L. (1987). Longitudinal change in three brief assessments of SDAT. *Journal of the American Geriatrics Society, 35,* 205–212.

Bergner, L., Hallstrom, A. P., Bergner, M., Eisenberg, M. S., & Cobb, L. A. (1985). Health status of survivors of cardiac arrest and of myocardial infarction controls. *American Journal of Public Health, 74,* 1321–1323.

Bergner, M. (1993). Development testing and use of the Sickness Impact Profile. In S. R. Walker and R. M. Rosser (Eds.), *Quality of Life Assessment: Key issues in the 1990's.* Boston: Kluwer Academic.

Bergner, M., Bobbit, R. A., Carter, W. B., & Gilson, B. S. (1981). The Sickness Impact Profile: Development and final revision of a health status measure. *Medical Care, 19,* 787–795.

Bergner, M., Bobbit, R. A., Pollard, W. E., Martin, D. P., & Gilson, B. S. (1976). The Sickness Impact Profile: Validation of a health status measure. *Medical Care, 14,* 57–67.

Blalock, J. E. (1989). A molecular basis for bidirectional communication between the immune and neuroendrocrine systems. *Physiological Reviews, 69,* 1–32.

Blessed, G., Tomlinson, B., & Roth, M. (1968). The association between quantitative measures of dementia and of senile change in the cerebral gray matter of elderly. *British Journal of Psychiatry, 114,* 797–811.

Bradburn, N. M. (1969). *The structure of psychological well-being.* Chicago: Aldine.

Brook, W. B., Jordan, J. S., Divine, G. W., Smith, K. S., & Neelon, F. A. (1990). The impact of psychologic factors on measurement of functional status: Assessment of the Sickness Impact Profile. *Medical Care, 28,* 793–804.

Bullinger, M. (1991). Quality of life: Definition, conceptualization and implications—A methodologist's view. *Theoretical Surgery, 6,* 143–148.

Cattell, R. B., Eber, H. W., & Tatsuoka, M. M. (1970). *The handbook for the sixteen personality factor questionnaire.* Champaign, IL: Institute for Personality and Ability Testing.

Christensen, A. J., Turner, C. W., Smith, T. W., Holman, J. M., & Gregory, M. C. (1991). Health locus of control and depression in end-stage renal disease. *Journal of Consulting and Clinical Psychology, 59,* 419–424.

Clark, D. A., Beck, A. T., & Stewart, B. (1990). Cognitive specificity and positive–negative affectivity: Complementary or contradictory views on anxiety and depression? *Journal of Abnormal Psychology, 99,* 148–155.

Clark, L. A., & Watson, D. (1988). Mood and the mundane: Relations between daily life events and self-reported mood. *Journal of Personality and Social Psychology, 54,* 296–308.

Clifford, P. A., Tan, S. Y., & Gorsuch, R. L. (1991). Efficacy of a self-directed behavioral health change program: Weight, body composition, cardiovascular fitness, blood pressure, health risk and psychosocial mediating variables. *Journal of Behavioral Medicine, 14,* 303–323.

Commission on Chronic Illness. (1957). *Chronic illness in the United States.* Cambridge, MA: Harvard University Press.

Comstock, G. W., & Helsing, K. J. (1976). Symptoms of depression in two communities. *Psychological Medicine, 6,* 551–564.

Conrady, L. J., Wish, J. R., Agre, J. C., Rodriguez, A. A., & Sperling, K. (1989). Psychologic characteristics of polio survivors: A preliminary report. *Archives of Physical Medicine Rehabilitation, 70,* 458.

Contrada, R. J., Leventhal, H., & O'Leary, A. (1991). Personality and health. In L. A. Pervin (Ed.), *Handbook of personality: Theory and research* (pp. 638–669). New York: Guilford Press.

Cook, W. W., & Medley, D. M. (1954). Proposed hostility and pharisaic–virtue scales for the MMPI. *Journal of Applied Psychology, 38,* 414–418.

Costa, P. T., & McCrae, R. R. (1985). Hypochondriasis, neuroticism, and aging: When are somatic complaints unfounded? *American Psychologist, 40,* 19–28.

Costa, P. T., & McCrae, R. R. (1987). Personality assessment in psychosomatic medicine. *Advances in Psychosomatic Medicine, 17,* 71–82.

Craven, J. L., Rodin, G. M., & Littlefield, C. (1988). The Beck Depression Inventory as a screening device for major depression in renal dialysis patients. *International Journal of Psychiatry in Medicine, 18,* 365–374.

Crisson, J. E., & Keefe, F. J. (1988). The relationship of locus of control to pain coping strategies and psychological distress in chronic pain patients. *Pain, 35,* 147–154.

Cummings, J., & Benson, F. (1986). Dementia of the Alzheimer type: An inventory of diagnostic clinical features. *Journal of the American Geriatrics Society, 34,* 12–19.

Daruna, J. H., & Morgan, J. E. (1990). Psychosocial effects on immune function: Neuroendocrine pathways. *Psychosomatics, 31,* 4–12.

De-Nour, A. K. (1982). Social adjustment of chronic dialysis patients. *American Journal of Psychiatry, 139,* 97–99.

Derogatis, L. R. (1975). *The Affects Balance Scale (ABS).* Baltimore: Clinical Psychometric Research.

Derogatis, L. R. (1977). *SCL-90-R: Administration, scoring and procedures manual—I.* Baltimore: Clinical Psychometric Research.

Derogatis, L. R. (1982). Self-report measures of stress. In L. Goldberger & S. Breznitz (Eds.), *Handbook of stress* (pp. 270–284). New York: Free Press.

Derogatis, L. R. (1983). *SCL-90-R: Administration, scoring and procedures manual–II.* Baltimore: Clinical Psychometric Research.

Derogatis, L. R. (1986). The Psychosocial Adjustment to Illness Scale (PAIS). *Journal of Psychosomatic Research, 30,* 77–91.

Derogatis, L. R. (1993). *BSI: Administration, scoring and procedures manual for the Brief Symptom Inventory II* (3rd ed.). Minneapolis, MN: National Computer Systems.

Derogatis, L. R. (1994). *SCL-90-R®: Administration, scoring and procedures manual—III* (3rd ed.). Minneapolis, MN: National Computer Systems.

Derogatis, L. R., Abeloff, M. D., & Melisaratos, N. (1979). Psychological coping mechanisms and survival in metastatic breast cancer. *Journal of the American Medical Association, 242,* 1504–1508.

Derogatis, L. R., & DellaPietra, L. (1994). Psychological tests in screening for psychiatric disorder. In M. Maruish (Ed.), *The use of psychological testing for treatment planning and outcome assessment* (pp. 22–54). Hillsdale, NJ: Erlbaum.

Derogatis, L. R., DellaPietra, L., & Kilroy, V. (1992). Screening for psychiatric disorder in medical populations. In M. Fava, G. Rosenbaum, & R. Birnbaum (Eds.), *Research designs and methods in psychiatry* (pp. 145–172). Amsterdam: Elsevier.

Derogatis, L. R., & Derogatis, M. F. (1990). *PAIS & PAIS-SR administration. Scoring and procedures manual—II.* Baltimore: Clinical Psychometric Research.

Derogatis, L. R., & Fleming, M. (in press). Psychosocial adjustment to illness scale: PAIS and PAIS-SR. In B. Spilker (Ed.), *Quality of life and pharmacoeconomics in clinical trials* (2nd ed.). New York: Raven Press.

Derogatis, L. R., & Lazarus, L. (1994). The SCL-90–R, Brief Symptom Inventory, and matching clinical rating scales. In M. Maruish (Ed.), *The use of psychological testing for treatment planning and outcome assessment* (pp. 217–248). Hillsdale, NJ: Erlbaum.

Derogatis, L. R., Lipman, R. S., Rickels, K., Uhlenhuth, E. H., & Covi, L. (1974). The Hopkins Symptom Checklist (HSCL). In P. Pinchot (Ed.), *Psychological measurements in psychopharmacology* (pp. 79–111). Basel, Switzerland: Karger.

Derogatis, L. R., & Lopez, M. (1983). *Psychosocial Adjustment to Illness Scale (PAIS and PAIS-R) scoring, procedures and administration manual—I.* Baltimore: Clinical Psychometric Research.

Derogatis, L. R., & Melisaratos, N. (1983). The Brief Symptom Inventory: An introductory report. *Psychological Medicine, 13,* 595–605.

Derogatis, L. R., & Meyer, J. K. (1979). A psychological profile of the sexual dysfunctions. *Archives of Sexual Behavior, 8,* 201–223.

Derogatis, L. R., Meyer, J. K., & Boland, P. (1981). Psychological profile of the female transsexual. *Journal of Nervous and Mental Disease, 169,* 157–168.

Derogatis, L. R., Meyer, J. K., & Vasquez, I. (1978). A psychological profile of the sexual dysfunctions. *Archives of Sexual Behavior, 8,* 201–223.

Derogatis, L. R., Morrow, G. R., Fetting, J., Penman, D., Piasetsky, S., Schmale, A. M., Henrichs, M., & Carnicke, C. M. (1983). The prevalence of psychiatric disorders among cancer patients. *Journal of the American Medical Association, 249,* 751–757.

Derogatis, L. R., & Rutigliano, P. J. (in press). Derogatis Affects Balance Scale (DABS). In B. Spilker (Ed.), *Quality of life and pharmacoeconomics in clinical trials.* New York: Raven Press.

Derogatis, L. R., & Spencer, P. M. (1982). *BSI administration and procedures manual—I.* Baltimore: Clinical Psychometric Research.

Derogatis, L. R., & Wise, T. N. (1989). *Anxiety and depressive disorders in the medical patient.* Washington, DC: American Psychiatric Press.

Deyo, R. A., Diehl, A. K., & Rosenthal, M. (1986). How many days of bed rest for acute low back pain? A randomized trial. *New England Journal of Medicine, 315,* 1064–1070.

Dick, J., Guiloff, R., Stewart, A., Blackstock, J., Bielawska, C., Paul, E., & Marsden, C. (1984). Mini-Mental State Examination in neurological patients. *Journal of Neurology, Neurosurgery, and Psychiatry, 47,* 496–499.

Dickson, L. R., Hays, L. R., Kaplan, O., Sherl, E., Abbot, S., & Schmitt, F. (1992). Psychological profile of somatizing patients attending the integrative clinic. *International Journal of Psychiatry in Medicine, 22,* 141–153.

Doyle, G., Dunn, S., Thadani., I., & Lenihan, P. (1986). Investigating tools to aid in restorative care for Alzheimer's patients. *Journal of Gerontological Nursing, 12,* 19–24.

Drory, Y., & Florian, V. (1991). Long-term psychosocial adjustment to coronary artery disease. *Archives of Physical Medicine and Rehabilitation, 72,* 326–331.

Escobar, J., Burnam, A., Karno, M., Forsythe, A., Landsverk, J., & Golding, J. (1986). Use of the Mini-Mental State Examination (MMSE) in a community population of mixed ethnicity: Cultural and linguistic artifacts. *Journal of Nervous and Mental Disease, 174,* 607–614.

Evans, D. L., McCartney, C. F., Haggerty, J. J., Nemeroff, C., Golden, R. N., Simon, J. B., Quade, D., Holmes, V., Droba, M., Mason, G. A., Fowler, C., & Raft, D. (1988). Treatment of depression in cancer patients is associated with better life adaptation: A pilot study. *Psychosomatic Medicine, 50,* 72–76.

Eysenck, H. J. (1959). *The manual of the Maudsley Personality Inventory.* London: University of London.

Eysenck, H. J. (1960). *The structure of human personality.* London: Methuen.

Eysenck, H. J. (1967). *The biological basis of personality.* Springfield, IL: Charles C Thomas.

Eysenck, H. J., & Eysenck, S. B. G. (1968). *Eysenck Personality Inventory.* San Diego, CA: Educational and Industrial Testing Service.

Faust, D., & Fogel, B. (1989). The development and initial validation of a sensitive bedside cognitive screening test. *Journal of Nervous and Mental Disease, 177,* 25–31.

Faustman, W., Moses, J., & Csernansky, J. (1990). Limitations of the Mini-Mental State Examination in predicting neuropsychological functioning in a psychiatric sample. *Acta Psychiatrica Scandinavica, 81,* 126–131.

Ferrans, C. E. (1990). Quality of life: Conceptual issues. *Seminars in Oncology Nursing, 6,* 248–254.

Fishback, D. (1977). Mental status questionnaire for organic brain syndrome, with a new visual counting test. *Journal of the American Geriatrics Society, 35,* 167–170.

Folks, D. G., Baker, D. M., Blake, D. J., Freeman, A. M., & Sokol, R. S. (1988). Persistent depression in coronary-bypass patients reporting sexual maladjustment. *Psychosomatics, 29,* 387–391.

Folstein, M., Folstein, S., & McHugh, P. (1975). Mini-Mental State. *Journal of Psychiatric Research, 12,* 189–198.

Foreman, M. (1987). Reliability and validity of mental status questionnaires in elderly hospitalized patients. *Nursing Research, 36,* 216–220.

Freeman, A. M., Fahs, J. J., Kolks, D. G., & Sokol, R. S. (1988). Cardiac transplantation: Clinical correlates of psychiatric outcome. *Psychosomatics, 29,* 47–54.

Frerichs, R. R., Aneshensel, C. S., & Clark, V. A. (1981). Prevalence of depression in Los Angeles County. *American Journal of Epidemiology, 113,* 691–699.

Friedman, H. S., & Booth-Kewley, S. (1987). The "disease-prone personality." *American Psychologist, 42,* 539–555.

Friedman, L. C., Baer, P. E., Nelson, D. V., Lane, M., Smith, F. E., & Dworkin, R. J. (1988). Women with breast cancer: Perception of family functioning and adjustment to illness. *Psychosomatic Medicine, 50,* 529-540.

Friedman, M., & Rosenman, R. H. (1959). Association of specific overt behavior pattern with blood and cardiovascular findings. *Journal of the American Medical Association, 169,* 1286–1296.

Funk, S. C., & Houston, B. K. (1987). A critical analysis of the Hardiness Scale's validity and utility. *Journal of Personality and Social Psychology, 53,* 572–578.

Garamoni, G. L., Reynolds, C. F., Thase, M. E., Frank, E., Berman, S. R., & Fasiczka, A. L. (1991). The balance of positive and negative affects in major depression: A further test of the states of mind model. *Psychiatry Research, 39,* 99–108.

Gatchel, R. J., Mayer, T. G., Capra, P., Barnet, J., & Diamond, P. (1986). Millon Behavioral Health Inventory: Its utility in predicting physical function in patients with low back pain. *Archives of Physical Medicine and Rehabilitation, 67,* 878–882.

Gilbar, O., & De-Nour, A. K. (1988). Adjustment to illness and dropout of chemotherapy. *Journal of Psychosomatic Research, 33,* 1–5.

Goldberg, D. (1972). *The detection of psychiatric illness by questionnaire.* Oxford, England: Oxford University Press.

Goldberg, D., & Hillier, V. F. (1979). A scaled version of the General Health Questionnaire. *Psychological Medicine, 9,* 139–145.

Goldberg, D., & Williams, P. (1988). *A user's guide to the general health questionnaire.* Windsor, England: Nfer-Nelson.

Goldfarb, C., Driesen, J., & Cole, D. (1967). Psychophysiologic aspects of malignancy. *American Journal of Psychiatry, 123,* 1545–1552.

Goldstein, D. A., & Antoni, M. H. (1989). The distribution of repressive coping styles among non-metastatic and metastatic breast cancer patients as compared to non-cancer patients. *Psychology & Health, 3,* 245–258.

Green, C. J., Millon, T., & Meagher, R. B., Jr. (1983). The MBHI: Its utilization in assessment and management of the coronary bypass surgery patient. *Psychotherapy and Psychosomatics, 39,* 112–121.

Greenwald, H. (1987). The specificity of quality of life measures among the seriously ill. *Medical Care, 25,* 642–651.

Haglund, R., & Schuckit, M. (1976). A clinical comparison of tests of organicity in elderly patients. *Journal of Gerontology, 31,* 654–659.

Hajek, V., Rutman, D., & Scher, H. (1989). Brief assessment of cognitive impairment in patients with stroke. *Archives of Physicial Medicine and Rehabilitation, 70,* 114–117.

Harkapaa, K., Jarvikoski, A., Mellin, G., & Hurri, H. (1991). Health locus of control beliefs and psychological distress a predictor for treatment outcome in low-back pain patients: Results of a 3-month follow-up of a controlled intervention study. *Pain, 46,* 35–41.

Hart, G. L., & Evans, R. W. (1987). The functional status of ESRD patients as measured by the Sickness Impact Profile. *Journal of Chronic Disease, 40* (Suppl. 1), 1175–1315.

Herzberg, F., Mathapo, J., Wiener, Y., & Wiesen, L. E. (1974). Motivation–hygiene correlates of mental health: An examination of motivational inversion in a clinical population. *Journal of Consulting and Clinical Psychology, 42,* 411–419.

Hochberg, M. C., & Sutton, J. D. (1988). Physical disability and psychosocial dysfunction in systemic lupus erythematosus. *Journal of Rheumatology, 15,* 959–964.

Hoehn-Saric, R. (1983). Affective profiles of chronically anxious patients. *Journal of Clinical Psychiatry, 5,* 43–56.

Holland, J. C., Morrow, G. R., Schmale, A., Derogatis, L. R., Stefanek, M., Berenson, S., Breitbart W., & Feldstein, M. (1990). A randomized clinical trial of alprazolam versus progressive muscle relaxation in cancer patients with anxiety and depressive symptoms. *Journal of Clinical Oncology, 49,* 1004–1011.

Houston, B. K., & Vavak, C. R. (1991). Cynical hostility: Developmental factors, psychosocial correlates, and health behaviors. *Health Psychology, 10,* 9–17.

Howard, K. I., Kopta, S. M., Krause, M. S., & Orlinsky, D. E. (1986). The dose-effect relationship in psychotherapy. *American Psychologist, 41,* 159–164.

Hull, J. G., Van Treuren, R. R., & Virnelli, S. (1987). Hardiness and health: A critique and alternative approach. *Journal of Personality and Social Psychology, 53,* 518–530.

Irvine, D., Brown, B., Crooks, J., Roberts, J., & Browne, G. (1991). Psychosocial adjustment in women with breast cancer. *Cancer, 67,* 1097–1117.

Jacobs, J., Berhard, M., Delgado, A., & Strain, J. (1977). Screening for organic mental syndromes in the medically ill. *Annals of Internal Medicine, 86,* 40–46.

Jenkins, C. D., Zyzanski, S. J., & Rosenman, R. H. (1979). *Manual for the Jenkins Activities Survey.* New York: Psychological Corporation.

Judd, B., Meyer, J., Rogers, R., Gandhi, S., Tanahashi, N., Mortel, K., & Tawakina, T. (1986). Cognitive performance correlates with cerebrovascular impairments in multi-infarct dementia. *Journal of the American Geriatrics Society, 34,* 355–360.

Kahn, R., Goldfarb, A., Pollack, M., & Peck, A. (1960). Brief objective measures for the determination of mental status in the aged. *American Journal of Psychiatry, 117,* 326–328.

Kobasa, S. C. (1979). Stressful life events, personality, and health: An inquiry into hardiness. *Journal of Personality and Social Psychology, 37,* 1–11.

Kobasa, S. C. (1982). The hardy personality: Toward a social psychology of stress and illness. In G. Sanders & J. Suls (Eds.), *Social psychology and health and illness* (pp. 3–32). Hillsdale, NJ: Erlbaum.

Kobasa, S. C., Maddi, S. R., & Covington, S. (1981). Personality and constitution as mediators in the stress–illness relationship. *Journal of Health and Social Behavior, 22,* 368–378.

Kobasa, S. C., Maddi, S. R., Pucetti, M. S., & Zola, M. A. (1985). Effectiveness of hardiness, exercise, and social support as resources against illness. *Journal of Psychosomatic Research, 29,* 525–533.

Kopta, S. M., Howard, K. I., Lowry, J. L., & Beutler, L. E. (1994). Patterns of symptomatic recovery in psychotherapy. *Journal of Consulting and Clinical Psychology, 62,* 1009–1016.

Kramer, M., German, P., Anthony, J., Von Korff, M., & Skinner, E. (1985). Patterns of mental disorders among the elderly residents of eastern Baltimore. *Journal of the American Geriatrics Society, 11,* 236–245.

Labbe, E. E., Myron, G., Fishbain, D., Rosomoff, H., & Rosomoff-Steele, R. (1989). Millon Behavioral Health Inventory norms for chronic pain patients. *Journal of Clinical Psychology, 45,* 383–390.

Lamping, D. L. (1981). *Psychosocial adaptation and adjustment to the stress of chronic illness.* Doctoral dissertation, Harvard University, Cambridge, MA.

Lamping, D. L. (1985). Assessment of health psychology. *Canadian Psychology, 26,* 121–139.

Langeluddecke, P., Baird, D., Hughes, C., Tennant, C., & Fulcher, G. (1989). A perspective evaluation of the psychosocial effects of coronary artery bypass surgery. *Journal of Psychosomatic Research, 33,* 37–45.

Langeluddecke, P., Tennant, C., Fulcher, G., Baird, D., & Hughes, C. (1989). Coronary artery bypass surgery: Impact upon the patient's spouse. *Journal of Psychosomatic Research, 33,* 155–159.

LaRue, A., D'Elia, L., Clark, E., Spar, J., & Jarvik, L. (1986). Clinical tests of memory in dementia, depression, and healthy aging. *Psychology and Aging, 1,* 69–77.

Lefcourt, H. M. (Ed.). (1981). *Research with the locus of control construct: Vol. 1. Assessment methods.* San Diego, CA: Academic Press.

Lesher, E., & Whelihan, W. (1986). Reliability of mental status instruments administered to nursing home residents. *Journal of Consulting and Clinical Psychology, 54,* 726–727.

Levy, S. M., Lee, J., Bagley, C., & Lippman, M. (1988). Survival Hazards Analysis in first recurrent breast cancer patients: Seven-year follow-up. *Psychosomatic Medicine, 50,* 520.

Libow, L. (1977). Senile dementia and pseudosenility: Clinical diagnosis. In C. Eisdorfer & R. Friedel (Eds.), *Cognitive and emotional disturbance in the elderly.* Chicago: Year Book Medical Publishing.

Libow, L. (1981). A rapidly administered, easily remembered mental status evaluation: FROMAJE. In L. S. Libow & F. T. Sherman (Eds.), *The core of geriatric medicine* (pp. 85–91). St. Louis, MO: Mosby.

Lumpkin, J. R. (1988). Establishing the validity of an abbreviated Locus of Control Scale: Is a brief Levenson's Scale any better? *Psychological Reports, 63,* 519–523.

Mackenzie, C. R., Charlson, M. E., DiGioia, D., & Kelley, K. (1986). Can the Sickness Impact Profile measure change? An example of scale assessment. *Journal of Chronic Disease, 39,* 429–438.

Maddi, S. R. (1990). *The personality construct of hardiness.* Unpublished manuscript.

Malt, U. F. (1989). The validity of the General Health Questionnaire in a sample of accidentally injured adults. *Acta Psychiatrica Scandinavica, 80*(Suppl. 355), 103–112.

Matthews, K. A. (1982). Psychological perspectives on the Type A behavior pattern. *Psychological Bulletin, 91,* 293–323.

Matthews, K. A. (1988). CHD and Type A behavior: Update on and alternative to the Booth-Kewley and Friedman quantitative review. *Psychological Bulletin, 104,* 373–380.

Matthews, K. A., Krantz, D. S., Dembroski, T. M., & MacDougall, J. M. (1982). Unique and common variance in structured interview and Jenkin's Activity Survey measures of the Type A behavior pattern. *Journal of Personality and Social Psychology, 42,* 303–313.

Mayou, R. (1990). Quality of life in cardiovascular disease. *Psychotherapy and Psychosomatics, 54,* 99–109.

McCartney, J., & Palmateer, L. (1985). Assessment of cognitive deficit in geriatric patients: A study of physician behavior. *Journal of the American Geriatrics Society, 33,* 467–471.

McCrae, R. R. (1991). The five-factor model and its assessment in clinical settings. *Journal of Personality Assessment, 57,* 399–414.

McDougall, G. (1990). A review of screening instruments for assessing cognition and mental status in older adults. *Nurse Practitioner, 15,* 18–28.

McLean, J. & Pietroni, P. (1990). Self-care: Who does best? *Social Science and Medicine, 30,* 591–596.

Mesulam, M., & Geschwind, N. (1976). Disordered mental status in the postoperative period. *Urologic Clinics of North America, 3,* 199–215.

Middelboe, T., Birket-Smith, M., Andersen, H. S., & Friis, M. L. (1992). Personality traits in patients with postconcussional sequelae. *Journal of Personality Disorders, 6,* 246–255.

Miller, T. R. (1991). The psychotherapeutic utility of the five-factors model of personality: A clinician's experience. *Journal of Personality Assessment, 57,* 415–433.

Millon, T., Green, C. J., & Meagher, R. B., Jr. (1979). The MBHI: A new inventory for the psychodiagnostician in medical settings. *Professional Psychology, 10,* 529–539.

Millon, T., Green, C. J., & Meagher, R. B., Jr. (1982a). *Millon Behavioral Health Inventory* (3rd ed.). Minneapolis, MN: National Computer Systems.

Millon, T., Green, C. J., & Meagher, R. B., Jr. (1982b). A new psychodiagnostic tool for clients in rehabilitation settings: MBHI. *Rehabilitation Psychology, 27,* 23–35.

Mischel, W. (1968). *Personality and assessment.* New York: Wiley.

Moguilner, M. E., Bauman, A., & De-Nour, A. K. (1988). The adjustment of children and parents to chronic hemodialysis. *Psychosomatics, 29,* 289–294.

Murawski, B. J., Penman, D., & Schmitt, M. (1978). Social support in health and illness: The concept and its measurement. *Cancer Nursing, 1,* 365–371.

Murphy, J. K., Sperr, E. V., & Sperr, S. J. (1986). Chronic pain: An investigation of assessment instruments. *Journal of Psychosomatic Research, 30,* 289–296.

Murphy, S. P. (1982). *Factors influencing adjustment and quality of life: A multivariate approach.* Doctoral dissertation, University of Illinois Medical Center, Chicago.

Nicassio, P. M., & Radojevic, V. (1993). Models of family functioning and their contribution to patient outcomes in chronic pain. *Motivation and Emotion, 17,* 295–316.

Nicassio, P. M., & Wallston, K. A. (1992). Longitudinal relationships among pain, sleep problems, and depression in rheumatoid arthritis. *Journal of Abnormal Psychology, 101,* 514–520.

Northhouse, L. L. (1988). Social support in patients' and husbands' adjustment to breast cancer. *Nursing Research, 37,* 91–95.

Okun, M. A., Zautra, A. J., & Robinson, S. E. (1988). Hardiness and health among women with rheumatoid arthritis. *Personality and Individual Differences, 9,* 101–107.

Oldenburg, B., MacDonald, G. J., & Perkins, R. J. (1988). Prediction of quality of life in cohort of end-stage renal disease patients. *Journal of Clinical Epidemiology, 41,* 555–564.

Parikh, R. M., Eden, D. T., Price, T. R., & Robinson, R. G. (1988). The sensitivity and specificity of the Center for Epidemiologic Studies Depression Scale in screening for post-stroke depression. *International Journal of Psychiatry in Medicine, 18,* 169–181.

Pert, C. B. (1986). The wisdom of the receptors: Neuropeptides, the emotions, and bodymind. *Advances, 3,* 8–16.

Pfeiffer, C. A., & Wetstone, S. L. (1988). Health locus of control and well-being in systemic lupus erythematosus. *Arthritis Care and Research, 1,* 131–138.

Pfeiffer, E. (1975). A short portable Mental Status Questionnaire for the assessment of organic brain deficit in elderly patients. *Journal of the American Geriatrics Society, 23,* 433–441.

Pollock, S. E., & Duffy, M. E. (1990). The Health-Related Hardiness Scale: Development and psychometric analysis. *Nursing Research, 39,* 218–222.

Powers, M. J., & Jalowec, A. (1987). Profile of the well-controlled, well-adjusted hypertensive patient. *Nursing Research, 36,* 106.

Rabins, P. V., Fitting, M. D., Eastham, J., & Fetting, J. (1990). The emotional impact in caring for the chronically ill. *Psychosomatics, 31,* 331–336.

Radloff, L. S. (1977). The CES-D Scale: A self-report depression scale for research in the general population. *Applied Psychological Measurement, 1,* 385–401.

Radloff, L. S., & Locke, B. Z. (1985). The community mental health assessment survey and the CES-D Scale. In M. M. Weissman, J. K. Meyers, & C. G. Ross (Eds.), *Community survey of psychiatric disorder* (pp. 177–189). New Brunswick, NJ: Rutgers University Press.

Rameizl, P. (1984). A case for assessment technology in long-term care: The nursing perspective. *Rehabilitation Nursing, 9,* 29–31.

Regier, D. A., Robert, M. A., Hirschfeld, M., Goodwin, F. K., Burke, J. D., Lazar, J. B., & Judd, L. L. (1988). The NIMH depression awareness, recognition, and treatment program: Structure, aims, and scientific basis. *American Journal of Psychiatry, 145,* 1351–1357.

Reisberg, B. (1984). Stages of cognitive decline. *American Journal of Nursing, 84,* 225–228.

Reisberg, B., Ferris, S., deLeon, M., & Crook, T. (1982). The Global Deterioration Scale for assessment of primary degenerative dementia. *American Journal of Psychiatry, 139,* 1136–1139.

Reisberg, B., Ferris, S., deLeon, M., & Crook, T. (1988). Global Deterioration Scale (GDS). *Psychopharmacology Bulletin, 24,* 661–663.

Reynolds, W. M., & Gould, J. W. (1981). A psychometric investigation of the standard and short-form Beck Depression Inventory. *Journal of Consulting and Clinical Psychology, 49,* 306–307.

Rhodewalt, F., & Zone, J. B. (1989). Appraisal of life change, depression, and illness in hardy and nonhardy women. *Journal of Personality and Social Psychology, 56,* 81–88.

Roberts, R. E., Rhoades, H. M., & Vernon, S. W. (1990). Using the CES-D Scale to screen for depression and anxiety: Effects of language and ethnic status. *Psychiatry Research, 31,* 69–83.

Roca, P., Klein, L., Kirby, S., McArthur, J., Vogelsang, G., Folstein, M., & Smith, C. (1984). Recognition of dementia among medical patients. *Archives of Internal Medicine, 144,* 73–75.

Rosenman, R. (1978). The interview method of assessment of the coronary-prone behavior pattern. In T. M. Dembroski, S. W. Weiss, J. L. Shields, S. G. Haynes, & M. Feinleib (Eds.), *Coronary-prone behavior.* New York: Springer-Verlag.

Rosenman, R. H., Brand, R. J., Jenkins, C. D., Friedman, M., Straus, R., & Wurm, M. (1975). Coronary heart disease in the Western Collaborative Group Study: Final follow-up experience of 8 1/2 years. *Journal of the American Medical Association, 233,* 872-877.

Roskam, S. (1986). *Application of a health locus of control typology approach towards predicting depression and medical adherence in rheumatoid arthritis.* Unpublished doctoral dissertation, Vanderbilt University, Nashville, TN.

Rothman, M. L., Hedrick, S. C., Bulcroft, K. A., Hickam, D. H., & Rubenstein, L. A. (1991). The validity of proxy-generated scores as measures of patient health status. *Journal of Medical Care, 29,* 115–124.

Rotter, J. B. (1954). *Social learning and clinical psychology.* Englewood Cliffs, NJ: Prentice Hall.

Rotter, J. B. (1966). Generalized expectancies for internal versus external control of reinforcement. *Psychological Monographs, 80*(1, Whole No. 609).

Rotter, J. B. (1982). *The development and applications of social learning theory.* New York: Praeger.

Rotter, J. B. (1990). Internal versus external control of reinforcement: A case history of a variable. *American Psychologist, 45,* 489–493.

Seltzer, A. (1989). Prevalence, detection and referral of psychiatric morbidity in general medical patients. *Journal of Royal Society Medicine, 82,* 410–412.

Shore, D., Overman, C., & Wyatt, R. (1983). Improving accuracy in the diagnosis of Alzheimer's disease. *Journal of Clinical Psychiatry, 44,* 207–212.

Shrout, P. E., & Yager, T. J. (1989). Reliability and validity of screening scales: Effect of reducing scale length. *Journal of Clinical Epidemiology, 42,* 69–78.

Strain, J. J., Fulop, G., Lebovits, A., Ginsberg, B., Robinson, M., Stern, A., Charap, P., & Gany, F. (1988). Screening devices for diminished cognitive capacity. *General Hospital Psychiatry, 10,* 16–23.

Strickland, B. R. (1989). Internal–external control expectancies: From contingency to creativity. *American Psychologist, 44,* 1–12.

Suls, J., & Rittenhouse, J. D. (1987). Personality and physical health: An introduction. *Journal of Personality, 55,* 155–167.

Teri, L., Larson, E., & Reifler, B. (1988). Behavioral disturbance in dementia of the Alzheimer type. *Journal of the American Geriatrics Society, 36,* 1–6.

Tosi, D. J., Judah, S. M., & Murphy, M. A. (1989). The effects of a cognitive experiential therapy utilizing hypnosis, cognitive restructuring, and developmental staging on psychological factors associated with duodenal ulcer disease: A multivariate experimental study. *Journal of Cognitive Psychotherapy, 3,* 273–290.

Turk, D. C., & Okifuji, A. (1994). Detecting depression in chronic pain patients: Adequacy of self-reports. *Behaviour Research and Therapy, 32,* 9–16.

Vingerhoets, A. J., & Assies, J. (1991). Psychoneuroendocrinology of stress and emotions: Issues for future research. *Psychotherapy and Psychosomatics, 55,* 69–75.

Wallston, B. S., & Wallston, K. A. (1978). Locus of control and health: A review of the literature. *Health Education Monographs, 6,* 107–117.

Wallston, B. S., Wallston, K. A., Kaplan, G. D., & Maides, S.A. (1976). Development and validation of the Health Locus of Control (HLC) Scale. *Journal of Consulting and Clinical Psychology, 44,* 580–585.

Wallston, K. A. (1993, August). Control of one's health: A 20-year focus on locus. Invited address at 103rd Annual Convention of the American Psychological Association, Toronto, Ontario, Canada.

Wallston, K. A., Wallston, B. S., & DeVellis, R. (1978). Development of the Multidimensional Health Locus of Control (MHLC) Scales. *Health Education Monographs, 6,* 160–170.

Wallston, K. A., Wallston, B. S., Smith, S., & Dobbins, C. J. (1987). Perceived control and health. *Current Psychological Research and Reviews, 6,* 5–25.

Watson, D. (1988). Intraindividual and interindividual analyses of positive and negative affect: Their relationship to health complaints, perceived stress and daily activities. *Journal of Personality and Social Psychology, 54,* 1020–1030.

Watson, D., Clark, L. A., & Carey, G. (1988). Positive and negative affectivity and their relation to anxiety and depressive disorders. *Journal of Abnormal Psychology, 89,* 346–353.

Watson, D., Clark, L. A., & Tellegen, A. (1988). Development and validation of brief measures of positive and negative affect: The PANAS Scales. *Journal of Personality and Social Psychology, 52,* 1063–1070.

Watson, D., & Tellegen, A. (1985). Toward a consensual structure of mood. *Psychological Bulletin, 98,* 219–235.

Weisberg, M. B., & Page, S. (1988). Millon Behavioral Health Inventory and perceived efficacy of home and hospital dialysis. *Journal of Social and Clinical Psychology, 6,* 408–422.

Weissman, M. M. (1975). The assessment of social adjustment: A review of techniques. *Archives of General Psychiatry, 32,* 357–365.

Weissman, M. M., Sholomskas, D., & John, K. (1981). The assessment of social adjustment: An update. *Archives of General Psychiatry, 38,* 1250–1258.

Wells, C. (1979). Pseudodementia. *American Journal of Psychiatry, 136,* 895–900.

Wells, K. B., Golding, J. M., & Burnham, M. A. (1988). Psychiatric disorders in a sample of the general population with and without chronic medical conditions. *American Journal of Psychiatry, 145,* 976–981.

Whitaker, A., Johnson, J., Shaffer, D., Rapoport, J., Kalikow, K., Walsh, B., Davies, M., Braiman, S., & Dolinsky, A. (1990). Uncommon trouble in young people: Prevalence estimates of selected psychiatric disorders in a nonreferred adolescent population. *Archives of General Psychiatry, 47,* 487–496.

Wilcoxon, M. A., Zook, A., & Zarski, J. J. (1988). Predicting behavioral outcomes with two psychological assessment methods in an outpatient pain management program. *Psychology and Health, 2,* 319–333.

Williams, R. B., Haney, T. L., Lee, K. L., Kong, Y., Blumenthal, J. A., & Whalten, R. E. (1980). Type A behavior, hostility, and coronary atherosclerosis. *Psychosomatic Medicine, 42,* 539–549.

Wolberg, W. H., Tanner, M. A., Malec, J. F., & Romsaas, E. P. (1989). Psychosexual adaptation to breast-cancer surgery. *Cancer, 63,* 1645–1655.

Wolf, T. H., Elston, R. C., & Kissling, G. E. (1989, Spring). Relationship of hassles, uplifts, and life events to psychological well-being of freshman medical students. *Behavioral Medicine,* 37–45.

Wolf, T. M., Von Almen, T. K., Faucet, J. M., Randall, H. M., & Franklin, F. A. (1991). Psychological changes during the first year of medical school. *Medical Education, 25,* 174–181.

World Health Organization. (1960). *Constitution of the World Health Organization.* Geneva, Switzerland: Author.

Zabora, J. R., Smith-Wilson, R., Fetting, J. H., & Enterline, J. P. (1990). An efficient method for psychosocial screening of cancer patients. *Psychosomatics, 31,* 192–196.

Zyzanski, S. J., Stanton, B. A., Jenkins, C. D., & Klein, M. B. (1981). Medical and social outcomes in survivors of major heart surgery. *Journal of Psychosomatic Research, 23,* 213–221.

Chapter

4

Neuropsychological Dysfunction: Research and Evaluation

Mark P. Kelly and Richard E. Doty

Clinical neuropsychology emerged as a discrete subspecialty in the late 1960s and early 1970s, marked by such developments as the founding of the International Neuropsychological Society, the establishment of the Division of Clinical Neuropsychology in the American Psychological Association, and the launching of the *Journal of Clinical Neuropsychology* (Benton, 1987). This rapidly growing field is concerned with the evaluation and treatment of the behavioral sequelae of cerebral dysfunction. Clinical neuropsychological evaluations reveal information needed for three major functions: diagnosis, clinical management, and research (Lezak, 1983). Diagnostic applications include

We gratefully acknowledge the assistance of Cheryl Torain in the preparation of this chapter.

identifying or localizing cerebral dysfunction, diagnosing different neurological and psychiatric disorders, and discriminating among neurological conditions. Clinical neuropsychology is historically rooted in this diagnostic tradition. The increasing accessibility of noninvasive anatomic brain-imaging methods has diminished its purely diagnostic role. Nevertheless, neuropsychological tests are often useful in evaluating conditions where neurodiagnostic procedures routinely fail to disclose a structural abnormality, including toxic and metabolic disorders and the sequelae of cardiac surgery (Benton, 1992).

Neuropsychological evaluations are increasingly used in clinical management. Precise information regarding a patient's pattern of cognitive strengths and weaknesses is essential for planning his or her effective rehabilitation. A comprehensive neuropsychological evaluation can help patients and families understand the consequences of brain dysfunction, which may be complex, unfamiliar, and confusing. Clearer understanding of the cognitive and emotional changes that follow brain damage can serve as a basis for counseling. Neuropsychological status is also pertinent to decisions involving living arrangements, educational plans, vocational choices, and legal matters. Serial assessment may be used to follow patients over time—to assess changes resulting from progression of disease, recovery from injury, or treatment.

Neuropsychological evaluations are also often used in diverse research protocols. Experimental neuropsychological studies have been valuable in elucidating basic brain behavior mechanisms. Clinical studies have charted the neurobehavioral manifestations of numerous diseases. Neuropsychological procedures have also been used to study the outcome of medication trials, surgical procedures, dialysis, electroconvulsive therapy, and cognitive remediation.

Clinical Neuropsychology: Relevance to Health Psychology and Clinical Behavioral Medicine

Both health psychology and behavioral medicine are concerned with the psychological correlates of wellness and disease and with applying techniques derived from behavioral science to prevention and management of physical illness (Schwartz & Weiss, 1977). Pomerleau (1979) has identified four principal aspects of clinical behavioral medicine: (a) direct modification of either overt behavior or physiological responses that compose a health problem, (b) interventions to improve compliance with treatment, (c) modification of behavioral risk factors for disease, and (d) modification of practitioner behavior. The first three activities involve techniques for modifying the behavior of patients who have either developed, or who are at high risk for developing, serious chronic illnesses. Many such illnesses result in varying degrees of neuropsychological impairment, whereas others serve as potent risk factors for frank neurological events. Because most health psychology and behavioral medicine interventions require active patient involvement, neuropsychological impairment may have serious ramifications for treatment planning. Through traditional neuropsychological assessment, the practitioner evaluates multiple cognitive parameters, including language skills, attention, memory, sensory and motor functioning, and performance on a variety of problem-solving tasks. Impairment in any of these areas could influence treatment planning in behavioral medicine. Choice of treatments, expected time frames for response, prognosis, and modifications of intervention strategies to accommodate deficits could all be influenced by a patient's neuropsychological status. In addition, behavioral medicine specialists, as frontline caregivers, are in a position to detect changes in behavior that may benefit from further neuropsychological or medical evaluation. Thus, practitioners working with medical patients can benefit from familiarity with neuropsychological techniques and the current state of knowledge regarding the specific neuropsychological correlates of chronic illness.

Our major objectives in this chapter are to review the neuropsychological aspects of a spectrum of chronic illnesses in adults and to provide guidelines to health psychologists for integrating neuropsychological services into their clinical practices. Neurological diseases—including multiple sclerosis, Parkinson's disease, and Alzheimer's disease—have received much attention in the neuropsychological literature, but we have chosen to focus here on systemic disorders. We have attempted to address those syndromes frequently encountered by health psychologists, and so the disorders we do cover tend to be those relatively common in the general population. This chapter is not an exhaustive review but a synopsis of the most pertinent information generated in the past 10 to 15 years. Availability of neuropsychological literature varies widely from disorder to disorder. Where it was possible, however, we have emphasized well-controlled studies in our discussions. For disorders where such studies were limited, group clinical studies, case studies, or information regarding neurological aspects are discussed. We conclude with comments about the potential utility of clinical neuropsychology for the health psychologist, including the potential use of screening techniques. For readers unfamiliar with neuropsychological tests, we have compiled a list of common test acronyms, full names, and attributes in the Appendix.

Neuropsychological Aspects of Chronic Illness

Hypertension

Etiology of hypertension is, in most cases, unknown. Hypertension without a demonstrated etiology is known as either *primary, essential,* or *idiopathic hypertension.* In cases where a specific cause can be identified, the condition is grouped under the label of *secondary hypertension.*

Virtually all studies comparing hypertensive patients to age-and-education-matched normotensive control patients have found poorer neuropsychological performance in the hypertensive group. For example, Shapiro, Miller, King, Ginchereau, and Fitzgibbon (1982) compared 41 patients with recently diagnosed mild hypertension to an equal number of controls on a battery of largely experimental measures of perceptual, cognitive, and psychomotor abilities. Hypertensive patients performed more poorly in tests from each area; none were taking antihypertensive medication. More recently, Waldstein, Ryan, Manuck, Parkinson, and Bromet (1991) evaluated 20 untreated hypertensive patients and 20 matched controls, using such tests as the SDLT and the WMS Visual Reproduction subtest.[1] Hypertensive patients performed more poorly on both of these measures. Studies by Elias and his colleagues (e.g., Elias, Robbins, Schultz, & Pierce, 1990; Elias, Robbins, Schultz, Streeten, & Elias, 1987), in which traditional procedures such as the HRB were used, yielded similar results. In the earlier Elias et al. (1987) study, 54 hypertensive patients and 54 matched controls were examined. Some hypertensive patients had been diagnosed with the disease for many years and were taking an-

[1] See the Appendix for definitions and attributes of tests cited throughout the chapter.

tihypertensive medication. Hypertensive patients with less education (averaging 13 years of education) performed more poorly than controls on a summary HRB measure (average impairment rating, or AIR) and on several individual HRB tests, whereas very highly educated hypertensive patients (averaging 17 years of education) performed as well as controls. Medication did not affect performance. In Elias et al.'s (1990) study, regression analysis was used to study HRB performance in 166 hypertensive patients and 135 normotensive controls. With age, sex, and education controlled for, hypertension was found to affect the AIR and several individual HRB measures. Blood pressure effects were larger in younger patients. All patients were tested off antihypertensive medication, but a history of medication use did not influence the results.

Does the neuropsychological impairment in hypertension increase with the disease duration? Results of two cross-sectional studies showed that patients with chronic hypertension performed no more poorly than those recently disagnosed (Francheschi, Tancredi, Smirne, Mercinelli, & Canal, 1982; Mazzuchi, Mutti, Poletti, Novarini, & Parma, 1986). Francheschi et al. found hypertensive patients' performance on such measures as the RPM, WMS, and Block Design of the WBI to be impaired, whereas in the Mazzuchi et al. study, impairment was seen on selected WAIS subtests and several memory measures. Within the group with chronic disease, those treated with antihypertensive medication performed better than those untreated. Researchers conducting recent longitudinal studies have also fairly consistently failed to find a progression of impairment over time (Elias, Robbins, Schultz, & Streeten, 1986; Elias, Schultz, Robbins, & Elias, 1989; R. Miller, Shapiro, King, Ginchereau, & Hosutt, 1984; Schultz, Elias, Robbins, Streeten, & Blakeman, 1986). Patients have been followed from intervals ranging from about 15 months to 10 years and have been examined with a variety of measures. Results of one study (R. Miller et al., 1984) suggested that patients receiving antihypertensive medications improved neuropsychologically over time, whereas untreated patients declined.

Two groups of researchers have commented that neuropsychological impairment in hypertension is subtle and, thus, unlikely to interfere with patients' domestic or vocational activities (Elias et al., 1987; R. Miller et al., 1984). To support this, Elias et al. noted that the proportion of hypertensive patients completing the HRB–AIR in the impaired range did not differ from controls. Conversely, Waldstein et al.

(1991) found that the performance of hypertensive patients was almost 1 standard deviation below that of controls on one of three measures and noted that this might well have clinical implications. Populations and measures in these studies varied, and further investigation is needed.

Several mechanisms have been proposed to explain the neuropsychological impairment inherent to hypertension, including cellular and metabolic changes in the central nervous system (Shapiro et al., 1982) and alterations related to subtle cerebral vascular disease (Franceschi et al., 1982).

Researchers have consistently found hypertension patients to perform more poorly than controls on a broad range of sensitive neuropsychological measures. Their degree of impairment appears to be subtle, and there has been no convincing evidence for progression over time. It has been suggested that treated patients tend to perform better than those who are not treated, but one must be careful not to overgeneralize. A plethora of medications have been used to treat hypertension, some of which may adversely affect cognition (e.g., McCaffrey, Ortega, Orsillo, Haase & McCoy, 1992). Implications of neuropsychological impairment for day-to-day performance, which would be of potential interest to the health psychologist, have not been studied directly. As with other conditions, the implications of neuropsychological deficits for daily life depend not only on the nature and degree of impairment but also on the specific demands placed on individual patients.

Diabetes Mellitus

Diabetes mellitus is characterized by chronic high blood glucose levels. Onset of Type I diabetes is most common during childhood and early adolescence. It is characterized by the inability to secrete insulin secondary to the destruction of pancreatic beta cells. As a result, carbohydrates cannot be metabolized and postprandial blood glucose levels rise dramatically if insulin is not administered. The etiology, although not fully understood, most probably arises from an interplay of genetic susceptibility and environmental insult (possibly viral), resulting in pancreatic inflammation and autoimmune-mediated destruction of beta cells. Type II diabetes most commonly occurs in obese individuals over age 40. Excessive insulin production related to chronic overeating is postulated as the major cause of Type II diabetes, which also results in beta cell damage (Foster, 1987; C. Ryan, 1988).

Most neuropsychological research has been focused on patients with Type I diabetes. C. Ryan, Williams, Orchard, and Finegold (1992) compared 75 Type I diabetic adults to 75 demographically similar, but nondiabetic controls, using a comprehensive battery comprising portions of the WAIS-R, WMS, HRB, and several other measures of psychomotor efficiency and memory. Diabetic patients performed more poorly than control subjects on measures of psychomotor efficiency and spatial information processing. Glycosylated hemoglobin values, which provide an estimate of diabetic control for the preceding 3 months (Foster, 1987), showed a weak association with psychomotor slowing and spatial information processing, whereas polyneuropathy was strongly associated with psychomotor efficiency. Prior severe hypoglycemia, age of onset, disease duration, and retinopathy were unrelated to performance. Using a somewhat smaller sample, Skenazy and Bigler (1984) studied patients with Type I diabetes and educationally similar controls, using the HRB, WAIS, and WMS. Diabetic patients performed more poorly on measures of psychomotor efficiency, Performance IQ, abstract reasoning, somatosensory function, and motor strength and speed. The authors created an index of diabetic severity based on illness duration, number of hospitalizations for either high or low blood sugar, number of diabetic comas, number of severe insulin reactions, and types of complications secondary to diabetes. Patients with more severe diabetes tended to perform more poorly on multiple neuropsychological measures evaluating sensory function, motor function, mental tracking, and language function. Skenazy and Bigler noted that the complications of diabetes (e.g., retinopathy and peripheral neuropathy) may affect reseachers' interpretations of performance.

Others have attempted to isolate factors associated with persistent neuropsychological impairment. Langan, Deary, Hepburn, and Frier (1991) studied 100 patients with Type I adult diabetes, using the WAIS-R and measures assessing memory and information-processing speed. Frequency of severe hypoglycemia was associated with poorer Performance IQ, several complex RT parameters, and a measure of rapid information processing. Findings were similar in a smaller study by Wredling, Levander, Adamson, and Lins (1990). They used the APTS (Levander & Elithorn, 1987) to compare two matched groups, each comprising 17 patients with Type I diabetes—one group with and the other without a history of severe recurrent hypoglycemia. The former performed more poorly on measures of motor coordination and speed, attention, complex perceptual ability, and planning. In contrast, Reichard, Berglund, Britz, Levander, and Rosenquist (1991) followed a group of 97 patients with Type I diabetes prospectively over 3 years, also using a portion of the APTS. They did not observe an association between the number of severe hypoglycemic episodes and neuropsychological performance. Thus, some, but not all, studies have indicated that severe episodic hypoglycemia is associated with persistent neuropsychological dysfunction. Holmes (1986) has suggested that early age of disease onset in combination with poor metabolic control results in subtle neuropsychological impairment in Type I diabetic men. However, she used the WAIS, achievement tests, and laboratory measures of RT and perception in studying only 27 patients, so these findings must be considered preliminary.

Additional studies have suggested that temporary alterations in blood glucose result in transient neuropsychological dysfunction. Holmes, Koepke, and Thompson (1986) used a repeatable battery to study 24 patients with Type I diabetes at three glucose levels. Choice RT and a go/no-go task were adversely affected by a low blood glucose level (55 mg/dl). Widom and Simonson (1990) have demonstrated impaired visuomotor speed in both diabetic patients and control subjects during experimentally induced hypoglycemia. Also, ramifications of transient hypoglycemia for day-to-day functioning have been addressed by Cox, Gonder-Frederick, Driesen, and Clarke (1991). Twenty-six Type I patients were evaluated in a driving simulator, and significant performance impairments were found during severe experimentally induced hypoglycemia.

Investigations have also revealed cognitive deficits in older Type II diabetic patients. U'Ren, Riddle, Lezak, and Bennington-Davis (1990) administered a battery assessing attention, mental speed, memory, and language to 19 patients with Type II diabetes and 19 healthy control subjects similar in age and education. Diabetic patients performed significantly more poorly on 7 of the 11 attention and memory tasks and on 1 of 2 language tests. Reaven, Thompson, Nahum, and Haskins (1990) studied 30 patients with Type II diabetes and 29 control subjects who were demographically similar, using portions of the WAIS-R, TMT, FTT, and other measures of abstract reasoning and memory. Here too, the diabetic patients performed more poorly on measures of memory and attention, and a deficiency in abstract reasoning was also found. Several neuropsychological measures were significantly related to glycosylated hemoglobin values and to patients' plasma glucose levels after fasting.

In summary, studies of neuropsychological impairment in Type I diabetes have most consistently found impairment on measures of attention and speeded-reasoning/information-proceessing tasks. Neuropsychological performance has generally been found to be related to disease severity, although not all studies have demonstrated a relationship to the number of severe hypoglycemic episodes. There is evidence that neuropsychological performance deteriorates acutely during hypoglycemia, as well as preliminary evidence that performance on a complex everyday task (e.g., driving) may be affected as a result. Type II diabetes has been less well studied, but there is some evidence to suggest that a broader range of abilities may be adversely affected by it than in Type I diabetes.

The underlying mechanism for neuropsychological impairment in diabetes is not well understood. Lack of glucose for cerebral metabolism resulting from hypoglycemia may be a cause in Type I diabetes. In Type II diabetes, direct cellular injury from hyperglycemia has been proposed. Both disorders are associated with blood vessel disease, which may result in cerebrovascular complications (U'Ren et al., 1990).

Chronic Obstructive Pulmonary Disease (COPD)

COPD is a condition involving the obstruction of airflow as a result of chronic bronchitis, emphysema, or both. Chronic bronchitis is characterized by hyperplasia and hypertrophy of the mucus-producing glands of the airways, resulting in increased tracheobronchial mucus production. Essentially, this narrows the airway, lowering airflow. Emphysema involves destruction of alveoli of the lungs, which diminishes the body's ability to oxygenate blood. Both conditions result in disruption of ventilation–perfusion matching and in reduction of arterial oxygen content (Ingram, 1987).

Several associated studies of neuropsychological function in COPD have been published during the past 10 years (Grant, Heaton, McSweeney, Adams, & Timms, 1982; Grant et al., 1987; McSweeney, Grant, Heaton, Prigatano, & Adams, 1985; Prigatano, Parsons, Wright, Levin, & Hawryluk, 1983). These studies have included large samples and controls matched for age, education, and socioeconomic status. Grant et al. (1982) used the HRB, WMS, and GP to study neuropsychological functioning in severe COPD. COPD patients performed significantly more poorly than the control subjects on both summary measures and in clinician ratings of performance, as well as on 11 of 14 key neuropsychological variables. Clinicians rated 77% of COPD patients and 46% of control subjects to have neuropsychological impairment, with 42% of COPD patients and only 14% of control subjects having moderate to severe impairment. Every clinically rated neuropsychological area of ability was poorer in the COPD patients than in control subjects, but the greatest differences were found on measures reflecting thought flexibility, abstraction, and complex perceptual-motor integration. Within the COPD group, several modest correlations confirmed the expected association between hypoxemia and neuropsychological impairment.

COPD patients with mild hypoxemia were examined by Prigatano et al. (1983). They used the HRB, supplemented by the LRNTB and portions of the WMS. Consistent with the results of Grant et al.'s (1982) study, Prigatano et al. reported that the COPD group performed more poorly than control subjects on HRB summary measures, although they found fewer significant differences on key neuropsychological variables. Most WMS and LRNTB parameters were also poorer in the COPD group. Overall, these COPD patients showed subtle impairment of abstract reasoning, memory, and speed of performance. Modest but significant correlations (with age and education effects partialed out) between HRB summary measures and partial pressure of oxygen in the arterial blood (PaO2) were found, suggesting that the level of blood oxygen is related to neuropsychological performance. Other analyses indicated that such factors as depression, general fitness, or motivation were unlikely to account for the impaired performance in the COPD group.

In Grant et al.'s 1987 study, groups from the two previously discussed studies were merged. A combined group of over 300 patients was divided into 3 subgroups (with mild, moderate, and severe hypoxemia) on the basis of PaO2 data. Factor-analytically derived ability scores showed a pattern of worsening impairment with progression of disease on three of the four factor scores (with verbal intelligence the exception). Similarly, the rate of neuropsychological impairment derived from HRB summary measures increased with disease severity.

On the basis of comparisons with healthy controls, Prigatano and Grant (1989) estimated the incidence of neuropsychological impairment to be less than 10% in mildly hypoxemic patients, 25% in moderately hypoxemic patients, and 40% in those with severe hypoxemia. A multiple regression analysis indicated that the degree of hypoxemia reliably predicted neuropsychological impairment.

The impact of neuropsychological impairment on day-to-day functioning and quality of life for those with COPD was studied by McSweeney et al. (1985), who, again, used the combined sample. Psychosocial and physical functioning were assessed with the Sickness Impact Profile, the Katz Adjustment Scale, the Profile of Mood States, and the Minnesota Multiphasic Personality Inventory (MMPI). Significant correlations were found between an HRB summary measure and most life-quality measures for COPD patients (but not for healthy control subects). Motor and psychomotor measures were related to physical mobility, self-care, socialization, and home management, whereas language tests correlated with ratings of communication. Neuropsychological status was more consistently related to activities of daily living and basic social role performance than to patients' emotional status.

Composite results suggest that neuropsychological impairment is common in COPD and that the rate and severity of impairment are related to progression of the disease. Verbal reasoning is relatively well preserved, but perceptual learning and problem solving, attention and mental speed, and simple motor functioning are more vulnerable. Preliminary evidence suggests that neuropsychological performance has a significant, albeit modest, influence on quality of life in this population. Knowlege of the neuropsychological aspects of COPD has been derived from a group of interrelated studies, however, placing limits on the generalizability of findings. These studies have also detected a high rate of clinically rated impairment in control subjects (e.g., 46% in Grant et al.'s [1982] study), raising the possibility that clinicians have a relatively low threshold for rating an individual as impaired.

Oxygen is a major resource for cerebral function, and the brain uses roughly 20% of total resting oxygen consumed by the body. Thus, it is not surprising that COPD would adversely affect neuropsychological performance (Prigatano & Levin, 1988). Evidence suggests that neurotransmitter synthesis is disrupted by hypoxia, providing one possible mechanism for neuropsychological impairment (Grant et al.,

1987). Diseases either associated with or exacerbated by COPD, including heart disease and generalized atherosclerosis, might also adversely affect neuropsychological functioning (Grant et al., 1982).

Cancer

Cancer remains a major source of morbidity and mortality in the United States (Silberberg & Lubera, 1989). The expanding role of health psychology in managing cancer patients has been highlighted by Spiegel, Bloom, Kraemer, and Gottheil (1989), who reported an 18-month survival advantage for cancer patients involved in a group treatment intervention in comparison with no-treatment control subjects.

Certain cancers affect the brain directly. There is substantial literature on the neurobehavioral sequelae of brain tumors, which, although beyond the purview of this chapter, has been covered recently by others (Berg, 1988). However, there are several nonmetastatic disorders of the brain resulting from carcinoma elsewhere in the body. Although these conditions are relatively uncommon, and no formal systematic neuropsychological studies of them exist, they may potentially be relevant to the health psychologist. Hence, we cover them here. In addition, because many treatments for cancer are potentially neurotoxic, there is some literature dealing with the neuropsychological concomitants of radiation and chemotherapy. These areas are also discussed.

Paraneoplastic syndromes are disorders that are caused by or associated with cancer but are not direct effects of primary or metastatic tumors. The incidence of paraneoplastic neurological syndromes in cancer patients is considerably less than 1% (Posner, 1989). Paraneoplastic syndromes may, in fact, precede the diagnosis of primary carcinoma. The most common paraneoplastic syndrome affecting the brain is paraneoplastic cerebellar degeneration. Patients with this disorder develop ataxia, dysarthria, and, at times, dysphagia. Pathological studies have indicated involvement of all parts of the cerebellum. Although the cerebral cortex is not usually involved, mild dementia has been reported in association with this syndrome. Immune-mediated damage to the nervous system has been postulated as the etiology (Posner, 1989). *Limbic encephalitis* is a relatively rare paraneoplastic disorder that is most often associated with lung cancer. Typically, the most striking neurobehavioral feature of the disorder is a severe impairment of recent memory, often accompanied by confusion, agitation, and anxiety or depression. Progression to global dementia is common, but the disorder sometimes remits spontaneously. Multiple brain areas may be affected, including the hippocampus, cingulate gyrus, piriform cortex, orbital aspects to the frontal lobe, and the amygdoloid nucleii. The pathogenesis is unknown (Posner, 1989). *Brain-stem* or *bulbar encephalitis* is a paraneoplastic disorder that is usually associated with encephalomyelitis elsewhere in the nervous system and that most commonly occurs among lung cancer patients. Signs of the disorder include diplopia, vertigo, dysarthria, and dysphagia. Pathological changes in the medulla and pons, along with perivascular infiltration, are present (Stefansson & Aranson, 1987).

Major treatments for cancer include chemotherapy and radiation. The objective of treatment is to kill or inactivate the cancer cells. During this process, however, normal tissue may also be damaged, and various neurological syndromes may result (Delattre & Posner, 1989). Several groups of neuropsychological researchers have attempted to evaluate the effects of chemotherapy and radiation in adult cancer patients.

J. Tucker et al. (1989) studied 17 patients with adult lymphoblastic leukemia and 7 with non-Hodgkins lymphoma who had undergone a regimen of prophylactic chemotherapy and central nervous system irradiation an average of 11.5 years earlier. These patients were drawn from an initial pool of 168 patients, 37 of whom had survived at the time of the study. Tucker et al. administered the WAIS, the RMT, and the NART. Median scores for all tests were in the average range, although there was considerable variability from patient to patient. Parth, Dunlap, Kennedy, Lane, and Ordy (1989) studied 20 bone-marrow transplant patients (of an initial sample of 44) prior to transplant and at 50 days, 100 days, and 1-year after transplant. Patients underwent a regimen of chemotherapy and total body radiation at the time of transplant. Three (of an initial 42) transplant donors, acting as control subjects, also completed the neuropsychological protocol, which was an experimental computerized battery. Patients performed more poorly than donors on several measures, especially early in the course of treatment. Results of these two studies were not conclusive, given the lack of reporting regarding critical patient characteristics (e.g., level of education), nonexistent or very small control groups, and the very high dropout rate. In the same period, P. Lee, Hung, Woo, Tai, and Choi (1989) compared 16 nasopharyngeal carcinoma patients treated with radiation an average of 5 1/2 years earlier with a group of recently diagnosed patients awaiting treatment. They used portions of the WAIS-R and WMS, as well as several other measures. The radiation treatment group performed more poorly on several measures, although a review of the report suggested that this group had less education, clouding interpretation of results. Previously, J. Lee et al. (1988) had also reported adverse neuropsychological effects of radiation therapy for lung cancer patients. Methodological details were not reported, so, once again, results must be viewed cautiously.

Although clinical descriptions of paraneoplastic disorders are available, these disorders are relatively uncommon in cancer patients. Formal neuropsychological studies of adult cancer patients (other than those of adults with primary brain tumors) are virtually nonexistent, whereas studies of the neuropsychological effects of cancer treatment suffer from serious methodological limitations. The neuropsychological aspects of cancer and its treatment have been better studied in children (Fletcher & Copeland, 1988), and more research with adults is sorely needed. In spite of this lack of empirical research, health psychologists may encounter cancer patients who they may suspect have cognitive dysfunction. The general guidelines for neuropsychological referral provided at the end of this chapter are applicable in such instances.

Systemic Lupus Erythematosus

Systemic lupus erythematosus (SLE) is a chronic remitting–relapsing, inflammatory disorder of unknown etiology. Onset is acute or insidious and principally involves the skin, joints, kidneys, and serosal membranes. Systemic symptoms are usually prominent and include fatigue, malaise, fever, anorexia, weight loss, and nausea. Nearly all patients with SLE develop arthralgias and myalgias, and most develop arthritis (Hahn, 1987). SLE may have a genetic predisposition and is thought to result from autoimmune disregulation. Treatment is symptomatic and often involves high doses of steroids, which can have significant behavioral side effects.

Estimates of the prevalence of central nervous system (or neuropsychiatric) involvement in SLE range from 14% to 75%; the wide range reflects variations in diagnostic criteria and study methodology (Carbotte, Denburg, & Denburg, 1992). Neuropsychiatric symptoms are broad ranging as well (Denburg, Carbotte, & Denburg, 1987; Ellis & Verity, 1979; Futrell, Schultz, & Millikan, 1992; Hay et al., 1992; Kirk,

Kertesz, & Polk, 1991; van Dam, Wekking, & Oomen, 1991). Carbotte et al. (1992) proposed dividing symptoms into major and minor groups. The major symptoms include cerebrovascular events, neuropathy, movement disorders, transverse myelitis, seizures, meningitis, organic brain syndrome, psychosis, and affective disorder. Symptoms that they categorized as minor are more subjective and include paresthesias or numbness, headache, cognitive complaints, mood swings, and adjustment disorders. These neuropsychiatric symptoms are not necessarily the result of long-standing disease; in fact, they are often present before or within the first year after diagnosis (Feinglass, Arnett, Dorsch, Zizic, & Stevens, 1976; van Dam et al., 1991).

The prevalence of cognitive impairment in SLE appears to be significant. Carbotte, Denburg, and Denburg (1986) found that approximately 66% of 62 female SLE patients showed cognitive impairment on a comprehensive neuropsychological battery. Impairment was roughly twice as prevalent in patients with current or past neuropsychiatric symptoms than in patients without such history. Other studies have also found a higher level of cognitive impairment in patients with a history of neuropsychiatric SLE (e.g., Denburg et al., 1987; Sonies, Klippel, Gerber, and Gerber, 1982). However, neither the level of psychological distress felt by patients nor the amount of their steroid medication has been shown to have a major negative influence on patients' performance on neuropsychological tests (Carbotte et al., 1986; Denburg et al., 1987; Ginsburg et al., 1992; Sonies et al., 1982). Similarly, the presence of systemic disease activity has not proved to be a significant factor affecting performance on neuropsychological tests, although qualitative evaluations have suggested that patients who are in an active phase of the disease may have more difficulty with cognitive control (Carbotte et al., 1992; Hay et al., 1992).

Studies using traditional neuropsychological batteries—including the WAIS, WMS, BVRT, RAVLT, RCF, COWA, and other measures of language and attention—converge in suggesting that memory and output speed are most consistently impaired in SLE (Carbotte et al., 1992; Hay et al., 1992; Sonies et al., 1982). These findings generally appear to reflect diffuse or multifocal impairment, as would be expected from the nature of SLE, and are generally mild in severity. Nevertheless, they may be practically significant: In Hay et al.'s study, 30% of working patients reported a decrease in work performance and 30% reported forgetfulness. Denburg et al. (1987) have also concluded that patients with SLE tend to be a heterogeneous group both clinically and neuropsychologically, mandating assessment of a broad domain of cognitive functions to detect deficits in individual patients.

The pathogenesis of neuropsychiatric SLE is not well understood. Currently, attention is being focused on the role of antineural–antibrain antibodies in the disease (Bluestein, 1984; Carbotte et al., 1992). Carbotte et al. have hypothesized five pathogenic mechanisms: (a) interference with neurotransmission, neuronal function, or both; (b) neuronal cell loss or lysis; (c) loss of neuronal plasticity and growth; (d) thrombosis, vasculopathy, or both; and (e) nervous system inflammation. As yet, however, no specific relationships have been definitively demonstrated.

Thyroid Dysfunction

Thyroid dysfunction may take the form of either a hyperthyroid or a hypothyroid state. The hyperthyroid condition is termed *Graves' disease,* or *thyrotoxicosis;* hypothyroidism in adults is often referred to as *Gull's disease,* or *myxedema.* Both conditions are much more common in women (7–10 times and 4–7 times, respectively) (Beckwith & Tucker, 1988) than in men. Onset of myxedema is often missed because it is so gradual.

Symptoms of hyperthyroidism have been quantified by Klein, Trzepacz, Roberts, and Levey (1988) in a rating scale that is shown in Exhibit 1.

In addition to those characteristics listed, emotional symptoms of depression, irritability, and anxiety, as well as cognitive manifestations, are often reported (Bommer, Eversmann, Pickardt, Leonhardt, & Naber, 1990; MacCrimmon, Wallace, Goldberg, & Streiner, 1979; Paschke et al., 1990; Rockey & Griep, 1980; Whybrow & Ferrell, 1974).

Mild, diffuse cognitive changes are generally reported in association with both acute and subclinical (i.e., normal peripheral thyroid hormone levels with suppressed thyroid stimulating hormone) hyperthyroidism. Researchers have also reported alterations in attention, concentration, and mental control (Alvarez, Gomez, Alavez, & Navarro, 1983; Paschke et al., 1990; Whybrow & Ferrell, 1974); in reasoning and abstraction (Bommer et al., 1990; Trzepacz, McCue, Klein, Greenhouse, & Levey, 1988); in psychomotor speed and dexterity (Bommer et al., 1990; Schlote et al., 1992; Zeitlhofer, Saletu, Stary, & Ahmadi, 1984); in word fluency (Bommer et al., 1990); and in memory (Bommer et al., 1990) among patients with hyperthyroidism. Most of these studies

Exhibit 1

Hyperthyroid Symptom Scale: Characteristics Measured and Response Scales

Nervousness

0 = *Absent*
1 = *Anxious only with stress*
2 = *Occasionally anxious at rest*
3 = *Often anxious, difficulty working or concentrating*
4 = *States freely that feels "very nervous most of the time"*

Sweating

0 = *Only with activity*
1 = *At rest but only in warm temperatures*
2 = *At rest in temperate climates, mainly involving the hands and intertriginous zones*
3 = *At rest involving many body areas*
4 = *Profusely diaphoretic almost constantly*

Heat tolerance

0 = *Normal temperature tolerance*
1 = *Periods of feeling warmer than those in the same room*
2 = *Significant difficulty with heat, requiring air conditioner constantly in the summertime*
3 = *Excessive difficulty with heat even in temperate climates*
4 = *Extreme difficulty with heat, does not feel comfortable even in cold weather as evidenced by lack of need for warm clothing or bed covers*

Hyperactivity

0 = *Normal activity level*
1 = *Increased activity level, increased productivity*
2 = *Increased productivity; decreased sleep time*
3 = *Performs some purposeless activity*
4 = *Frequent episodes of purposeless activity; unable to sit still during examination*

Tremor: Examination of outstretched hands

0 = *Absent*
1 = *Barely perceptible*
2 = *Tremor demonstrated readily on examination*
3 = *Marked tremor but able to perform fine motor skills*
4 = *Hands shake excessively, difficulty performing fine motor skills*

Exhibit continues

Exhibit 1 (contd.)

Weakness

0 = *Normal strength*
1 = *Subjective weakness but with normal exercise tolerance*
2 = *Decreased exercise tolerance to near maximal activity*
3 = *Decreased tolerance to stair climbing or arising from chair*
4 = *Extreme weakness such that patient can barely lift objects or walk up stairs*

Hyperdynamic precordium

0 = *Normal precordium activity and apical impulse*
1 = *Tachycardia, 90 beats per minute with normal apical impulse*
2 = *Tachycardia, 90 beats per minute with increased apical impulse*
3 = *Tachycardia, 110 beats per minute with increased apical impulse*
4 = *Tachycardia, 110 beats per minute, apical impulse and carotid upstroke both increased, systolic outflow murmur*

Diarrhea

0 = *1 bowel movement (BM) per day; formed stool*
1 = *2–4 formed BMs per day*
2 = *1–4 loose stools per day*
3 = *4 formed BMs per day*
4 = *4 loose stools per day*

Appetite

0 = *Appetite normal, no weight loss*
1 = *Appetite normal, weight loss*
2 = *Appetite increased, no weight loss*
3 = *Appetite increased, weight loss*
4 = *Appetite decreased, weight loss*

Assessment of daily function (degree of incapacitation)

0 = *Normal (none)*
1 = *Minimal impairment (10%)*
2 = *Mild impairment (30%)*
3 = *Moderate impairment (60%)*
4 = *Severe impairment (90%)*

Total score

Note. From "Symptom Rating Scale for Assessing Hyperthyroidism," by I. Klein, P. Trzepacz, M. Roberts, and G. Levey, 1988, *Archives of Internal Medicine, 148,* p. 388.

were conducted outside of the United States, often with measures not routinely used here. Several studies have shown evidence of cognitive improvement after treatment, even when initial performance was not significantly poorer than that of control subjects (MacCrimmon et al., 1979; Trzepacz, McCue, Klein, Greenhouse, & Levey, 1988; Wallace, MacCrimmon, & Goldberg, 1980; Zeitlhofer et al., 1984). Although results have not been entirely consistent, some researchers have found significant correlations between measures of thyroid function and test performance (Bommer et al., 1990; MacCrimmon et al., 1979; Trzepacz, McCue, Klein, Levey, & Greenhouse, 1988; D. Tucker, Penland, Beckwith, & Saustead, 1984; Zeitlhofer et al., 1984). Others have speculated that thyroid status may interact with age to amplify cognitive effects in older patients (Bommer et al., 1990; Wallace et al., 1980). Also, despite improvement in thyroid status, residual effects may remain, especially in patients with subclinical hyperthyroidism (Bommer et al., 1990). There is also evidence that after a return to a euthyroid state, a patient may take several months to recover, and even then residual cognitive effects may remain (Bommer et al., 1990; MacCrimmon et al., 1979).

Hypothyroidism can result from a variety of disorders (e.g., Gull's disease and Hashimoto's disease; Greer, 1983). It has received less attention in the literature than hyperthyroidism. Hypothyroidism may be more prevalent in elderly people and is one cause of reversible dementia (Osterweil et al., 1992). Symptoms can have insidious onset and include lethargy, constipation, intolerance to cold, and muscle stiffness and cramps. Later signs include slower intellectual and motor activity, reduced appetite, weight gain, hair loss, dry skin, impaired hearing, sleep apnea, and myxedema.

The cognitive effects of hypothyroidism are less well documented than those of hyperthyroidism. However, impairment has been reported on measures of recent memory, concentration, simple arithmetic, and mental flexibility (Whybrow & Ferrell, 1974). In a more recent study, Osterweil et al. (1992) examined hypothyroidism in an older population and found no differences from control subjects for patients with minimal hypothyroidism, in contrast with those who had overt hypothyroidism. However, differences between the hypothyroid patients (minimal and overt combined) and control subjects were found overall on 6 of the 15 measures: constructional praxis, verbal learning and retention, verbal fluency, attention, and psychomotor speed. Measures of mental control and flexibility also approached significance. Improvement was seen with treatment, and little additional improvement occurred beyond the point at which a stable euthyroid state was achieved (i.e., the fifth month in the study), although the most seriously affected patients were not available for follow-up.

In summary, the effects of hyperthyroid and hypothyroid states on neuropsychological performance are similar and appear to reflect a diffuse effect on the central nervous system. The primary areas affected are concentration, recent memory and learning, verbal fluency, mental flexibility, and problem solving. The mechanisms through which altered thyroid hormone levels affect cognition and behavior are not well understood. Although the effects on neuropsychological tests appear similar, the underlying mechanisms (i.e., hypometabolic vs. hypermetabolic states) may be quite different.

Either directly or indirectly, thyroid hormones do affect multiple metabolic processes, including those of the central nervous system. A recent hypothesis has implicated beta adrenergic receptors as particularly important in mediating the effects of thyroid function on brain activity (Beckwith & Tucker, 1988). Effects of thyroid hormone level on mood support the beta adrenergic hypothesis. In addition, the catecholamines have been implicated as mediators in recent models of attention and memory (McGaugh, 1983), processes that have been observed to be affected by altered thyroid hormone levels.

Renal Failure and Dialysis

The effects of renal failure or end-stage renal disease, include hypothermia, hypertriglyceridemia, increased serum insulin, acidosis, increased plasma parathyroid hormone, bone disease, fluid retention, atrial hypertension, anemia, endocrine disturbances, gastrointestinal abnormalities, and neurological and cognitive disturbances (Arieff, 1981; Brenner & Lazarus, 1987). Treatment for renal failure often involves dialysis.

Neuropsychological effects of uremia, resulting from untreated renal failure, may include reduced mental alertness, fatiguability, intellectual impairment, decreased concentration, memory deficits, reduced perceptual-motor coordination, and personality changes (Arieff, 1981). In addition to the effects of end-stage renal disease itself, two dialysis-related syndromes have been identified: (a) dialysis disequilibrium syndrome and (b) dialysis dementia, also called *progressive dialysis encephalopathy.* The former is largely controlled by attention to the techniques of dialysis, such as frequency of sessions and blood-flow rates (Hart & Kreutzer, 1988; Lazarus & Kjellstrand, 1981). The latter is progressive and usually fatal. Initial symptoms of progressive dialysis encephalopathy include mild stuttering or stammering and motor aphasia occurring transiently during or immediately following dialysis (Alfrey, 1986; Victor & Martin, 1987). Aluminum toxicity has been implicated as a causal factor, and its incidence has decreased greatly with the increased control of aluminum levels during treatment (Alfrey, 1986; Hart & Kreutzer, 1988).

Numerous researchers have investigated the effects of the uremic state on patients' neuropsychological functioning. Osberg, Meares, McKee, and Burnett (1982) reviewed earlier studies and noted a consistent trend for Verbal IQ scores in uremic patients to be from 5 to 14 points above Performance IQ scores, with Digit Symbol and Block Design subtests consistently below average. Neuropsychological effects of uremia have been documented in several studies (Bosch & Schlebusch, 1991; Hagberg, 1974; McKee, Burnett, Raft, Batten, & Bain, 1982; J. Ryan, Souheaver, & DeWolfe, 1981; Souheaver, Ryan, & DeWolfe, 1982; Teschan et al., 1979). Impaired performance on TMT, HCT, TPT, Sensory Perceptual Examination, and Spatial Relations of the HRB as well as visual and verbal recall and RT have been found. In addition, Teschan et al. found that indexes of renal failure (e.g., blood urea nitrogen and serum creatine) were correlated with neuropsychological performance. In general, impairment in patients capable of being tested has been mild to moderate and diffuse, and their verbal ability is relatively preserved. Patients have shown the most consistently impairment on measures dealing with higher level cognitive processes, that is, those requiring sustained attention, mental flexibility, psychomotor speed, and spatial perception.

Dialysis has been shown to at least partially alleviate the neuropsychological effects of end-stage renal disease, although some studies have suggested that it has residual effects. The long-term effects of dialysis have also been investigated. Hagberg (1974) evaluated 23 patients before dialysis and then again at 6 and 12 months after dialysis. Results indicated improvement in all areas retested (Vocabulary, Paired Associates, WBI Block Design, Visual Retention, Memory for Designs, RT, and Mirror Test), and many patients scored at average levels by 12 months. Teschan et al. (1979) reported improvement among their subjects on numerous measures following dialysis (e.g., auditory short-term memory, RT, sustained attention, and TMT). However, dialyzed groups still performed worse than control groups on most measures, and additional improvement was noted in dialyzed patients who subsequently had kidney transplants. J. Ryan et al. (1981) used an extensive array of tests based on the HRB to assess uremic patients, dialysis patients, and well-matched medical-psychiatric control subjects. They found fewer deficits in dialysis patients than in uremic patients; however, dialysis patients were still impaired relative to control subjects on 7 of 10 measures. Improvement after dialysis has largely been noted to occur in the first 12 months or so after dialysis begins (Hagberg, 1974; McKee et al., 1982; Teschan et al., 1979).

Dialysis does not completely reverse the effects of renal failure (Lazarus & Kjellstrand, 1981). The presence of anemia or elevated parathyroid hormone levels may affect neuropsychological functioning (Brown et al., 1991; Gilli & DeBastiani, 1983; Marsh et al., 1991; Wolcott, Marsh, LaRue, Carr, & Nissenson, 1989). In addition, hypertension or hypertriglyceridemia have been suggested as causal factors in dialysis-related encephalopathy (Lazarus & Kjellstrand, 1981). Dialysis-related complications, such as infections and side effects of drugs used in the procedure, can also adversely affect patients' neuropsychological functioning over time. Neuropsychological data for longer periods of time have been mixed (Gilli & DeBastiani, 1983; Ziesat, Logue, & McCarty, 1980). However, the majority of evidence has suggested little additional deterioration over time, despite continued impairment in levels of performance (Brancaccio, Damasso, Spinnler, Sterzi, & Vallar, 1981; Jackson, Warrington, Roe, & Baker, 1987; Ratner, Adams, Levin, & Rourke, 1982; Wolcott et al., 1988).

Researchers have also probed the nature of inter- and intrasession variation in neuropsychological performance in dialysis patients, with equivocal results. For example, there may be a period after dialysis during which neuropsychological performance is diminished (Lewis, O'Neill, Dustman, & Beck, 1980) as the body readjusts. Subjects tested during a dialysis session may also demonstrate reduced performance on cognitive tasks (Smith & Winslow, 1990). These areas remain to be more thoroughly investigated.

Liver Disease

The liver serves a multitude of anabolic, catabolic, and storage functions. Diseases that affect the liver may significantly affect multiple metabolic activities, including protein synthesis; glucose formation; detoxification of ammonia, various hormones, and drugs; storage of glycogen and some vitamins; and maintenance of normal visceral blood flow (Podolsky & Isselbacher, 1987). The liver is also a primary regulator of plasma cholesterol and other fats and removes a variety of foreign materials from circulation.

Two primary liver disorders are discussed here: portal-systemic encephalopathy (PSE) and Wilson's disease (WD). Although many diseases affect the liver, their cognitive effects may be collectively summarized under the general term *PSE*. Neuropsychological effects of liver disorders other than WD appear to be similar, regardless of the specific underlying etiology. WD also affects the liver directly, but its distinctive properties and treatability merit specific attention.

WD is a relatively rare autosomal recessive disorder involving an inability of the liver to metabolize copper. As a result, copper accumulates in the liver, brain (especially the basal ganglia), and other organs. Onset of this illness can range from early childhood to young adulthood. Early neurological manifestations include tremor bradykinesia, dysarthria, dysphagia, hoarseness, and, less frequently, choreic movements or dystonic posturing. Sensory functioning is generally spared. WD responds well to treatments that reduce copper absorption by the body. Neuropsychiatric manifestations may be present and include subtle changes such as argumentativeness and excessive emotionality. Overt depression, paranoia, and psychosis can occur in more advanced cases (Scheinberg, 1987).

Medalia and her colleagues (Isaacs-Glaberman, Medalia, & Scheinberg, 1989; Medalia, Galynker, & Scheinberg, 1992; Medalia, Isaacs-Glaberman, & Scheinberg, 1988) have performed a series of investigations into the neuropsychological functioning of patients with WD. Results from these investigations have indicated that levels of performance on tasks requiring psychomotor speed are reduced for neurologically involved patients. Mild memory differences were also present and were felt to be primarily related to retrieval problems, although other researchers could not confirm these findings (Lang, Muller, Claus, & Druschky, 1990). Generally, verbal abilities showed little effect from the disease. Lang et al. also noted mild differences on a variety of neuropsychological measures in WD patients in comparison with control subjects, particularly for perceptual speed. Those patients with neurological signs appeared to be most affected on neuropsychological measures. Although WD appears to respond well to treatment, the long-term neuropsychological effects of the disease require further exploration.

When damage to the liver severely reduces its ability to function, PSE may result (Tarter, Edwards, & Van Thiel, 1988). The pathogenesis of PSE is not fully understood, and its severity may range from mild to extreme degrees. Neuropsychological testing has proved to be a sensitive indicator of PSE (Hockerstedt et al., 1990; Tarter, Hegedus, Van Thiel, Edwards, & Schade, 1987). Researchers have reported performance on neuropsychological tests to correlate with blood levels of ammonia, amino acids, and albumin (Gilberstadt et al., 1980; Marchesini et al., 1980) and with computerized tomography abnormalities (Bernthal et al., 1987) in patients who have cirrhosis. Differences between cirrhosis patients, control subjects, or published norms have been found for a variety of neuropsychological measures (e.g., BVRT; various RT measures; TM–Part B; and tests of attention, concentration, and spatial capacity; Moore et al., 1989; Tarter, Arria, Carra, & Van Thiel, 1987; Tarter, Carra, Switala, & Van Thiel, 1987; Weissenborn et al., 1990).

Recent studies examining the effects of liver transplantation on patients with hepatic encephalopathy (i.e., PSE; Hockerstedt et al., 1990; Powell et al., 1990; Tarter, Switala, Arria, Plail, & Van Thiel, 1990) have clearly illustrated pretransplant decrements in comparison with control subjects—primarily in the areas of visuoconstructive and psychomotor skills, short-term recall, and static ataxia. Several months after the transplant, improvement was documented in comparison with pretransplant levels. Pretransplant deficits noted were initially mild and generally improved after transplant, although some very mild decrements appeared to remain. Tarter et al. included a chronic disease control group (with Crohn's disease) and attributed some of the deficits to the nonspecific effects of chronic disease.

Little research exists exploring quality of life for cirrhotic patients. Gazzard, Price, and Dawson (1986) reported that 19 of 29 portal–caval shunt patients who averaged 9 years postshunt were considered very difficult to deal with by close relatives: 12 reported deterioration in their marriages, 8 had retired, and 7 had given up hobbies. The researchers pointed out that these patients exhibited characteristics similar to those of leukotomy patients described in the literature.

Tarter et al. (1984) found that cirrhotic patients who were not alcoholics were unable to fully meet the demands of daily living.

Schomerus et al. (1981) found deficits in neuropsychological performance that were judged severe enough to interfere with driving in 85% of 40 cirrhotic patients with portal hypertension, even though patients were selected because they had shown no clinical signs of PSE. Deficits were more severe in alcoholic cirrhotic patients. In summary, neuropsychological deficits involving psychomotor performance, visuoconstructive ability, and memory are found in many patients who have liver dysfunction. Little research has focused on higher level cognitive ability, such as problem solving (Tarter, Carra, et al., 1987), however. Neuropsychological measures are relatively sensitive indicators of hepatic encephalopathy with several studies indicating higher sensitivity than the electroencephalogram.

HIV Infection and AIDS

The first cases of AIDS were reported in 1981. AIDS is caused by infection with HIV. Individuals infected with HIV present clinically with a spectrum of conditions ranging from asymptomatic seropositive status to full-blown AIDS. The Centers for Disease Control have developed a four-tiered classification system for HIV and AIDS: Stage 1 describes individuals with acute infection, Stage 2 those with asymptomatic infection, Stage 3 those with generalized lymphadenopathy, and Stage 4 those with symptomatic AIDS. Centers for Disease Control figures indicate that about 250,000 cases of AIDS have been diagnosed in the United States since 1981, with roughly 1 to 2 million persons estimated to be HIV infected (Curran, 1992).

Neurological complications of HIV infection are frequent and variable. Disruption of the immune system by HIV may give rise to multiple brain disorders, including opportunistic infections and neoplasms. Also common is brain dysfunction resulting from metabolic changes because of the failure of other organ systems in the body. Several disorders, including the AIDS dementia complex and aseptic meningitis, appear to relate directly to the effects of HIV. Susceptibility to neurological complications is greatest in the later stages of the illness (Price, 1992).

AIDS dementia complex was first described by Price and his colleagues in 1986 (Navia, Jordan, & Price, 1986). Early clinical descriptions have emphasized impairment of memory, concentration, and psychomotor speed as initial symptoms. AIDS dementia complex typically appears following the onset of other clinical manifestations of

AIDS, and it is progressive. Recent data have suggested that 7% to 8% of patients with AIDS suffer from HIV encephalopathy—a disorder described in similar, but not identical, terms to AIDS dementia complex (Janssen, Nwanyanwu, Selik, & Sten-Green, 1992). Comprehensive neuropsychological characterization of this complex has yet to be accomplished.

Recent neuropsychological studies of HIV patients have typically focused on samples of patients with either AIDS and AIDS-related complex (Stage 4, as described above) or asymptomatic HIV patients (Stages 2 or 3). Using a subsample from the Multicenter AIDS Cohort Study, E. Miller et al. (1990) administered a focused battery of neuropsychological tests (TM, Digit Span of the WAIS-R, COWA, GP, SDMT, and RAVLT) to 84 HIV-positive Stage 4 outpatients and to 769 seronegative control subjects. When age and education were covaried, the Stage 4 group performed more poorly than the control group on two psychomotor tests: TM and SDMT. Depending on the cutoff criteria used, between 8% and 14.5% of Stage 4 patients showed neuropsychological impairment relative to control subjects. In a related study with a somewhat smaller sample, E. Miller, Satz, and Visscher (1991) found a series of simple and choice RT measures to be more sensitive to impairment in Stage 4 patients than the standard neuropsychological battery (with the only impaired measure in the traditional battery being the RAVLT). Depression could not account for the deficits detected.

Other studies of symptomatic HIV-positive patients, although involving more comprehensive batteries, have used smaller samples. In another project of the Multicenter AIDS Cohort Study, Van Gorp, Miller, Satz, and Visscher (1989) evaluated 34 HIV-positive Stage 4 patients (20 with AIDS and 14 with AIDS-related complex and 13 control subjects, using an abbreviated WAIS-R; subtests of the WMS; and several other measures of language, memory, attention, and psychomotor speed. Patients with AIDS-related complex were unimpaired relative to control subjects. Patients with AIDS had lower WAIS-R Verbal, Performance, and Full Scale IQ scores than did control subjects, as well as poorer performance on some measures of cognitive flexibility and motor speed and of memory. Overall, results suggested that patients with AIDS showed most consistent deficits on measures of nonverbal memory and timed psychomotor tasks. Reinvang, Froland, and Skripeland (1991) evaluated 21 patients with AIDS and 18 control subjects (acute leukemia patients) with the WAIS-R, TMT, GP, and several measures of learning and memory. Patients with AIDS showed impairment on the WAIS-R Performance IQ, selected WAIS-R subtests, GP, and TM. Roughly one half of the patients with AIDS scored 2 standard deviations and more from published norms on two or more tests. Timed motor, psychomotor, and nonverbal reasoning tasks were particularly sensitive to AIDS-related cognitive changes.

Researchers conducting neuropsychological studies of symptomatic HIV patients have deliberately attempted to exclude those with gross neurological illness (e.g., opportunistic central nervous system infections or tumors) and substance abuse. The presence and variety of neuropsychological impairment in clinically referred patients may, however, be much more variable. Several authors (e.g., Kaemingk & Kaszniak, 1989; Reinvang et al., 1991)—citing clinical, neuropsychological, and pathological evidence—have suggested that AIDS dementia complex has many attributes of a subcortical dementia syndrome.

The presence of neuropsychological impairment in individuals who have asymptomatic HIV infections (Stages 2 and 3) is a subject of controversy. Many studies, including those involving the Multicenter AIDS Cohort Study sample, have found no evidence for impairment in asymptomatic patients (Clifford, Jacoby, Miller, Seyfried, & Glickman, 1990; Janssen et al., 1989; E. Miller et al., 1991; E. Miller et al., 1990; Reinvang et al., 1991; Selnes et al., 1990). Others have found evidence for cognitive decline (Grant, Atkinson, et al., 1987; Wilkie, Eisdorfer, Morgan, Loewenstein, & Szapocznik, 1990). This issue will no doubt undergo further study, but composite evidence suggests that significant cognitive decline in asymptomatic patients is relatively infrequent and that neuropsychological impairment is more common in the later stages of infection.

The ramifications of HIV-related cognitive changes for patients' day-to-day functioning have yet to be formally studied. The importance of empirical data to address this issue has been underscored by the role that neuropsychological studies have played in public policy and personnel decisions involving patients with this illness (Harter, 1989).

To summarize, AIDS is a relatively new disorder with great potential to affect neurological functioning both directly and indirectly. There has been an explosion of information about this disease, and knowledge of the neuropsychological aspects of AIDS is evolving rapidly. Given the many ways in which AIDS may affect brain function, the psychologist in clinical practice may encounter a variety of neuropsychological syndromes, including frank dementia, focal neuropsychological disturbances, or more subtle cognitive impairment. Significant cognitive decline in asymptomatic HIV patients appears to be relatively infrequent. Clinicians, including neuropsychologists and health psychologists alike, must recognize the formidable potential of this disease to cause serious psychological distress that may also disrupt cognitive functioning. The implications of HIV-related cognitive changes for day-to-day functioning are likely to be the subject of scientific scrutiny over the next several years.

Clinical Implementation

As the foregoing brief reviews illustrate, neuropsychological complications of chronic illness are not uncommon. Formal neuropsychological examination is appropriate whenever cognitive impairment is suspected. Neuropsychological consultation is typically most useful when a concise referral has been formulated. The following is a list of common and appropriate referral questions: Does the patient show signs of cognitive impairment? Is the cognitive complaint most likely the result of cerebral dysfunction or psychopathology? Does the patient have deficits significant enough to interfere with his or her ability to work or live independently? Has the patient shown changes in cognition following a baseline evaluation?

The evaluation usually will begin with review of medical records to provide a context in which to interpret test data and to alert the examiner to any special conditions (e.g., visual impairment or paralysis) that might affect choice of procedures or interpretation of results. The review can also provide precise information about current treatments that may affect performance.

A second component of the evaluation involves gathering information about current symptoms and the context for referral as well as demographic, social, medical, and psychiatric history. These data are ordinarily obtained during a patient interview and, at times, are supplemented with information provided by other sources. Performance on neuropsychological tests can be affected by a host of variables not related to cerebral pathology, including age, education, and occupational experience (Heaton, Grant, & Matthews, 1986). Certain skills, particularly those involving motor strength, may also be affected by the patient's sex. Furthermore, a patient may have a history of developmental or psychiatric disorders that may substantially alter the neuropsychologist's interpretation of certain tests. Thus, a detailed history is critical to adequate evaluation.

The core feature of the examination involves administration and interpretation of a comprehensive battery of standardized tests. In a thorough evaluation, a psychologist will examine a broad range of cognitive, perceptual, and motor functions, both to address functional brain integrity and to provide information about a broad range of skills and abilities. Because the behavioral expression of cerebral dysfunction varies as a function of the location, type, severity, and chronicity of the responsible lesions, neuropsychological evaluations are necessarily multidimensional. Several standard test batteries have been devised, but none is universally accepted. Neuropsychologists frequently assemble test batteries suited to the condition and demographic characteristics of their patient, as well as the nature of the referral question. Such batteries can be used flexibly, with modifications made on the basis of clinical need (Lezak, 1983).

Although they vary in terms of the tests used, comprehensive neuropsychological examinations should typically assess a domain of cognitive, sensory, and motor abilities, such as the following: (a) receptive and expressive language; (b) elementary and complex motor abilities; (c) sensory function—including tactile, visual, and auditory receptive abilities; (d) attention, concentration, and mental flexibility; (e) learning and memory, (f) intellectual processes—including verbal, numerical, spatial, and sequential reasoning abilities; and (g) abstract concept formation. Neuropsychological assessment of a patient with chronic illness would appropriately address performance in the above areas. Examples of more specific tests that have commonly been used to assess those with chronic illness can be found in the Appendix. For more exhaustive information regarding specific tests, see the texts by Lezak (1983) and by Spreen and Strauss (1991). In many settings, neuropsychological evaluations routinely include a formal assessment of psychopathology. Because individuals with chronic illness are at risk for developing depression and other psychiatric disturbances (e.g., Faulstick, 1987), and because emotional status may affect neuropsychological performance (Lezak, 1983), we strongly recommend that formal assessment of psychopathology be included in any examination of chronically ill patients.

Comprehensive neuropsychological evaluations are time-consuming and are not always readily available. In some situations, the health psychologist may be responsible for evaluating unselected cases to identify those for whom further neuropsychological examination would be useful and some type of screening battery would be desirable. There are at least two approaches to screening. First, one or more brief tests highly sensitive to brain damage can be administered (Lezak, 1983). A more time-consuming alternative is to use a "minibattery," made up of tests chosen to briefly sample a range of functions (e.g., Golden, 1976; Goldstein, Tarter, Shelley, & Hegedus, 1983).

The selection of tests composing a screening battery for possible neuropsychological impairment may vary from setting to setting, depending on such factors as the precise reason for screening; the amount of time that can be allocated to test administration; the type and degree of expected impairment; and patient characteristics, including age, educational background, overall health status, and stamina (see chap. 3 in this volume for specific cognitive-screening measures). The foregoing review suggests that neuropsychological impairment associated with chronic illness may, in many instances, be subtle. If the goal of brief screening is to detect possible impairment meriting further investigation, then short tests highly sensitive to brain dysfunction may be useful. Examples of such tests include the TMT, SDMT, and the SCWT. Each is well validated and can be administered under most circumstances in about 10 minutes, and each has been used in studies of patients with chronic illness. Age- and education-adjusted norms have recently become available for the TM, which may further enhance the value of this measure as a screening device (Heaton, Grant, & Matthews, 1991).

In studies reviewed for this chapter, patients tended (with some exceptions) to be young or, especially, middle-aged adults. Yet, some clinical settings serve primarily geriatric patients, where the co-occurrence of primary central nervous system disease (e.g., Alzheimer's disease or stroke) with chronic systemic illness may be a consideration. In addition, some chronic systemic illnesses, if untreated, may cause or contribute to causation of frank delirium or dementia. Again, see chapter 3 in this volume, on psychological assessment, for a discussion of screening techniques for more pronounced cognitive impairment.

Although screening techniques may be helpful in some settings, there are perils in their use. Tests highly sensitive to brain damage may also be affected by other variables, including age and education. Because many individuals who have a chronic illness may be elderly, this is of substantial importance. Uncritical use of standard cutoff scores to detect cerebral dysfunction may be extremely misleading. For example, Davies (1968) administered TM to 80 healthy normal controls in their 70s and found approximately 90% to be misclassified as brain damaged by standard cutoff scores. Tests sensitive to cerebral dysfunction may also be affected by psychiatric disorders (Lezak, 1983). Screening instruments additionally fail to account for the myriad behavioral manifestations that may accompany neurological illness. Adams and Heaton (1990) have cautioned against using brief screening techniques for such disorders as AIDS and HIV, where the neuropsychological correlates are not known in detail. If screening techniques are used, the availability of age- and education-appropriate normative data is critical. As with any other psychological test, screening measures should be administered, scored, and interpreted only by individuals who are fully qualified and trained. Health psychologists who use screening techniques are encouraged to seek the assistance of a clinical neuropsychologist to aid with such issues as test selection, identification of an appropriate normative database, and training in test administration and scoring. The clinical neuropsychologist may also provide input regarding quality control and program evaluation in a screening situation. Ongoing availability of a trained neuropsychologist to consult in such matters as interpretation of results and the timing of referral for more extended evaluation is also recommended.

Future Needs and Developments

As neuropsychologists play a greater role in evaluating the chronically ill patient, the research needs become more substantial. Most chronic illnesses have not been thoroughly studied. Investigators designing neuropsychological studies would do well to review the guidelines postulated by Parsons and Prigatano (1978) for conducting neuropsychological research. They emphasized including adequate controls for age, education, socioeconomic status, and gender, as well as having appropriately trained personnel to administer tests. In preparing this chapter, we reviewed a number of papers that, although sophisticated from a medical standpoint, regrettably either failed to take these factors into account or did not provide adequate descriptive information. Results were therefore confounded or uninterpretable. The underlying mechanisms of neuropsychological impairment in chronic illnesses remain largely unknown. Identification of these mechanisms and studies relating neuropsychological variables to both disease-specific physiological measures and neuroimaging techniques (e.g., magnetic resonance imaging, positron-emission tomography, and single-photon-emission computed tomography) would also be valuable. Better understanding of these mechanisms may result in improvements in the treatment of impaired individuals or in the prevention of impairment. The impact of neuropsychological impairment on patients' day-to-day activities and quality of life has only begun to be studied empirically and remains yet another worthwhile area of investigation.

Standard approaches to detecting neuropsychological impairment in patients with chronic illnesses are lacking for most disorders. Butters et al. (1990) recently proposed extended and brief neuropsychological batteries to study AIDS- and HIV-related cognitive changes. These batteries, although assessing a range of abilities, emphasize those neuropsychological abilities that research has shown are most likely to be compromised by the disease. This approach has great appeal and, if successful, may serve as a model on which to structure the examination of patients with other chronic illnesses. Additionally, current neuropsychological techniques were developed and validated on groups of patients with primary neurological disease, so development of entirely new techniques for patients with chronic illness is highly desirable. Along these lines, the superior sensitivity of reaction time measures in the recent study of HIV-related cognitive changes (E. Miller et al., 1991) is intriguing; however, greater standardization and development of normative databases is imperative before such tasks can be used clinically. Brief, repeatable neuropsychological examinations may be especially useful for documenting disease progression or treatment effects among patients with chronic illnesses. Initial evidence has suggested that computerized tasks, which allow for control of practice effects, could be extremely helpful, and their development should be encouraged (Kay, 1991).

Chronic illness is becoming more prevalent as technical advances in medicine improve the ability to sustain life. Systemic disease may be associated with physical, emotional, and cognitive disability. Because cognitive disorders may substantially affect adjustment and quality of life, involvement of neuropsychologists with patients who have chronic illnesses is likely to increase.

REFERENCES

Adams, K., & Heaton, R. (1990). Statement concerning the NIMH neuropsychological battery. *Journal of Clinical and Experimental Neuropsychology, 12,* 960–962.

Alfrey, A. (1986). Dialysis encephalopathy. *Kidney International, 29,* S53–S57.

Alvarez, M., Gomez, A., Alavez, E., & Navarro, D. (1983). Short communication: Attention disturbance in Graves' disease. *Psychoneuroendocrinology, 8,* 451–454.

Arieff, A. (1981). Neurological complications of uremia. In B. Brenner & R. Rector (Eds.), *The kidney* (pp. 2306–2343). Philadelphia: W. B. Saunders.

Beckwith, B., & Tucker, D. (1988). Thyroid disorders. In R. Tarter, D. Van Thiel, & K. Edwards (Eds.), *Medical neuropsychology* (pp. 197–221). New York: Plenum.

Benton, A. (1987). Evolution of a clinical specialty. *Clinical Neuropsychologist, 1,* 5–8.

Benton, A. (1992). Clinical neuropsychology: 1960–1990. *Journal of Clinical and Experimental Neuropsychology, 14,* 407–417.

Berg, R. (1988). Cancer. In R. Tarter & D. Van Thiel (Eds.), *Medical neuropsychology* (pp. 265–290). New York: Plenum.

Bernthal, P., Hays, A., Tarter, R., Van Thiel, D., Lecky, J., & Hegedus, A. (1987). Cerebral CT scan abnormalities in cholestatic and hepatocellular disease and their relationship to neuropsychologic test performance. *Hepatology, 7,* 107–114.

Bluestein, H. (1984). Antineuronal antibodies in the pathogenesis of neuropsychiatric manifestations of systemic lupus erythematosus. In P. Behan & F. Spreafico (Eds.), *Neuroimmunology* (pp. 157–165). New York: Raven Press.

Bommer, M., Eversmann, T., Pickardt, R., Leonhardt, A., & Naber, D. (1990). Psychopathological and neuropsychological symptoms in patients with subclinical and remitted hyperthyroidism. *Klinische Wochenschrift, 68,* 552–558.

Bosch, B., & Schlebusch, L. (1991). Neuropsychological deficits associated with uremic encephalopathy: A report of 5 patients. *South African Medical Journal, 79,* 560–562.

Brancaccio, D., Damasso, R., Spinnler, H., Sterzi, R., & Vallar, G. (1981). Does chronic kidney failure lead to mental failure? A neuropsychologic survey of self-sufficient outpatients. *Archives of Neurology, 38,* 757–758.

Brenner, B. M., & Lazarus, J. M. (1987). Chronic renal failure: Pathophysiologic and clinical considerations. In E. Braunwald, K. Isselbacher, R. Petersdorf, J. Wilson, & A. Fauci (Eds.), *Principles of internal medicine* (pp. 1155–1162). New York: McGraw-Hill.

Brown, W., Marsh, J., Wolcott, D., Takushi, R., Carr, C., Higa, J., & Nissenson, A. (1991). Cognitive function, mood, and P3 latency: Effects of the amelioration of anemia in dialysis patients. *Neuropsychologia, 29,* 35–45.

Butters, N., Grant, I., Haxby, J., Judd, L., Martin, A., McClelland, J., Pequegnat, W., Schacter, D., & Stover, E. (1990). Assessment of AIDS-related cognitive changes: Recommendations of the NIMH workshop on neuropsychological assessment approaches. *Journal of Clinical and Experimental Neuropsychology, 12,* 973–978.

Carbotte, R., Denburg, S., & Denburg, J. (1986). Prevalence of cognitive impairment in systemic lupus erythematosus. *Journal of Nervous and Mental Disease, 174,* 357–364.

Carbotte, R., Denburg, S., & Denburg, J. (1992). Cognitive dysfunction and systemic lupus erythematosus. In R. Lahita (Ed.), *Systemic lupus erythematosus* (pp. 865–881). New York: Churchill Livingstone.

Clifford, D., Jacoby, R., Miller, J., Seyfried, W., & Glickman, M. (1990). Neuropsychometric performance of asymptomatic HIV-infected subjects. *AIDS, 4,* 767–774.

Cox, D., Gonder-Frederick, L., Driesen, N., & Clarke, W. (1991). Driving performance of Type I patients during euglycemia, moderate and severe hypoglycemia. *Diabetes, 40,* 557A.

Curran, J. (1992). Epidemiology of HIV infection and AIDS. In J. Wyngaarden, L. Smith, & J. Bennett (Eds.), *Textbook of medicine* (pp. 1918–1925). Philadelphia: W. B. Saunders.

Davies, A. (1968). The influence of age on Trail Making Test performance. *Journal of Clinical Psychology, 24,* 96–98.

Delattre, J., & Posner, J. (1989). Medical complications of chemotherapy and radiation therapy. In M. Aminoff (Ed.), *Neurology in general medicine* (pp. 365–387). New York: Churchill Livingstone.

Denburg, S., Carbotte, R., & Denburg, J. (1987). Cognitive impairment in systemic lupus erythematosus. *Journal of Clinical and Experimental Neuropsychology, 9,* 323–339.

Elias, M., Robbins, M., Schultz, N., & Pierce, T. (1990). Is blood pressure an important variable in research on aging and neuropsychological test performance? *Journal of Gerontology, 45,* 128–135.

Elias, M., Robbins, M., Schultz, N., & Streeten, D. (1986). A longitudinal study of neuropsychological test performance for hypertensive and normotensive adults: Initial findings. *Journal of Gerontology, 41,* 503–505.

Elias, M., Robbins, M., Schultz, N., Streeten, D., & Elias, P. (1987). Clinical significance of cognitive performance in hypertensive patients. *Hypertension, 9,* 192–197.

Elias, M., Schultz, N., Robbins, M., & Elias, P. (1989). A longitudinal study of neuropsychological performance by hypertensives and normotensives: A third measurement point. *Journal of Gerontology, 44,* 25–28.

Ellis, G., & Verity, M. (1979). Central nervous system involvement in systemic lupus erythematosus: A review of neuropathologic findings in 57 cases, 1957–1977. *Seminars in Arthritis and Rheumatism, 8,* 212–221.

Faulstick, M. (1987). Psychiatric aspects of AIDS. *American Journal of Psychiatry, 144,* 551–556.

Feinglass, E., Arnett, F., Dorsch, C., Zizic, T., & Stevens, M. (1976). Neuropsychiatric manifestations of systemic lupus erythematosus: Diagnosis, clinical spectrum, and relationship to other features of the disease. *Medicine, 55,* 323–339.

Fletcher, J., & Copeland, D. (1988). Neurobehavioral effects of central nervous system prophylactic treatment of cancer in children. *Journal of Clinical and Experimental Neuropsychology, 10,* 495–537.

Foster, D. (1987). Diabetes mellitus. In E. Braunwald, K. Isselbacher, R. Petersdorf, J. Wilson, & A. Fauci (Eds.), *Principles of internal medicine* (pp. 1778–1797). New York: McGraw-Hill.

Francheschi, M., Tancredi, O., Smirne, S., Mercinelli, A., & Canal, N. (1982). Cognitive processes in hypertension. *Hypertension, 4,* 226–229.

Futrell, N., Schultz, L., & Millikan, C. (1992). Central nervous system disease in patients with systemic lupus erythematosus. *Neurology, 42,* 1649–1657.

Gazzard, B., Price, H., & Dawson, A. (1986). Detection of hepatic encephalopathy. *Postgraduate Medical Journal, 62,* 163–166.

Gilberstadt, S., Gilberstadt, H., Zieve, L., Buegel, B., Collier, R., & McClain, C. (1980). Psychomotor performance defects in cirrhotic patients without overt encephalopathy. *Archives of Internal Medicine, 140,* 519–521.

Gilli, P., & DeBastiani, P. (1983). Cognitive function and regular dialysis treatment. *Clinical Nephrology, 19,* 188–192.

Ginsburg, K., Wright, E., Larson, M., Fossel, A., Albert, M., Schur, P., & Liang, M. (1992). A controlled study of the prevalence of cognitive dysfunction in randomly selected patients with systemic lupus erythematosus. *Arthritis and Rheumatism, 35,* 776–782.

Golden, J. (1976). The identification of brain damage by an abbreviated form of the Halstead-Reitan Neuropsychological Battery. *Journal of Clinical Psychology, 32,* 821–826.

Goldstein, G., Tarter, R., Shelley, C., & Hegedus, A. (1983). The Pittsburgh Initial Neuropsychological Testing System (PINTS). *Journal of Behavioral Assessment, 5,* 227–238.

Grant, I., Atkinson, J., Hesselink, J., Kennedy, C., Richman, D., Spector, S., & McCutchon, J. (1987). Evidence for early central nervous system involvement in the Acquired Immune Deficiency Syndrome (AIDS) and other human immunodeficiency virus infections. *Annals of Internal Medicine, 107,* 828–836.

Grant, I., Heaton, R., McSweeney, A., Adams, K., & Timms, R. (1982). Neuropsychologic findings in hypoxemic chronic obstructive pulmonary disease. *Archives of Internal Medicine, 142,* 1470–1476.

Grant, I., Prigatano, G., Heaton, R., McSweeney, A., Wright, E., & Adams, K. (1987). Progressive neuropsychologic impairment and hypoxemia. *Archives of General Psychiatry, 44,* 999–1006.

Greer, M. A. (1983). Disorders of the thyroid. In J. H. Stein (Ed.), *Internal medicine* (pp. 1738–1759). Boston: Little, Brown.

Hagberg, B. (1974). A prospective study of patients in chronic hemodialysis: Predictive value of intelligence, cognitive deficit and ego defense structures in rehabilitation. *Journal of Psychosomatic Research, 18,* 151–160.

Hahn, B. H. (1987). Systemic lupus erythematosus. In E. Braunwald, K. Isselbacher, R. Petersdorf, J. Wilson, & A. Fauci (Eds.), *Principles of internal medicine* (pp. 1418–1423). New York: McGraw-Hill.

Hart, R., & Kreutzer, J. (1988). Renal systems. In R. Tarter, D. Van Thiel, & K. Edwards (Eds.), *Medical neuropsychology* (pp. 99–120). New York: Plenum.

Harter, D. (1989). Neuropsychological status of asymptomatic individuals seropositive to HIV-1. *Annals of Neurology, 26,* 589–591.

Hay, E., Black, D., Huddly, A., Creed, F., Tomenson, B., Bernstein, R., & Holt, P. (1992). Psychiatric disorder and cognitive impairment in systemic lupus erythematosus. *Arthritis and Rheumatism, 35,* 411–416.

Heaton, R., Grant, I., & Matthews, C. (1986). Differences in neuropsychological test performance associated with age, education, and sex. In I. Grant & K. Adams (Eds.), *Neuropsychological assessment of neuropsychiatric disorders* (pp. 100–120). New York: Oxford University Press.

Heaton, R., Grant, I., & Matthews, C. (1991). *Comprehensive norms for an expanded Halstead-Reitan battery: Demographic correlations, research findings, and clinical applications.* Odessa, FL: Psychological Assessment Resources.

Hockerstedt, K., Kajaste, S., Isonienie, H., Muuronen, A., Raininko, R., Seppalainen, A.-M., & Hilborn, M. (1990). Tests for encephalopathy before and after liver transplantation. *Transplantation Proceedings, 22,* 1576–1578.

Holmes, C. (1986). Neuropsychological profiles in men with insulin dependent diabetes. *Journal of Consulting and Clinical Psychology, 54,* 386–389.

Holmes, C., Koepke, K., & Thompson, R. (1986). Simple versus complex performance impairments at three blood glucose levels. *Psychoneuroendocrinology, 11,* 353–357.

Ingram, R. (1987). Chronic bronchitis, emphysema, and airways obstruction. In E. Braunwald, K. Isselbacher, R. Petersdorf, J. Wilson, J. Martin, & A. Fauci (Eds.), *Principles of internal medicine* (pp. 1987–2095). New York: McGraw-Hill.

Isaacs-Glaberman, K., Medalia, A., & Scheinberg, I. (1989). Verbal recall and recognition abilities in patients with Wilson's disease. *Cortex, 25,* 353–361.

Jackson, M., Warrington, F., Roe, C., & Baker, L. (1987). Cognitive function in hemodialysis patients. *Clinical Nephrology, 27,* 26–30.

Janssen, R., Nwanyanwu, O., Selik, R., & Sten-Green, J. (1992). Epidemiology of human immunodeficiency virus encephalopathy in the United States. *Neurology, 42,* 1472–1476.

Janssen, R., Saykin, A., Cannon, L., Campbell, J., Pinksy, P., Hessal, N., O'Malley, P., Lifson, A., Doll, L., Rutherford, G., & Kaplan, J. (1989). Neurological and neuropsychological manifestations of HIV infection: Association with AIDS-related complex but not asymptomatic HIV-1 infection. *Annals of Neurology, 26,* 592–600.

Kaemingk, K., & Kaszniak, A. (1989). Neuropsychological aspects of human immunodeficiency virus infection. *Clinical Neuropsychologist, 3,* 309–326.

Kay, G. (1991). Repeated testing applications employing computer-based performance assessment measures. *Journal of Clinical and Experimental Neuropsychology, 13,* 50.

Kirk, A., Kertesz, A., & Polk, M. (1991). Dementia with leukoencephalopathy in systemic lupus erythematosus. *Canadian Journal of Neurological Sciences, 18,* 344–348.

Klein, I., Trzepacz, P., Roberts, M., & Levey, G. (1988). Symptom rating scale for assessing hyperthyroidism. *Archives of Internal Medicine, 148,* 387–390.

Lang, C., Muller, D., Claus, D., & Druschky, K. (1990). Neuropsychological findings in treated Wilson's disease. *Acta Neurologica Scandinavia, 81,* 75–81.

Langan, S., Deary, I., Hepburn, D., & Frier, B. (1991). Cumulative impairment following recurrent severe hypoglycemia in adult patients with insulin treated diabetes mellitus. *Diabetologia, 34,* 337–344.

Lazarus, J. M., & Kjellstrand, C. M. (1981). Dialysis: Medical aspects. In B. M. Brenner & F. C. Rector, Jr. (Eds.), *The kidney* (pp. 2490–2543). Philadelphia: W. B. Saunders.

Lee, J., Sheer, D., Valdivaseo, D., Jeffries, T., Umsawadi, W., Murphy, W., Yung, J., Licciardello, J., & Hong, W. (1988). Long term effects of brain irradiation and chemotherapy on neuropsychologic performance in patients with lung cancer. *Proceedings of the American Association of Cancer Research, 29,* 218.

Lee, P., Hung, B., Woo, E., Tai, P., & Choi, D. (1989). Effects of radiation therapy on neuropsychological functioning in patients with nasopharyngeal carcinoma. *Journal of Neurology, Neurosurgery, and Psychiatry, 52,* 488–492.

Levander, S., & Elithorn, A. (1987). *APT Manual.* Trondheim, Norway: Department of Psychiatry and Behavioral Medicine, University of Trondheim.

Lewis, E., O'Neill, W., Dustman, R., & Beck, E. (1980). Temporal effects of hemodialysis on measures of neural efficiency. *Kidney International, 17,* 357–363.

Lezak, M. (1983). *Neuropsychological assessment.* New York: Oxford University Press.

MacCrimmon, D., Wallace, J., Goldberg, W., & Streiner, D. (1979). Emotional disturbance and cognitive deficits in hyperthyroidism. *Psychosomatic Medicine, 41,* 331–340.

Marchesini, G., Zoli, M., Dondi, C., Cecchini, L., Angiolini, A., Bianchi, B., & Pisi, E. (1980). Prevalence of subclinical hepatic encephalopathy in cirrhotics and relation to plasma amino acid imbalance. *Digestive Diseases and Science, 35,* 763–768.

Marsh, J., Brown, W., Wolcott, D., Carr, C., Harper, R., Schweitzer, S., & Nissenson, A. (1991). HuEPO treatment improves brain and cognitive function of anemic dialysis patients. *Kidney International, 39,* 155–163.

Mazzuchi, A., Mutti, A., Poletti, A., Novarini, A., & Parma, M. (1986). Neuropsychological deficits in arterial hypertension. *Acta Neurologica Scandinavia, 73,* 619–627.

McCaffrey, R., Ortega, A., Orsillo, S., Haase, R., & McCoy, G. (1992). Neuropsychological and physical side effects of metroprolol in essential hypertensives. *Neuropsychology, 6,* 225–238.

McGaugh, J. L. (1983). Preserving the presence of the past: Hormonal influences on memory storage. *American Psychologist, 38,* 161–174.

McKee, D., Burnett, G., Raft, D., Batten, P., & Bain, K. (1982). Longitudinal study of neuropsychological functioning in patients on chronic hemodialysis: A preliminary report. *Journal of Psychosomatic Research, 26,* 511–518.

McSweeney, A., Grant, I., Heaton, R., Prigatano, G., & Adams, K. (1985). Relationship of neuropsychological status to everyday functioning in healthy and chronically ill patients. *Journal of Clinical and Experimental Neuropsychology, 7,* 281–291.

Medalia, A., Galynker, I., & Scheinberg, I. (1992). The interaction of motor, memory and emotional dysfunction in Wilson's disease. *Biological Psychiatry, 31,* 823–826.

Medalia, A., Isaacs-Glaberman, K., & Scheinberg, I. (1988). Neuropsychological impairment in Wilson's disease. *Archives of Internal Medicine, 45,* 502–504.

Miller, E., Satz, P., & Visscher, B. (1991). Computerized and conventional neuropsychological assessment of HIV-1 infected homosexual men. *Neurology, 41,* 1608–1616.

Miller, E., Selnes, O., McArthur, J., Satz, P., Becker, J., Cohen, B., Sheridan, K., Machado, A., VanGorp, W., & Visscher, B. (1990). Neuropsychological performance in HIV-1 infected homosexual men: The Multicenter AIDS Cohort Study (MACS). *Neurology, 40,* 197–203.

Miller, R., Shapiro, A., King, H., Ginchereau, E., & Hosutt, J. (1984). Effect of antihypertensive treatment on the behavioral consequences of elevated blood pressure. *Hypertension, 6,* 203–208.

Moore, J., Dunk, A., Crawford, J., Deans, H., Besson, J., DeLacey, G., Sinclair, T., Mowat, N., & Brunt, P. (1989). Neuropsychological deficits and morphological MRI brain scan abnormalities in apparently healthy nonencephalopathic patients with cirrhosis. *Journal of Hepatology, 9,* 319–325.

Navia, B., Jordan, B., & Price, R. (1986). The AIDS dementia complex: I. Clinical features. *Annals of Neurology, 19,* 517–524.

Osberg, J., Meares, G., McKee, D., & Burnett, G. (1982). Intellectual functioning in renal failure and chronic dialysis. *Journal of Chronic Diseases, 35,* 445–457.

Osterweil, D., Syndulko, K., Cohen, S., Pettler-Jennings, P., Hershman, J., Cummings, J., Tourtelotte, W., & Soloman, D. (1992). Cognitive function in non-demented older adults with hypothyroidism. *Journal of the American Geriatrics Society, 40,* 325–335.

Parsons, O., & Prigatano, G. (1978). Methodological considerations in clinical neuropsychological research. *Journal of Consulting and Clinical Psychology, 46,* 608–619.

Parth, P., Dunlap, W., Kennedy, R., Lane, N., & Ordy, J. (1989). Motor and cognitive testing of bone marrow transplant patients after chemoradiotherapy. *Perceptual and Motor Skills, 68,* 1227–1241.

Paschke, R., Harsch, I., Schlote, B., Vardarli, I., Schaaf, L., Kaumeier, S., Teuber, J., & Usadel, K. (1990). Sequential psychological testing during the course of autoimmune hyperthyroidism. *Klinische Wochenschrift, 68,* 942–950.

Podolsky, D. K., & Isselbacher, K. J. (1987). Derangements of hepatic metabolism. In E. Braunwald, K. Isselbacher, R. Petersdorf, J. Wilson, & A. Fauci (Eds.), *Principles of internal medicine* (pp. 1309–1315). New York: McGraw-Hill.

Pomerleau, O. (1979). Behavioral medicine: The contribution of experimental analysis of behavior to medical care. *American Psychologist, 34,* 654–663.

Posner, J. (1989). Paraneoplastic syndromes involving the nervous system. In M. Aminoff (Ed.), *Neurology and general medicine* (pp. 341–364). New York: Churchill Livingstone.

Powell, E., Peneler, M., Chalk, J., Parkin, P., Strong, R., Lynch, S., Kerlin, P., Cooksley, W., Cheng, W., & Powell, L. (1990). Improvement in chronic hepatocerebral degeneration following liver transplantation. *Gastroenterology, 98,* 1079–1082.

Price, R. (1992). Neurologic complications of HIV infection. In J. Wyngaarden, L. Smith, & J. Bennett (Eds.), *Textbook of medicine* (pp. 1928–1932). Philadelphia: W. B. Saunders.

Prigatano, G., & Grant, I. (1989). Neuropsychological correlates of COPD. In A. McSweeney & I. Grant (Eds.), *Chronic obstructive disease: A behavioral perspective.* New York: Marcel Dekker.

Prigatano, G., & Levin, D. (1988). Pulmonary system. In R. Tarter, D. Van Thiel, & K. Edwards (Eds.), *Medical neuropsychology* (pp. 11–26). New York: Plenum.

Prigatano, G., Parsons, O., Wright, E., Levin, D., & Hawryluk, G. (1983). Neuropsychological test performance in mildly hypoxemic patients with chronic obstructive pulmonary disease. *Journal of Consulting and Clinical Psychology, 51,* 108–116.

Ratner, D., Adams, K., Levin, N., & Rourke, B. (1982). Effects of hemodialysis on the cognitive and sensory-motor functioning of the adult chronic hemodialysis patient. *Journal of Behavioral Medicine, 6,* 291–311.

Reaven, G., Thompson, L., Nahum, D., & Haskins, E. (1990). Relationship between hyperglycemia and cognitive function in older NIDDM patients. *Diabetes Care, 13,* 16–21.

Reichard, P., Berglund, A., Britz, A., Levander, S., & Rosenquist, V. (1991). Hypoglycemic episodes during intensified insulin treatment: Increased frequency but no effect on cognitive function. *Journal of Internal Medicine, 229,* 9–16.

Reinvang, I., Froland, S., & Skripeland, V. (1991). Prevalence of neuropsychological deficit in HIV infection. Incipient signs of AIDS dementia complex in patients with AIDS. *Acta Neurologica Scandinavia, 83,* 289–293.

Rockey, P. H., & Griep, R. J. (1980). Behavioral dysfunction in hyperthyroidism. *Archives of Internal Medicine, 140,* 1194–1197.

Ryan, C. (1988). Neurobehavioral disturbances associated with disorders of the pancreas. In R. Tarter, D. Van Thiel, & K. Edwards (Eds.), *Medical neuropsychology* (pp. 121–158). New York: Plenum.

Ryan, C., Williams, T., Orchard, T., & Finegold, D. (1992). Psychomotor slowing associated with distal symmetrical polyneuropathy in adults with diabetes mellitus. *Diabetes, 41,* 107–113.

Ryan, J., Souheaver, G., & DeWolfe, A. (1981). Halstead-Reitan test results in chronic hemodialysis. *Journal of Nervous and Mental Diseases, 169,* 311–314.

Scheinberg, H. I. (1987). Wilson's disease. In E. Braunwald, K. Isselbacher, R. Petersdorf, J., Wilson, J. Martin, & A. Fauci (Eds.), *Principles of internal medicine* (pp. 1636–1638). New York: McGraw-Hill.

Schlote, B., Nowotny, B., Schaaf, L., Kleinbohl, D., Schmidt, R., Teuber, J., Paschke, R., Vardarli, I., Kaumeier, S., & Usadel, K. (1992). Subclinical hyperthyroidism: Physical and mental state of patients. *European Archives of Psychiatry and Clinical Neuroscience, 241,* 357–364.

Schomerus, H., Hamster, W., Blunch, H., Reinhard, U., Mayer, K., & Dolle, W. (1981). Latent portasystemic encephalopathy: Nature of cerebral functional defects and their effect on fitness to drive. *Digestive Diseases and Sciences, 26,* 622–630.

Schultz, N., Elias, M., Robbins, M., Streeten, D., & Blakeman, N. (1986). A longitudinal study of hypertensives on the Wechsler Adult Intelligence Scale: Initial findings. *Journal of Gerontology, 41,* 169–175.

Schwartz, G., & Weiss, S. (1977). What is behavioral medicine? *Psychosomatic Medicine, 36,* 377–381.

Selnes, O., Miller, E., McArthur, J., Gordon, B., Munaz, A., Sheridan, K., Fox, R., Saah, A., & Multicenter AIDS Cohort Study. (1990). HIV infection: No evidence of cognitive decline during asymptomatic stages. *Neurology, 40,* 204–208.

Shapiro, A., Miller, R., King, H., Ginchereau, E., & Fitzgibbon, K. (1982). Behavioral consequences of mild hypertension. *Hypertension, 4,* 355–360.

Silberberg, E., & Lubera, J. (1989). Cancer statistics, 1989. *Ca-A Cancer Journal for Clinicians, 39,* 3–20.

Skenazy, J., & Bigler, E. (1984). Neuropsychological findings in diabetes mellitus. *Journal of Clinical Psychology, 40,* 246–258.

Smith, B., & Winslow, E. (1990). Cognitive changes in chronic renal patients during hemodialysis. *ANNA Journal, 17,* 283–287.

Sonies, B., Klippel, J., Gerber, R., & Gerber, L. (1982). Cognitive performance in systemic lupus erythematosus. *Arthritis and Rheumatism, 25*(Suppl.), S80.

Souheaver, G., Ryan, J., & DeWolfe, A. (1982). Neuropsychological patterns in uremia. *Journal of Clinical Psychology, 38,* 490–496.

Spiegel, D., Bloom, J., Kraemer, H., & Gottheil, E. (1989, October 14). Effect of psychosocial treatment on survival of patients with metastatic breast cancer. *Lancet,* pp. 888–891.

Spreen, O., & Strauss, E. (1991). *A compendium of neuropsychological tests.* New York: Oxford University Press.

Stefansson, K., & Aranson, B. (1987). Neurologic manifestations of systemic neoplasia. In E. Braunwald, K. Isselbacher, R. Petersdorf, J. Wilson, J. Martin, & A. Fauci (Eds.), *Principles of internal medicine* (pp. 1600–1604). New York: McGraw-Hill.

Tarter, R., Arria, A., Carra, J., & Van Thiel, D. (1987). Memory impairments concomitant with nonalcoholic cirrhosis. *International Journal of Neuroscience, 32,* 853–859.

Tarter, R., Carra, J., Switala, J., & Van Thiel, D. (1987). Sequential concept formation capacity in subclinical (latent) portal-systemic encephalopathy. *International Journal of Neuroscience, 32,* 891–894.

Tarter, R., Edwards, K., & Van Thiel, D. (1988). Neuropsychological dysfunction due to liver disease. In R. Tarter, D. Van. Thiel, & K. Edwards (Eds.), *Medical neuropsychology* (pp. 75–97). New York: Plenum.

Tarter, R., Hegedus, A., Van Thiel, D., Edwards, N., & Schade, R. (1987). Neurobehavioral correlates of cholestatic and hepatocellular disease: Differentiation according to disease specific characteristics and severity of the identified cerebral dysfunction. *International Journal of Neuroscience, 32,* 901–910.

Tarter, R., Hegedus, A., Van Thiel, D., Schade, R., Gavaler, J., & Starzl, T. (1984). Non-alcoholic cirrhosis associated with neuropsychological dysfunction in the absence of overt evidence of hepatic encephalopathy. *Gastroenterology, 86,* 1421–1427.

Tarter, R., Switala, J., Arria, A., Plail, J., & Van Thiel, D. (1990). Subclinical hepatic encephalopathy: Comparison before and after orthotopic liver transplantation. *Transplantation, 50,* 632–637.

Teschan, P., Ginn, H., Bourne, J., Ward, J., Hamel, B., Nunnally, J., Musso, M., & Vaughn, W. (1979). Quantitative indices of clinical uremia. *Kidney International, 15,* 676–697.

Trzepacz, P., McCue, M., Klein, I., Greenhouse, J., & Levey, G. (1988). Psychiatric and neuropsychological response to propranolol in Graves' disease. *Biological Psychiatry, 23,* 678–688.

Trzepacz, P., McCue, M., Klein, I., Levey, G., & Greenhouse, J. (1988). A psychiatric and neuropsychological study of patients with untreated Graves' disease. *General Hospital Psychiatry, 10,* 49–55.

Tucker, D., Penland, J., Beckwith, B., & Saustead, H. (1984). Thyroid function in normals: Influences on the electroencephalogram and cognitive performance. *Psychophysiology, 22,* 72–78.

Tucker, J., Prior, P., Green, C., Ede, G., Stevenson, J., Gawler, J., Jamal, G., Charlesworth, M., Thakkar, C., Patel, P., & Lister, T. (1989). Minimal neuropsychological sequelae following prophylactic treatment of the central nervous system in adult leukemia and lymphoma. *Cancer, 60,* 775–780.

U'Ren, K., Riddle, M., Lezak, M., & Bennington-Davis, M. (1990). The mental efficiency of the elderly person with Type 2 diabetes mellitus. *Journal of the American Geriatric Society, 38,* 505–510.

van Dam, A., Wekking, E., & Oomen, H. (1991). Psychiatric symptoms as features of systemic lupus erythematosus. *Psychotherapy and Psychosomatics, 55,* 132–140.

Van Gorp, W., Miller, E., Satz, P., & Visscher, B. (1989). Neuropsychological performance in HIV-1 immunocompromised patients: A preliminary report. *Journal of Clinical and Experimental Neuropsychology, 11,* 763–773.

Victor, M., & Martin, J. B. (1987). Nutritional and metabolic diseases of the nervous system. In E. Braunwald, K. Isselbacher, R. Petersdorf, J. Wilson, J. Martin, & A. Fauci (Eds.), *Principles of internal medicine* (pp. 2000–2011). New York: McGraw-Hill.

Waldstein, S., Ryan, C., Manuck, S., Parkinson, D., & Bromet, E. (1991). Learning and memory function in men with untreated blood pressure elevation. *Journal of Consulting and Clinical Psychology, 59,* 513–517.

Wallace, J., MacCrimmon, D., & Goldberg, W. (1980). Acute hyperthyroidism: Cognitive and emotional correlates. *Journal of Abnormal Psychology, 89,* 519–527.

Weissenborn, K., Scholz, M., Hinrichs, H., Wiltfang, J., Schmidt, F., & Kunkel, H. (1990). Neuropsychological assessment of early hepatic encephalopathy. *Electroencephalography and Clinical Neurophysiology, 75,* 289–295.

Whybrow, P., & Ferrell, R. (1974). Thyroid state and human behavior: Contributions from a clinical perspective. In A. J. Prange (Ed.), *The thyroid axis, drugs, and behavior* (pp. 5–28). New York: Raven Press.

Widom, B., & Simonson, D. (1990). Glycemic control and neuropsychologic function during hypoglycemia in patients with insulin dependent diabetes mellitus. *Annals of Internal Medicine, 112,* 904–912.

Wilkie, F., Eisdorfer, C., Morgan, R., Loewenstein, D., & Szapocznik, J. (1990). Cognition in early human immunodeficiency virus infection. *Archives of Neurology, 47,* 433–440.

Wolcott, D., Marsh, J., LaRue, A., Carr, C., & Nissenson, A. (1989). Recombinant human erythropoietin treatment may improve quality of life and cognitive function in chronic hemodialysis patients. *Journal of Kidney Diseases, 14,* 478–485.

Wolcott, D., Wellisch, D., Marsh, J., Schaeffer, J., Landsverk, J., & Nissenson, A. (1988). Relationship of dialysis modality and other factors to cognitive function in chronic dialysis patients. *American Journal of Kidney Diseases, 12,* 275–284.

Wredling, R., Levander, S., Adamson, V., & Lins, P. (1990). Permanent neuropsychological impairment after recurrent episodes of severe hypoglycemia in men. *Diabetologia, 33,* 152–157.

Zeitlhofer, J., Saletu, B., Stary, J., & Ahmadi, R. (1984). Cerebral function in hyperthyroid patients. *Neuropsychobiology, 11,* 89–93.

Ziesat, H., Logue, P., & McCarty, S. (1980). Psychological measurement of memory deficits in dialysis patients. *Perceptual and Motor Skills, 50,* 311–318.

Appendix

Commonly Used Neuropsychological Tests

Abbreviation	Test name	Description
	General Intellectual Ability	
WBI	Wechsler Bellevue Intelligence Scale	Most commonly used neuropsychological test, consisting of 11 subtests yielding summary scores of Verbal, Performance, and Full Scale IQ
WAIS	Wechsler Adult Intelligence Scale	
WAIS-R	Wechsler Adult Intelligence Scale–Revised	
SILS	Shipley Institute for Living Scale	Paper-and-pencil test consisting of vocabulary and verbal abstraction subtests
PPVT	Peabody Picture Vocabulary Test	Multiple-choice test of receptive vocabulary
NART	New Adult Reading Test	Oral reading test used to assess premorbid intellectual level
	Memory and Learning	
WMS	Wechsler Memory Scale	Tests assessing orientation, attention, and verbal and nonverbal recent memory; Russell revision incorporates delayed recall trials on WMS; WMS-R is updated version
WMS-R	Wechsler Memory Scale–Revised	
BVRT	Benton Visual Retention Test	Test evaluating immediate visual recall of geometric figures

Appendix continues

Appendix (contd.)

Abbreviation	Test name	Description
	Memory and Learning *(contd.)*	
DS	Digit Supraspan	Test evaluating number of trials needed to learn a string of numbers
SDLT	Symbol Digit Learning Test	Test requiring learning and retention of symbol and digit associations
RMT	Recognition Memory Test	Memory test evaluating recognition memory for words and unfamiliar faces
RAVLT	Rey Auditory Verbal Learning Test	Word list learning task with five learning trials and delayed recall following interference
	Reasoning and Conceptualization	
RPM	Raven's Progressive Matrices	Multiple-choice visual pattern matching and analogy test with three versions of increasing difficulty: Colored, Standard, and Advanced
HCT	Halstead Category Test	Nonverbal test of deductive reasoning and concept formation
WCST	Wisconsin Card Sorting Test	Nonverbal card-sorting task requiring deductive reasoning, concept formation, and set switching
GPT	Gorham Proverbs Test	Test involving interpretation of proverbs
	Language	
COWA	Controlled Oral Word Association Test	Test requiring production of as many words as possible in 60 seconds beginning with a letter of the alphabet

Abbreviation	Test name	Description
	Language *(contd.)*	
BN	Boston Naming Test	Task of confrontation naming
TT	Token Test	Test of receptive language requiring execution of increasingly complex commands
	Visuospatial and Constructional	
RCF	Rey-Osterrieth Complex Figure	Test that entails copying a complex geometric figure; recall trial or trials may be included
	Motor	
PP	Purdue Pegboard	Measure involving placement of pegs into holes with left, right, and then both hands
GP	Grooved Pegboard	Measure evaluating placement of pegs with ridges into slotted holes
FTT	Finger Tapping Test	Timed assessment of index finger tapping speed
TPT	Tactual Performance Test	Test requiring placement of 10 variously shaped blocks into a form board while blindfolded; recall of shape and location is assessed
RT	Reaction Time	Test assessing response speed to stimuli that may be either simple or complex
	Attention and Concentration	
TMT	Trail Making Test	Paper-and-pencil task involving connecting dots containing seqeuntially ordered stimuli

Appendix (contd.)

Abbreviation	Test name	Description
	Attention and Concentration *(contd.)*	
SSPT	Speech Sounds Perception Test	Paced and lengthy phoneme-discrimination task
SRT	Seashore Rhythm Test	Paced and lengthy rhythm-pattern discrimination task
SCWT	Stroop Color and Word Test	Test evaluating the ability to shift perceptual set to conform to changing stimulus demands
SDMT	Symbol Digit Modalities Test	Measure similar to WAIS-R Digit Symbol subtest
DL	Dichotic Listening	Test involving perception and recall of simultaneously presented words
	Batteries	
HRB	Halstead Reitan Battery	Battery of five core tests (TPT, SSPT, SRT, HCT, FTT) yielding seven scores: An impairment index equal to the proportion of scores below a cutoff is calculated.
LNNB	Luria-Nebraska Neuropsychological Battery	Battery of 11 subtests measuring a wide range of neuropsychological functions
APTS	Automated Psychological Test System	Computerized neuropsychological battery developed in Scandinavia
LRNTB	Lafayette Repeatable Neuropsychological Test Battery	Brief battery with alternative forms developed for repeatable assessment, portions of which are taken from the HRB

Chapter

5

Ethnocultural Influences in Evaluation and Management

Kathleen Young and Nolan Zane

Increasing ethnic and cultural diversity in the United States creates a challenge for researchers and practitioners alike. From 1980 to 1990—in contrast to the non-Hispanic White population's growth of 6%—the African American population grew 13.2%, to nearly 30 million; the Asian American population doubled to 7.3 million; the Latino American population grew 53% to 22.4 million; and the American Indian, Inuit, or Aleut population grew 38% to nearly 2 million (U.S. Bureau of the Census, 1991). In some cases, much of the growth of ethnic populations can be attributed to high rates of immigration into the United States (O'Hare & Felt, 1991). As such, non-White ethnic

The preparation of this chapter was supported in part by Grant R01-MH44331 from the National Research Center on Asian American Mental Health.

groups make up almost 25% of the population of the United States. Although the ethnic diversity varies by region—nearly 43% of the population of California, as opposed to 2% of the population of Maine, consists of non-White ethnic groups—there is clearly a demographic trend toward ethnic diversity in this country. It is both a challenge to and the responsibility of researchers and practitioners to acknowledge and incorporate this diversity into research and practice.

Ethnocultural and sociocultural factors have consistently been implicated in illness behavior. As Mechanic (1978) noted, illness behavior involves processes by which people monitor their bodies, recognize and interpret symptoms, respond to reduce the perceived distress or dysfunction, and seek help from professional health care providers or indigenous healers. Given that illness is a subjective experience in which discontinuities of an intrapersonal and social nature are attended to, processed, and acted on (Barondess, 1979), it is important to consider the specific cultural context that defines the parameters of these experiences. This is especially salient when one is considering chronic illness behavior and processes. Blackwell and Gutmann (1986) have conceptualized chronic illness as a syndrome with the following features: development of disability that is disproportionate to the detectable disease, search for disease validation, appeal for physician responsibility, development of attitudes of personal vulnerability and entitlement, avoidance of health roles and adoption of sick roles, and use of interpersonal behaviors to maintain sick roles. It is evident that many of these behaviors and attitudes can be differentially developed and reinforced depending on the specific sociocultural context in which they occur. Despite this recognition of culture as an important influence on illness, there still remains a great need for more informative research and theory on how culture shapes and defines illness experiences. Moreover, health psychology continues to be challenged by the issue of how to effectively address cultural issues in health care interventions. Our purpose in this chapter is thus (a) to review research and theory on how cultural variables affect the process and phenomenology of chronic illness behavior, (b) to propose a model for reconceptualizing ethnocultural factors with respect to illness behavior, and (c) to discuss implications of developing more culturally responsive health interventions in caring for chronically ill people from culturally diverse backgrounds.

Problems of Definition: Race, Ethnicity, Culture, and Social Class

Researchers and practitioners have not always agreed on means by which the impact of culture ought to be considered. One of the problems has been that of definition (see Betancourt & Lopez, 1993, for an excellent discussion of this issue). *Race, ethnicity,* and *culture* are frequently, but often erroneously, used interchangeably, because of less than clear definitions and actual variations in usage by different authors (see, e.g., Draguns, 1989; McGoldrick, 1982; Root, 1992; Shweder, 1990). Because of the lack of agreement in defining these terms, we begin with a brief outline of how these terms have been used and how they are used in this chapter. *Race* has usually been conceived of as a biological category, in which certain biological traits, such as skin color, are passed on from one generation to another through heredity; yet race is undoubtedly a social construction as well (see Spickard, 1992). *Ethnicity* may pertain to race, but it has also been used to designate those who share a common culture or nationality. Definitions of *culture* are too numerous to detail, but for the purposes of this chapter, culture will entail (but is not limited to) socially shared and negotiated beliefs and practices that are transmitted from one generation to the next. Thus, race, ethnicity, and culture may or may not overlap. This is especially important in regard to immigrant ethnic groups; for these, acculturation and generational status may be better predictors of behaviors than ethnicity alone. It is important for researchers or practitioners to avoid treating individuals of a particular ethnic or cultural group as if they all have had the same background and to determine the extent to which an individual is similar, or different from, a particular group.

Other variables frequently confounded with race, ethnicity, or culture relate to socioeconomic status (SES). Yet, because of the history of racial discrimination, or unequal opportunities for ethnic groups in the United States and other countries, low SES is associated in some groups with ethnic group status. It is thus not always easy to separate the influences of SES from the influences of culture (see, e.g., Betancourt & Lopez, 1993). To avoid misattributing to ethnicity those effects that may actually be caused by low SES, researchers must control for such factors as income, occupational status, and educational level.

Conceptual Framework for Examining Cultural Influences on Illness

The theoretical and practical importance of examining cultural variables has long been recognized (e.g., Fabrega, 1974; Kleinman, 1980; Mechanic, 1986). What has been more challenging is the development of theoretical approaches that clearly articulate and frame the specific processes by which cultural variables affect the phenomenology of illness. There have been many discipline-specific attempts to investigate the impact of cultural factors on illness. Notable among these have been qualitative anthropological research projects, investigations into social epidemiology, and studies of psychological factors that influence the illness process (see, e.g., Hugh & Vallis, 1986). More recently, there has been research investigating ethnic variation in physiological processes and vulnerabilities (e.g., K. M. Lin, Poland, & Nagasaki, 1993). Exhibit 1 shows a categorical, domain-specific arrangement of the biological, cognitive, linguistic, psychological–emotional, and social factors that psychologists should consider when working with ethnically and culturally diverse patients. Because of discipline-specific investigations, and because there have been few integrative theoretical frameworks to guide this research, the empirical work examining cultural influences on illness often has appeared fragmented and nonprogrammatic.

In one of the more promising and comprehensive efforts toward better articulating the impact of cultural variables, Angel and Thoits (1987) have proposed a process-oriented model of how cultural influences affect illness labeling, symptom evaluation, and help seeking. The model focuses on cognitive processes and schemas that mediate the illness experience. Culture is hypothesized to influence four major processes with respect to illness: (a) attentional processes in response to physical or emotional change, (b) interpretation of the change, (c) acting on symptoms, and (d) relabeling and reevaluation.

Although it is quite informative, Angel and Thoits's (1987) model appears to have several features that require greater elaboration or modification. First, how individuals interpret the importance or significance of a particular state can be greatly affected by the social feedback that they receive about these experiences. The evaluation or appraisal is also affected by the amount of social resources that people perceive they have. Both of these processes involve social supports.

Exhibit 1

Considerations in Working With Ethnically and Culturally Diverse Patients

Biological

- Ethnic differences in physiology (e.g., lactose intolerance)
- Drug metabolism and efficacy differences due to physiological differences
- Drug metabolism and efficacy differences due to differences in dietary practices

Cognitive

- Attentional focus (inward or outward)
- Outcome and self-efficacy expectations
- Health schemas surrounding the believed causes of illness (e.g., natural or supernatural or individual or extraindividual), norms for symptom expression, and help seeking

Linguistic

- Competence in expression and comprehension of language used during medical visit
- Cultural idioms of distress

Psychological–Emotional

- Use of psychological dimension (e.g., mind–body dualism or psychophysical holism)
- Cultural patterns of emotional expression, self-disclosure
- Culturally preferred presentation of discontinuity (physical or emotional)
- Ego-focused versus other-focused emotions

Social

- Familial-social support network as a resource
- Social input, feedback, and social comparisons
- Interdependent versus independent social structure
- Culturally sanctioned pathways to care and preferred treatments
- Alternative indigenous health networks
- Accessibility of health care (cost, insurance, and language)

As such, the inclusion or focus on social supports as an important cultural influence on the interpretation process appears warranted. Second, outcome and self-efficacy expectations have been identified as important cognitive variables in help-seeking and coping behaviors.

Moreover, cultural norms in help-seeking and coping preferences would be expected to influence these expectations. Identifying the role of these two types of expectancies may facilitate the articulation of cultural effects on the coping and help-seeking processes.

Third, the model's emphasis on cognitive structures and decision making implies a linear, rational set of processes that are affected by cultural factors. However, health attitudes and actions often have not been adequately captured by rational, decision-making models of behavior. What appears to be lacking is an idea of the overall process by which these four types of experiences are interrelated in terms of a person's functioning. The model emphasizes how individuals perceive and assess discrepancies in their experience and then act to reduce these discrepancies. Carver and Scheier (1981) described these processes as reflecting the self-regulatory functions of human behavior. Thus, perhaps the processes reflected within this model can be conceptualized as self-regulatory functions in which an individual's culture can affect a number of processes or states—namely, the four previously mentioned. In this way, one can use self-regulation theory to make certain predictions about how ethnocultural variables may influence health behaviors and responses.

Finally, and perhaps most important, is that focusing on cognitive factors, despite clarifying certain intrapsychic processes, leaves out a significant part of the literature on cultural variables: the anthropological, sociological, and biological research. In this chapter, we attempt to integrate the many perspectives provided by these different disciplines. Table 1 shows Angel and Thoits's (1987) model as we have revised it to highlight the previously mentioned cultural variables and the self-regulatory process in health behaviors. It should be noted that the ethnocultural factors mentioned are not meant to represent a complete list of all of the possible ethnocultural factors that may affect the illness experience. The factors listed were chosen, in some cases, for their usefulness in illustrating the model. Moreover, there may be wide variability in the empirical bases among the factors that appear in the table, especially because there are differences in the methods and histories of the disciplines from which these factors have emerged. Furthermore, although we recognize that several of the more global factors, such as health schemas, may affect the illness experience at several different stages outlined in the model, for the purposes of clarity we have categorized the ethnocultural factors according to the domain in which we believed they would have the most impact.

Table 1

Ethnocultural Influences on the Illness Process

State or process	Ethnocultural factor
Vulnerability to becoming ill	physiological responsivity genetics diet exposure to stressful life events exposure to disease agents
Attention to state of discontinuity	self-monitoring emotional sensitivity cognitive filtering
Interpretation of state of discontinuity	health schemas and explanatory models symptom experience culture-bound syndromes symptom differences
Response to illness state	personal coping symptom presentation and stigma help seeking social support and networks health care resources mainstream health services alternative or indigenous practices
Response to health care intervention	working relationship between the patient and care provider cultural incongruities in the process of treatment problem conceptualization modes of care and treatment treatment goals drug metabolism bicultural functioning
Relabeling and reevaluation	social feedback functional criteria

Note. From "The Impact of Culture on the Cognitive Structure of Illness," by R. Angel and P. Thoits, 1987, *Culture, Medicine, and Psychiatry, 11*, p. 474. Copyright 1987 by Kluwer Academic Publishers. Adapted with permission.

Essentially, the model hypothesizes how culture affects different aspects of the illness experience. First, culture can influence a person's vulnerability to illness. An increasing number of studies (e.g., Myers, 1993) have documented ethnic differences in people's physiological responsivity to stress and other environmental stimuli. These differences in physiological responsivity may significantly affect an individual's propensity to become ill. Other research (e.g., Harburg et al., 1973) has found that certain ethnocultural groups may be exposed to stressful life events and disease agents at a higher rate than others. It is thus important to add an earlier stage in the illness process to Angel and Thoits's (1987) model to represent such important pre-illness variables as genetics, physiological responses, and exposure to factors in the environment that can increase an individual's vulnerability to become ill.

The next step in the process of the illness experience involves attention to or recognition by the individual that something has changed in either an emotional or physical manner. Essentially, the individual experiences a state of discontinuity (L. Eisenberg, 1977). The attentional processes that determine how this information is processed can be influenced by the manner in which people are socialized in their particular culture to monitor their bodily and emotional states. For example, Tanaka-Matsumi and Marsella (1976) found that, in a word association study, Japanese Nationals associated more external referent and somatic terms to the word *depression* and White Americans associated terms that referred to internal mood states.

Once a state of discontinuity is experienced, this experience must be evaluated and interpreted to determine whether it constitutes a symptom or sign of an impending disorder. As Angel and Thoits (1987) noted, once something is recognized as a symptom, other evaluations follow concerning the seriousness, cause, responsibility, and prognosis of the disease. A person's culture affects this interpretation process in at least two ways. First, the judgments made about symptoms and the underlying disorder rely greatly on health and illness schemas and the beliefs that a culture emphasizes (Kleinman, 1980). For example, Kinzie (1985) noted that many Southeast Asians have a folk tradition in which illness is believed to be caused by physiological factors or supernatural forces (e.g., the consequence of offending a deity or spirit). Such people may be less likely to differentiate between psychological, physiological, and supernatural causes of illness. Second, these judgments often are made on the basis of feedback from others within the same sociocultural group. In other words, the interpretation of a symptom or an evaluation of an impending disease frequently incorporates social input and social comparisons. Cultural norms and attitudes concerning symptom expression, the amount of distress to be tolerated, the relative frequency that the symptom has been experienced by others, and so on, significantly affect how individuals interpret their symptoms and understand the presumed underlying disease.

These interpretations can induce individuals to respond to the identified illness, which can include pursuing a course of action to reduce symptoms and remediate the underlying disease. At this stage in the process of the illness experience, personal coping and help-seeking efforts come into play. Individuals use a variety of strategies depending on their evaluations of symptoms, perceived resources, perceived barriers to these resources, self-efficacy in self-help, and the personal response costs associated with each of these alternatives. The help-seeking process has probably received the most attention in the research conducted on culture and health (e.g., T. Lin, Tardiff, Donetz, & Goresky, 1978; H. Neighbors, 1985; Rogler, Malgady, & Rodriguez, 1989). For example, Asian Americans have been found to differ from White Americans in help-seeking behaviors for emotional difficulties. They are less likely to request outside help for these difficulties, turning first to their families for help and then to outside agencies or mainstream services as a last resort (Tracey, Leong, & Glidden, 1986). Indigenous health care and support systems as well as the formal medical system become involved in this help-seeking process. However, it is important to note that these systems may not be mutually exclusive or even conflictual in terms of providing competing sources of care or help. In fact, Hoang and Erickson (1985) have observed how one system of care can be used for one health care problem, whereas the other system may be used for another problem.

Once a source of help has been identified and obtained, a variety of ethnocultural factors can affect an individual's response to the recommended treatment. On a physiological level, ethnic differences have been found in the metabolism of certain drugs; thus, the pharmacokinetic efficacy of drug treatments is an important consideration. Cultural differences in provider and patient roles, problem conceptualization, the desired health state, and the means by which health is to be obtained can all affect treatment compliance.

Throughout this process, individuals reappraise their situations on the basis of their experiences with care providers and with others in their communities. The process of reevaluation is similar to the appraisal process, except it is additionally affected by the experiences garnered in the previous stages. For example, an illness interpretation or intervention might increase self-monitoring, which, in turn, is likely to affect the processes of relabeling and reevaluation. Influences from the mainstream medical health care system and those from the patient's community support system, which can include indigenous health care practices, largely determine how a person reassesses his or her medical outcomes. This interaction between the former and latter constitutes an important process that has seldom received empirical attention.

Vulnerability to Illness

Physiological Responsivity and Genetics

Although most of this chapter is focused on ethnocultural factors, advances in the study of ethnic variation in biological processes should be noted, because biological differences may underlie ethnic differences both in the occurrence rates of certain diseases and in physiological responsivity (in terms of drug response and reactivity to other environmental stimuli) for a particular group. Although at this time biopsychosocial research has not revealed the complex interconnections between physiological, psychological, and social constructs, we provide a brief discussion of the trends in cross-ethnic biological research for the practitioner to consider, with hopes that future research can integrate the different levels of analysis.

Cross-cultural epidemiological studies have found ethnic differences in the mortality rates, incidence, and prevalence of many diseases. One such recent study in Los Angeles found that the mortality rates of African Americans, Euro-Americans, and Hispanic Americans were more than twice that of Asian Americans (Frerichs, Chapman, & Maes, 1984). Other research has revealed ethnically linked genetic disorders, such as sickle-cell anemia, in those whose ancestors originated in sub-Saharan Africa; Tay-Sachs disease in Ashkenazi Jews; and cystic fibrosis in American Pueblo Indians. Even many of the more common diseases such as hypertension, heart disease, and cancer have been found to manifest cross-ethnic variation (Cruikshank & Beevers, 1989; K. M. Lin, Poland, & Nagasaki, 1993; Polednak, 1989).

Newly articulated biopsychosocial models are currently being developed to formulate and clarify the relationship between biological and psychosocial factors in autonomic reactivity among African Americans (N. B. Anderson, 1989; N. B. Anderson, McNeilly, & Myers, 1991). Epidemiological studies have found that African Americans are at higher risk for hypertension than Euro-Americans. Biologically oriented research on the pathophysiology of hypertension in African Americans has suggested that ethnic differences in cardiovascular and neuroendocrine reactivity to stress and in sodium retention and excretion may form the biological vulnerability underlying the incidence and prevalence of hypertension among African Americans (Myers, 1993). Evolutionary hypotheses have been proposed that suggest that—at another time and in a different environment—sodium retention may have been adaptive where salt was scarce, such as in West Africa (Grim & Wilson, 1989; Jackson, 1991). At the same time, other researchers have been investigating possible psychosocial factors for hypertension in African Americans, such as lower socioeconomic status and membership in an oppressed minority group, in addition to such sociocultural factors as having diets high in salt and fat. Thus, advances in different disciplines are converging on the same phenomena. It is hoped that biopsychosocial models can integrate these different levels of analysis by clarifying the points at which they intersect.

Diet

One's vulnerability to illness may be affected by one's nutritional consumption. Just as culture influences dietary practices, it can affect nutritional status. Although ethnocultural influences are most obvious from well-articulated food taboos, such as the Islamic and Jewish prohibitions of eating pork, or the Hindu prohibition of eating beef, cultures do also shape dietary preferences. For example, the condiments that Asians consume in a traditional diet—such as soy sauce, fish sauces, bean sauces, dried salted fish, and pickled vegetables—tend to be extremely high in sodium (Chew, 1983). Likewise, many people in the United States consume diets high in sugar, animal fat, salt, and processed foods. These cultural preferences for particular foods often affect nutritional status and increased risk for some diseases.

Exposure to Stressful Life Events

Individuals from certain ethnic minority groups may be more vulnerable to illness because they have a history of exposure to the stress associated with war (e.g., refugees), anti-ethnic violence, racism, or cultural adjustment. Medical practitioners are often unaware of the health-risk status of many Southeast Asian refugees. Community and clinical studies have indicated, however, that many Southeast Asian refugees experience serious and prolonged trauma as a result of mass exodus from their homeland (Meinhardt, Tom, Tse, & Yu, 1986; Mollica, Wyshak, & Lavelle, 1987). Empirical investigations over the past decade have consistently shown that Southeast Asian refugees, having endured extreme hardships—such as war, torture, and the death of loved ones—are particularly at high risk for developing posttraumatic stress disorder (Kinzie et al., 1990; Kroll et al., 1989). Posttraumatic stress is especially chronic and debilitating for Southeast Asians because many refugees reexperience the traumatic events and persistently engage in attempts to deny or avoid the trauma.

It should be noted that differential exposure to stress among ethnocultural groups is not limited to traumatic experiences. Ethnic minority individuals may also become more vulnerable to illness because they experience higher levels of chronic stress associated with daily hassles (Rowlison & Felner, 1988) and such ordeals as communicating in a nonnative language (e.g., English); coping with discrimination and prejudice; and adjusting to new cultural lifestyles, vocations, and gender roles.

Exposure to Disease Agents

The relationship between health and socioeconomic status has been well documented (Dutton, 1986; Marmot, Kogevinas, & Elston, 1987). Individuals in lower socioeconomic classes have significantly higher rates of both morbidity and mortality when compared with upper-class individuals (Marmot et al., 1987). Low SES is associated with many health-risk problems, such as high levels of stress, unsafe occupations (entailing exposure to hazardous chemicals or conditions; Palinkas, 1987), obesity, alcohol consumption, and smoking (Marmot et al., 1987). Because in some groups low SES is associated with ethnicity, it is important to attempt to delineate (if possible) ethnocultural and socioeconomic status effects. Recent studies (e.g., Healy, 1994) have shown that ethnic minority communities in the United States, even those that are not of lower SES, bear a "disproportionate burden" of hazardous waste facilities and environmental pollutants, which is likely to increase their vulnerability to illness. Moreover, some minority communities that rely on fishing to supplement their diets may be inadvertently accumulating higher than recommended levels of harmful toxins (Healy, 1994).

As outlined at the beginning of this chapter, part of the increasing ethnic and cultural diversity in the United States is due to increased immigration. Immigrants may come from countries where certain diseases are more prevalent; thus, they and their communities may have an increased likelihood of exposure to disease agents or to being disease carriers. For example, the distribution of chronic carriers of the hepatitis-B virus differs globally: Seventy-five percent of disease carriers live in Asia (R. S. Hann, 1994). Chronic infection with the hepatitis-B virus may lead to hepatitis, hepatocellular carcinoma, and chronic liver disease. Studies have suggested that foreign-born Asian Americans are more likely to be carriers of hepatitis than American-born Asians (R. S. Hann, 1994). Similarly, immigrants from Third World countries may have had a higher exposure to infectious diseases, such as tuberculosis, cholera, or typhoid, or to such parasitic infestations as hookworm infestation, pinworms (enterobiasis), and malaria (R. S. Hann, 1994), and they may unwittingly expose others in their communities to disease. Thus, the health professional should keep in mind that in some immigrant ethnic communities individuals may have increased exposure to disease agents that may be uncommon in the general U.S.-born population.

Attention to State of Discontinuity

As outlined in the conceptual framework (Exhibit 1), one of the initial stages in the process of an illness experience is the individual's immediate reaction to an objective physiological change.[1] Even though

---

[1] At this point it is important to acknowledge that even the organization of this chapter and the provision for an "objective physiological change" reflects our own Western cultural health schema, which assumes that illness begins with a discrete physiological process rather than with an interpersonal or supernatural (or other) process.

a physiological change occurs, given the amount of sensory input that continuously presents itself to an individual, not all information can be attended to. There are, after all, individual differences in the awareness of bodily sensations (Miller, Murphy, & Buss, 1981). The information that an individual attends to depends in part on his or her cognitive "filters," which select input for attention not only on the basis of signal strength, but also on the basis of the familiarity—and thus meaningfulness—of the signal to the individual's cognitive schemas. Signals that are consistent with—and hence, familiar and meaningful to—an individual's existing cognitive schema are more likely to be attended to or to be processed more quickly than signals that are not consistent with existing schemas (McHugh & Vallis, 1986). These cognitive schemas are, in part, culturally determined because cultures create their own thresholds and criteria of what is to be considered (physiologically) relevant. (Such criteria are probably based on culture-specific health and illness belief systems, which might include taxonomies of symptom clusters.) Cultures may also differ in the socialization of people's attention to and the significance they ascribe to internal states (Angel & Thoits, 1987) or in the extent to which people direct attention to various types of sensations.

Ethnic differences in attentional processes, whether arising from biological factors or from cultural socialization of attention to bodily sensations, may influence the experience of emotion and vice versa. Emotional states often serve as "markers" to a person that a state of discontinuity exists. Some researchers have argued that differences in the expression of emotions result in differences in physiological reactivity. For example, Pennebaker (1985) has suggested that denying or suppressing emotions increases autonomic reactivity. Because cultures prescribe the normative expression of a variety of behaviors, it is not surprising that there is cultural variation in the construction and expression of emotion (Ekman, 1993; Kleinman & Kleinman, 1991; Lutz & White, 1986), and this variability may influence attentional processes. Cultural values may underlie differences in experienced emotions, or in the significance that individuals attribute to the experience of their emotions. Markus and Kitayama (1991) have argued that cultures that encourage independence foster ego-focused emotions such as anger and pride, whereas cultures that value interdependence foster such emotions as shame and sympathy that place others as the main focus. They suggested that these two cultural orientations (independence vs. interdependence) may result in differences in the emotional experience of the individual. For example, those from cultures valuing independence may experience the emotion of pride more often than those from "interdependent" cultures.

Interpreting the State of Discontinuity

Once the objective physiological change is recognized as a change from a previous state, an individual must evaluate this change within the context of his or her preexisting knowledge base. First, the importance or seriousness of the change is likely to be appraised; if the change is judged to be serious or to be a symptom of something serious, then this may impel the individual to take some kind of action. Culture influences this process because an individual obtains knowledge through his or her culture, and this culturally acquired knowledge is likely to be organized into health schemas.

Health Schemas and Explanatory Models

To make sense out of their illness experience, individuals often have what has been called "explanatory models" (Kleinman, 1980) of what is happening to them. Explanatory models may include an individual's ideas about the etiology, severity, course, outcome, and most effective treatment for his or her illness. An individual's particular explanatory model is embedded within a larger framework comprised of that individual's cognitive schema of health and illness. Schemas of health and illness may display significant cultural variation, such that although an individual from one culture may consider a particular objective physiological phenomenon as normal, an individual from another culture may consider that same phenomenon a symptom of a disease process. For example, Heggenhougen and Shore (1986) reported that many villagers in Malaysia believed that having intestinal worms was normal and that the absence of worms would indicate that something was wrong.

The assumptions embedded within the Western health schema are most obvious when they are contrasted with health schemas from other cultures. In a comparison of the Western health and illness schema with that of many other world cultures, Landrine and Klonoff (1992) suggested that in the Western schema, an illness is conceived of as a discrete event, even a "reified entity," experienced by an individual. The causes of the illness can be described as "natural," and would include genes, viruses, bacteria, or stress. By contrast, other cultures may conceive of an illness as extending beyond the individual—as an interpersonal process rather than something contained within one individual—and the causes of illness may be interpersonal or supernatural (such as punishment from the gods for social transgressions). For example, from the perspective of illness as an interpersonal process, the illness of one member of a family may be conceived as being caused by the moral transgressions of another family member. In some cultures, illnesses are commonly viewed as being caused by God or other supernatural entities. In a review of the culturally constructed theories of the causes of illness in nearly 200 cultures, Murdock (1980) found that most cultures endorse supernatural causes of illness and that only a few cultures consider illness to result from natural factors.

Cultural variation in health and illness schemas may amplify the usual discrepancies between the health schemas of a patient and his or her practitioner (Leventhal, Meyer, & Nerenz, 1980). For example, in one study comparing the health beliefs of Mexican Americans, mainstream nurse practitioners, and individuals representing the predominant American view about the cause and treatment of chest pain, Mexican Americans were found to have distinctly different, culture-specific beliefs (Kosko & Flaskerud, 1987). Mexican Americans' beliefs about the cause and preferred treatment of chest pain reflected a culture-specific health schema in which some illnesses are thought to result from an imbalance between the humors of the body (blood, phlegm, black bile, and yellow bile) in which treatments of "hot" and "cold" foods or medicines are thought to restore humoral balance (Foster, 1981). Mexican Americans were more likely to believe that chest pain resulted from a fright experience or as a punishment from God, whereas nurse practitioners and individuals from the predominant culture were more likely than Mexican Americans to believe that chest pain was a symptom of heart trouble. Furthermore, Mexican Americans were more likely to endorse taking hot liquids for chest pain and to consider good health a matter of luck (Kosko & Flaskerud, 1987). Thus, cultural schemas of health and illness may have a significant effect on the patient's interpretation of and the meaning given to an objective physiological change, and health schema differences can thereby affect practitioner–patient communication and understanding.

Symptom Experience

There are at least two aspects of symptomatology: (a) the patient's symptom experience and (b) his or her symptom presentation, through which the variety of the individual's symptom experience is selectively expressed. The individual's symptom experience is largely determined by both objective physiological problems and his or her preexisting health schemas. By comparison, symptom presentation is affected by such sociocultural factors as stigma and social role expectations, as well as by the help-seeking situations themselves. In the next section we focus on the symptom experience. The cultural factors affecting symptom presentation are discussed later.

Culture-bound syndromes. The anthropological literature provides many examples of what could be considered either cultural differences in symptom experience or culture-bound syndromes, depending on one's perspective. The problem for cross-cultural researchers and practitioners alike is to determine the meaning of cultural variation in symptom manifestation. One approach has been to assert that, despite cultural variation in the manifestation of symptoms, there are underlying disease processes that are universal. Examples of this approach would be the classification of culturally constellated symptoms into Western taxonomies, such as categorizing what is known as *amok* in Malaysia or the Philippines as a reactive psychosis with homicidal features (Kleinman, 1988) or *ataques de nervios* in the Latino community as acute dissociative responses, acute conversion symptoms, or acute schizophrenic turmoil (Guarnaccia, DeLaCancela, & Carrillo, 1989). Kleinman (1988) has labeled the imposition of one culture's diagnostic categories onto individuals in another culture a "category fallacy," although he maintains that certain psychiatric diagnoses, such as organic brain disorders and manic–depressive psychoses, are cross-culturally valid.

In contrast to the universalistic perspective, another approach maintains that the expression of culturally constellated symptomatology constitutes "an integral and patterned aspect of the emotional and cognitive experience of specific cultural groups" (Koss, 1990, p. 6). From this perspective, the practice of categorizing culturally varying symptom patterns into the taxonomies developed by one culture is also the imposition of a particular, culturally constituted value system over another such belief system. Because a gap between the two systems is likely, this process results in the loss of important, culturally unique aspects of a culture's illness experience.

Symptom differences. Researchers have suggested that socially constructed, internalized norms of behavior are important in symptom manifestation. For instance, social modeling has been found to influence physiological reactivity (Craig, 1987). In the seminal study of male patients hospitalized for back pain and spinal lesions in New York, Zborowski found differing cultural norms in the experience of pain (Zborowski, 1969, 1978): In comparison with White American men, Jewish and Italian men were very vocal in expressing their pain, whereas Irish men were stoic and tended to deny pain. Yet even though both Jewish and Italian men voiced their pain, they differed in that the Italian men wanted the pain to stop immediately, whereas Jewish men were most concerned about how the pain might affect their future. Although certain aspects of Zborowski's studies have been criticized, other studies have corroborated his main finding and have further elaborated the notion of ethnic variation in how pain is experienced. Different ethnic groups have been found to vary in their experiences of pain, in psychological distress in reaction to pain, and in the impact of pain on their daily functioning (see, e.g., Lipton & Marbach, 1984; Weisenberg, Kreindler, Schachat, & Werboff, 1975). It is likely that these differences are due to differing cultural expectations in the manifestation and management of pain: Some cultures may value and reinforce a stoicism in pain expression, whereas others may encourage or tolerate vocal complaints or expansive expressions of pain. As cultures provide guidelines of normative behavior for members, they also socialize particular patterns of behavior that will be perceived and attended to by members of the culture as illnesses. Thus, at the very least, culture-specific symptomatology is meaningful within that culture's context as a way of manifesting distress. In this case, it may be helpful for health care providers to inquire beyond patients' physical symptoms, to gain a better understanding of the cultural schema that underlies particular symptom patterns.

Response to Illness State

Given that there can be significant cultural variation in health and illness schemas, it is not surprising that culture may also influence patterns of personal coping, symptom presentation, and patterns of help seeking.

Personal Coping

Most people experience chronic illnesses and the symptoms associated with these illnesses as major stressful life events. Lazarus and Folkman (1984) distinguished between the two modes of personal coping: problem-focused and emotion-focused coping. The former refers to direct efforts by the individual to change the person–environment relationship so that the source of stress is modified or eliminated. In contrast, *emotion-focused coping* refers to responses by the individual that control or mitigate the emotional reactions often elicited by the stressor. The primary function of emotion-focused coping is to maintain emotional equilibrium, whereas the major function of problem-focused coping is to manage the stressor itself. Chronic illnesses are often perceived as threatening or harmful situations in which there are few opportunities for beneficial change. In these situations, Folkman and Lazarus (1980) have indicated, individuals tend to use emotion-focused modes of coping because they lack the ability to directly alter the situation. However, even within this general context of personal coping, research has suggested that sociocultural factors can influence the specific type of emotion-focused coping used. Castro and Miranda (1985) studied differences in response to stress among Mexican Americans and White Americans. Although the latter evinced a higher level of knowledge about the relationship between stress and illness, the former used more stress-reducing, emotion-focused efforts (in terms of time-out periods for relaxation) to reduce stress. The investigators noted that in Mexican American culture, relaxation is seen as an effective and adaptive way of coping with daily stress. Seagall and Wykle (1988) found that African American respondents of all ages reported using their religious faith as a common way of coping with the distress caused by certain stressors. Little empirical work has examined coping among Asian Americans, but Mau and Jepson (1990) have suggested that Asian Americans may cope differently with certain emotional problems in comparison with Whites because of ethnic differences in appraising problems. In their study, Asian Americans were less likely to perceive certain psychosocial difficulties as "problems" because of their greater acceptance of eccentric and deviant behaviors.

Symptom Presentation and Stigma

An important factor that is likely to influence how an individual acts on his or her symptoms is the negative value associated with a particular illness. *Stigma* is a social label that negatively transforms the way others view the individual (Goffman, 1963). Because illnesses are embedded within cultural belief systems that include the likely causes of the illness, some illnesses may carry particular kinds of stigma. For example, in some cultures, sexually transmitted diseases carry a stigma, perhaps because the disease is believed to result from immoral or socially undesirable behavior. The afflicted individual may be perceived as responsible for or deserving of the ailment, and social ostracism may result (Gruman & Sloan, 1983; Jones et al., 1984). Another factor affecting social rejection is the perceived threat that the illness poses to other people (Jones et al., 1984). Both the actual risk (e.g., with highly infectious diseases) and the culturally constructed fears of contamination or contagion surrounding particular diseases affect how other individuals will treat the sick person. In the United States, interventions ranging from temporary quarantine to enforced separation from the rest of society for life (e.g., such as in leper colonies) have been used for a variety of conditions because of cultural beliefs about the threat or contagiousness of particular diseases. Currently, the stigma associated with AIDS arises from both culturally based moral judgments and fears of contamination.

Because individuals are aware of the cultural schemas for some, particularly stigmatized, illnesses, the negative moral or physically threatening connotations associated with an illness and its attendant social impact are likely to influence their response to symptoms of a suspected illness. An individual may thus try to conceal symptoms from others (Jones et al., 1984) or to ignore or deny symptoms, because an acknowledgment of the symptoms may entail stigmatization by his or her social group. An individual may be less likely to consult with significant others about the symptoms and to seek professional care. Furthermore, because stigma can extend to members of an individual's family (Goffman, 1963), individuals may act not only to protect themselves but also to protect significant others from stigma. Alternatively, a person may seek help but present with symptoms that may not entail as much social stigma. For example, the stigma regarding mental illness has been socially constructed and maintained in many cultures, including that of dominant U.S. culture (Blackwell, 1967).

Individuals may present physical symptoms to a health care provider, rather than symptoms that would entail a mental illness, in order to seek help but, at the same time, avoid stigmatization.

Help Seeking

The experience of symptoms or expressed distress may or may not be related to help-seeking behavior. Simply because an individual expresses a significant amount of distress, it does not necessarily follow that he or she will take action to alleviate the symptoms, nor is it easy to predict what kind of action he or she will take. Given the variation in the ways that cultures conceptualize the causes of illnesses and constrain symptom expression, cultural variability in help seeking or culturally different approaches to treatment should not be surprising. Angel and Cleary (1984) found that even though less acculturated Mexican Americans reported more symptoms than non-Hispanic Whites, they were less likely to seek help for their reported symptoms. Whether an individual will ignore the symptoms, self-treat, self-medicate, or seek lay, indigenous, or mainstream medical advice can be more accurately understood by attending to his or her health schema. If an individual has a clearly articulated understanding of the presumed illness and a range of culturally shaped prescriptives of the appropriate actions to undertake, then he or she will likely act within the range of culturally provided alternatives.[2]

As discussed earlier, it is well known that there is ethnic variation in patterns of mainstream health care utilization. Sociocultural factors, including socioeconomic status (income, employment), education and literacy, health insurance status, immigration status, social networks and social support systems, and familiarity with the mainstream U.S. health care system affect the utilization of health care services (May-

[2] For example, in one culture, the culturally normative responses to certain symptoms may include staying home from work, lying in bed and resting, drinking lots of fluids, taking one's temperature, swallowing aspirin every 4 hours, and seeing a physician. An individual may choose among these as appropriate actions given the symptoms. However, actions appropriate in other cultures for the same symptoms—burning incense, meditating, praying, or going to see an herbalist—may not be within the range of an individual's schema; thus, it is not likely that these actions would be considered.

eno & Hirota, 1994). Further, as with most motivated behavior, within each group there are likely to be culturally sanctioned patterns of help-seeking and pathways to care for particular illnesses. In some cases, indigenous health care providers will be sought out prior to, or in addition to, mainstream care.

Social Support and Networks

There are cultural differences in the role family and significant others play in the interpretation of the patient's manifest symptoms, which in turn influence the initiation of help seeking or pathways to care. One study, which compared White, Chinese, and Native American psychiatric patients' pathways to mainstream psychiatric care found distinctly different help-seeking patterns between the ethnic groups (T. Lin et al., 1978). Individual White patients experienced symptoms, consulted with significant others to interpret their symptoms, reviewed and evaluated possible health or mental health care resources, and sought help among those resources, consistent with Mechanic's (1982) illness behavior model. In contrast, Native American patients were usually referred for psychiatric care by the criminal justice system or social service agencies, suggesting that psychiatric care was more imposed on, than sought by, the individual Native American patient. Chinese patients were rarely found to be referred by legal or social service agencies and were most often brought in for care by their families; however, once in the psychiatric system, Chinese patients were found to exhibit severe psychiatric symptoms, suggesting that the individual's family had attempted to manage his or her difficulties prior to seeking mainstream psychiatric care. Thus, in contrast with White patients' patterns of help seeking, Chinese patients' entry into mainstream psychiatric care would be considered delayed. However, if each patient were understood in terms of his or her cultural context—for individual decision making, familial care, court referrals, and other sociocultural constructs—then the impact of these cultural variables would clarify the reasons for the different help-seeking patterns.

Mainstream Health Services

The mainstream health care system in the United States is complex and sometimes expensive. Acquiring access to health care services, along with negotiating one's way through the system, can be a difficult process even for those who regularly use mainstream health care. Sociocultural factors have a large impact on mainstream health service use. As discussed earlier, some ethnic groups are overrepresented in the low SES strata. Numerous studies have documented the effect of socioeconomic factors on access to or use of mainstream health services. For example, low income, unemployment, lack of medical insurance, and low educational achievement have been shown to decrease the likelihood that an individual will have access to mainstream care (Chavez, 1984; Mayeno & Hirota, 1994). One study revealed that, even among individuals with identified chronic illnesses, a significant proportion of ethnic minorities and those with low income or lacking health insurance had not visited a physician that year (Freeman et al., 1987). Thus, it is not surprising that there are ethnic group differences in the use of mainstream health services.

For immigrants, language may be a barrier to effective access and use if the patient has only limited English proficiency and there are no translators available to facilitate communication between the care provider and the patient. Moreover, these patients may have concerns about their immigration status and may fear that use of the health care system may result in deportation. Such fears are based in fact: Immigrants can be denied U.S. residency if the Immigration and Naturalization Service judges them likely to become dependent on public assistance (Mayeno & Hirota, 1994).

Even though the barriers to health care for ethnic minorities and those of lower SES have long been recognized, and despite legislative mandates to provide linguistically accessible services, the majority of the mainstream health care system has taken only minimal steps to respond to these access needs. However, some programs have directly targeted ethnic minority or low SES individuals, providing translators; bilingual and bicultural staff; and community outreach, culturally competent, and culturally acceptable services. Given the current national health care reform and funding constraints, at this time it is unclear whether mainstream health care will continue to make accommodations for ethnically and culturally diverse people.

Alternative or Indigenous Health Care Practices

In the United States, a variety of alternative resources are available and coexist with mainstream health care systems. In some communities, culturally constituted care systems comprising indigenous folk healers—such as herbalists, acupuncturists, bone setters, *curanderas*, root doctors, *espiritistos*, shamans, *kahunas*, faith healers, psychic healers, and spiritual advisors—provide treatments consistent with a specific culture's particular health and illness schema (Fabrega, 1974; Freund & McGuire, 1991; Harwood, 1981). It should be emphasized that the use of indigenous healers varies, depending on an individual's exposure or access to these resources, availability and belief in a particular cultural health schema, and acculturation to traditional or mainstream health systems (Landrine & Klonoff, 1992). Furthermore, the use of indigenous healers may result from factors other than culturally based treatment preferences. Many researchers have noted a kind of medical pluralism in developing countries, because there may be great variability in the access to or availability of mainstream medical and indigenous health care (Heggenhougen & Shore, 1986; Leslie, 1977). Thus, recent immigrants may use indigenous healers not because of underlying cultural beliefs that these treatments are the most appropriate, but because they are the most accessible—in terms of availability, communication, geographic location, or cost—and because these factors were used to determine outside consultation in previous help-seeking attempts. It should also be noted that it is not solely members of ethnic and cultural minority groups who seek alternative health care. In a national telephone survey of English-speaking adults in the United States, Eisenberg and colleagues (D. M. Eisenberg et al., 1993) found that a third of the respondents admitted to using unconventional therapies.[3] These were generally used to supplement, rather than as a substitute for, mainstream medical care and were most often used for chronic conditions (D. M. Eisenberg et al., 1993).

[3] *Unconventional medicine* was defined by the researchers as medical interventions not usually taught at U.S. medical schools or available at U.S. hospitals. The unconventional therapies specified in the study included relaxation techniques, chiropractics, massage, imagery, spiritual healing, commercial weight-loss programs, lifestyle diets, herbal medicine, megavitamin therapy, self-help groups, energy healing, biofeedback, hypnosis, homeopathy, acupuncture, folk remedies, exercise, and prayer.

Response to Health Care Intervention

Patient–Care Provider Working Relationship

Even if a person can access services, cultural differences between the patient and care provider can create problems that can mitigate the effectiveness of treatment. A critical factor in determining how patients respond to health interventions is the type and quality of the relationship that develops between patients and their health care professionals. There is a growing appreciation of the fact that effective medical and health care practices result from the successful application of certain medical techniques and procedures and that this application must be conducted within the context of a successful working alliance. Research has consistently shown that cultural differences between patients and care providers can adversely affect treatment outcomes (e.g., Sue, Fujino, Hu, Takeuchi, & Zane, 1991; Sue & Zane, 1987; Zane & Sue, 1991). Lack of a good working relationship because of cultural differences between patients and care providers can lead to numerous problems that can mitigate treatment efficacy. Some of these include (a) limited self-disclosure by the patient, which impedes adequate assessment and diagnosis; (b) cultural biases of the care provider that complicate assessment, diagnosis, and treatment planning; (c) treatment compliance difficulties that truncate the impact of treatment; and (d) inappropriate use of interpreters and translators by health care personnel that creates confusion in role relationships and complicates assessment and treatment. Of these, it appears that assessment and treatment compliance can be most dramatically affected by cultural incongruities between the patient and care provider.

Assessment. Prior to and while establishing a working relationship with a client, the care provider must evaluate the client to make treatment decisions. In the case of psychiatric diagnosis in particular, clinician bias during the assessment process has been the subject of debate and numerous investigations (for reviews, see Abramowitz & Murray, 1983; H. W. Neighbors, Jackson, Campbell, & Williams, 1989; Sattler, 1977). For example, many studies have reported a higher prevalence of schizophrenia and a lower prevalence of mood disorders among African Americans in comparison with Whites. In exploring this phenomenon, investigators have suggested that the effect of race on the psychiatric diagnosis of African Americans may be due to misdiagnoses resulting from racial bias (H. W. Neighbors et al., 1989), errors in clinical judgment (which can include both underpathologizing and overpathologizing; Lopez, 1989), or the use of diagnostic instruments that have not been validated on non-White populations (Brislin, Lonner, & Thorndike, 1973).

Assessment biases are critical to recognize, because diagnoses are usually linked to treatment recommendations. A recent study of the Los Angeles County mental health system found that African American and Asian American clients were more likely to be diagnosed as psychotic than Whites, whereas Latinos were less likely to be diagnosed as psychotic (Flaskerud & Hu, 1992b). Moreover, Whites and Asian Americans were more likely to be diagnosed with major affective disorders than African Americans or Latinos. Flaskerud and Hu (1992a) found that diagnosis, SES, and primary language (English or non-English) were significantly related to the treatment modality provided (i.e., whether a patient would receive therapy with or without medication). Clients who had a psychotic diagnosis, had low SES, or preferred a non-English language were more likely to be treated with medication and had fewer therapy sessions with their primary therapist (Flaskerud & Hu, 1992a). This suggests that diagnostic considerations can and do influence treatment decisions.

Treatment compliance. Treatment compliance depends somewhat on the extent to which the individual incorporates new information into a preexisting schema, or—as may be the case when existing schemas are qualitatively different from that advised—constructs a new schema. Because compliance with most treatment recommendations usually takes effort and a reorganization of some aspects of an individual's daily routine, patients will evaluate the practitioner's recommendations on a variety of dimensions before acting on them (Freund & McGuire, 1991). For instance, the patient may assess whether there might be a less difficult or invasive alternative treatment. He or she may evaluate whether the doctor or the recommended treatment appears credible or likely to help the problem. He or she may compare a mainstream recommendation with recommendations from lay or indigenous healers. And, finally, the patient may modify the recommended treatment (with or without practitioner input). Treatment compliance is likely to be greater if practitioners' recommendations are consistent with patients' preexisting health schemas. Even though patients may be motivated to comply with recommended treatment regimens, they may not remember the treatment if they do not share the same health schema (Steffensen & Colker, 1982). Support from others in the patient's social or familial network can also influence compliance (Heggenhougen & Shore, 1986).

Cultural competence. Some research has suggested that the treatment process is enhanced when patients and care providers are from the same cultural backgrounds. For example, a study examining mental health services found that ethnic match (which can imply cultural match) between clients and therapists was associated with longer stays in treatment, lower dropout rate (i.e., dropout after one session), and better treatment outcome (Sue et al., 1991). This suggests that ethnic or cultural match between a patient and a care provider may facilitate the development of a successful working alliance. However, the proportion of ethnic health care providers is not commensurate with each groups' proportional representation in the overall population of the United States (Association of American Medical Colleges, 1989; Bureau of Health Professions, 1984). For example, although African Americans composed 11.7% of the U.S. population in 1980, only 2.6% of physicians at that time were African American (Bureau of Health Professions, 1984; U.S. Bureau of the Census, 1991). Because, at this time, it is not only infeasible but also impossible to provide an ethnic match between ethnic minority patients and care providers, it is important that available care providers learn to work with patients who are ethnically, and perhaps culturally, different.

The need for health care providers to work more effectively with ethnic minority patients has been referred to as an issue of cultural competence. *Cultural competence* is defined as having the skills, attitudes, and experiences that enable a person to function effectively in different cultural contexts (Lynch & Hanson, 1992). At a minimum, there are three aspects of cultural competence. First, the care provider must have *cognitive competence*; that is, he or she must have adequate knowledge of a cultural group's lifestyle, values, normative behaviors, customs, traditional roles, and so on. Most professional health care training programs that do emphasize cultural diversity issues have focused training on the development of cognitive competence. However, there are aspects of cultural competence that go beyond this acquisition of knowledge about different cultures and ethnic minority groups. A second aspect of cultural competence involves affective competence. *Affective competence* refers to one's ability to feel or to empathize with what others feel and experience. For example, many ethnic minorities do not believe that certain White people have sufficient affective (emotional) competence to truly empathize with them as people of minority status who must seek help in a mainstream health clinic. Finally, cultural competence requires that care providers have *role competence,* or the ability to carry out appropriate role performances with their ethnic minority patients. This third aspect of cultural competence is considered to be the most difficult type of competence to develop. Often it is the lack of role competence that hinders the development of good working relationships between patients and care providers.

Cultural Incongruities in the Process of Treatment

All three aspects of competence are important, but it is often difficult to clearly state how a care provider can go about becoming culturally competent. In other words, What are the role behaviors, attitudes, and values that the provider must learn to be culturally competent in a particular culture? Obviously, this task is not an easy one that can be completed in a short period of time. Sue and Zane (1987) have formulated a heuristic model for guiding practitioners' efforts to develop more cultural competence. Cultural differences greatly influence how people communicate with each other, especially when this communication centers on solving a problem between the two parties. Unfortunately, even when a person has obtained knowledge about another person's culture or has learned certain customary ways of relating to that person, communication problems still persist. This is because both knowledge and techniques are necessary but not sufficient for effective intercultural communication. Knowing cultural knowledge and cultural techniques is inadequate because both are somewhat removed or distal from the interpersonal processes that take place between people from different cultures. For example, knowledge of a patient's culture is considered to be an essential aspect of culture-responsive service. However, even knowledge of ethnic minority culture may not always facilitate effective services. Health care staff may act on insufficient knowledge or overgeneralize what they have learned about culturally dissimilar groups in a literal and stereotypical fashion. For example, simply knowing that *personalismo* constitutes an important aspect of Hispanic interpersonal relations does not inform staff about how this dynamic specifically affects gestures during the initial stages of a developing interpersonal relationship.

One important interpersonal process that affects the working alliance is credibility. *Credibility* is defined as the patient's belief in the effectiveness of the care provider and the treatment. It has been found to be an important predictor of treatment efficacy (Kazdin & Wilcoxon, 1976). Sue and Zane (1987) have hypothesized that cultural incongruities have a great impact on treatment and care provider credibility. They believe that at least two factors are important in enhancing credibility: ascribed status and achieved status. *Ascribed status* is one's position or role as assigned by others or according to cultural norms. For example, in traditional East Asian cultures, teachers have more ascribed status and credibility than lawyers and health care professionals. Credibility can also be achieved. *Achieved credibility* refers to the skills and actions of health professionals in their work with ethnic minority patients. Ascribed and achieved credibility obviously are related, but each tends to have distinct implications for health service use. A practitioner's lack of ascribed credibility may be the primary reason that a patient initially does not use health services, whereas decrements in a practitioner's achieved credibility may better explain less frequent use and more problems related to poor relations with ethnic minority users. According to the proposed model, service-relevant cultural differences can occur in three aspects of achieved credibility that can adversely affect the developing working relationship between patients and care providers: problem conceptualization, modes of health care, and treatment goals.

Problem conceptualization. A shared conceptual system between patient and care provider is critical to the process of delivering culturally responsive health services. If the patient's health needs and problems are conceptualized by the care provider in a manner that is incongruent with the patient's belief systems and personal constructs (Frank, 1961), then the credibility of the practitioner may be diminished. Cultures differ in the explanatory models they use to account for health and illness. And, as Meichenbaum (1976) noted, when difficulties in problem conceptualization occur, patients are less likely to engage in treatment assignments and procedures.

Modes of care and treatment. Cultural incongruities can arise over the type of tasks or modes of health care that are considered appropriate and necessary to promote a cure or remediation of a particular health problem. In other words, the health care techniques and procedures used to respond to the patient's health needs may run counter to certain cultural norms or violate certain role relationships considered important in a particular ethnic culture. For example, some health clinics serving Asian communities have found that certain mentally ill Asian clients avoid using the psychotropic medication prescribed to them because they believe it will cause an imbalance in their bodies between hot and cold substances. In Asian medicine, the goal is to balance hot and cold substances for health, and imbalance creates illnesses. From this perspective, taking psychotropic medication that is perceived as a hot substance may paradoxically cause more illness.

Treatment goals. Even when there is cultural congruence between patients and care providers in problem conceptualization and modes of health care, patients may still stop using health services because they feel that the treatment has been unsuccessful. It is possible that ethnic minority patients are applying different criteria to judge services than are commonly applied by health care professionals. In Western medicine, great emphasis is placed on removing subjective distress experienced by the patient. In contrast, other cultures place less importance on the elimination of personal distress and greater importance on returning the patient to a productive social role in his or her community (T. Murase & Johnson, 1974).

Sue and Zane's (1987) model provides one way of conceptualizing the process of how cultural differences can affect the working alliance between patients and their care providers. The three areas identified as affecting achieved credibility should be considered as working hypotheses that can serve to alert care providers to potential problems of role competence.

Drug Metabolism

Recent research in medical genetics (see Polednak, 1989) and pharmacology (see Kalow, 1989, 1991; Kalow, Goedde, & Agarwal, 1986) has demonstrated significant ethnic variation in biological processes and drug responsivity. For example, ethnic variation in the flushing response to alcohol can be traced to genetic differences in the particular enzymes involved in the metabolism of alcohol, such as aldehyde dehydrogenase (Agarwal & Goedde, 1990; Yoshida, 1993). In one study, 80% of Asians and nearly 50% of Native Americans who had not been preexposed to alcohol flushed in response to alcohol, in comparison with only 10% of Whites (Wolff, 1972). Genetic research into ethnic differences in alcohol metabolism has found ethnic group differences in the incidence of genomic mutation in several aldehyde dehydrogenase isozymes, and there has been some speculation about the role of the aldehyde dehydrogenase genotype and the incidence and prevalence of ethnic differences in alcohol-related problems (see Yoshida, 1993, for a comprehensive review of recent research). K. M. Lin et al. (1993), among others, have argued that some of the ethnic variation in enzyme systems may have evolved for adaptive purposes. For example, glucose-6-dehydrogenase deficiency among those whose ancestors came from malaria-infested regions might be of selective adaptive value, because this deficiency is also associated with an increased resistance to malaria.

Ethnic differences have been found in the metabolism, and thus efficacy, of prescribed drugs (Wood & Zhou, 1991). For example, the efficacy of the betablocker propranolol in treating hypertension has been found to vary by ethnicity. Among Blacks, propranolol was often ineffective (Moser & Lunn, 1981). By contrast, the effective dosage for treating hypertension in Chinese was found to be much lower than that required for Whites (Zhou et al., 1989). Thus, possible ethnic differences in drug responsivity should be considered in the treatment of ethnic patients.

In addition to the previously discussed bases of ethnic differences in metabolism, diet has been demonstrated to influence the effectiveness of some drugs (e.g., K. E. Anderson, Conney, & Kappas, 1982; Pantuk, Pantuk, Kappas, Conney, & Anderson, 1991) and the incidence and prevalence of disease in cross-cultural and cross-national studies as well as among immigrant groups (see Kolonel, 1988). The sociocultural aspects of diet are most clearly seen in studies detailing the effects of acculturation and the accompanying dietary changes on rates of disease or on pharmacokinetics in some ethnic groups. There have been studies documenting the relationship between a culture's diet and certain diseases (Polednak, 1989). For example, in cultures with diets high in animal fat—such as in the United States, where fat makes up nearly 40% of caloric intake (Weisberger, 1991)—there is a higher incidence of colorectal cancer (Howson, Hiyama, & Wynder, 1986) and breast cancer (Goodwin & Boyd, 1987). Traditional Chinese and Japanese diets contain less than half the fat of Western diets, and researchers have suggested that the increase in colorectal and breast cancer among Chinese and Japanese Americans may be attributable, in part, to their change from traditional, low-fat diets to American high-fat diets. Other studies have shown that when immigrants change from their original culture's dietary habits to eat a Western diet their responses to certain drugs become more similar to those of Western Whites (Mucklow et al., 1980, 1982). In one study, which compared the metabolism of antipyrine in Whites and East Indians living in Britain with that of East Indians living in India, researchers found that the pharmacokinetics of antipyrine in East Indian Britons who maintained a traditional Indian vegetarian diet were similar to East Indians living in India, whereas the pharmacokinetic profile of East Indians who ate meat was more similar to that of the British Whites (Desai et al., 1980; Dollery, Fraser, Mucklow, & Bulpitt, 1979).

Bicultural Functioning

In the United States, increasing multiculturalism provides a context in which there are a variety of behavioral and sociopsychological alternatives available to the individual whose ethnicity or culture differs from that of the majority. It may be useful for practitioners to be aware of various ways that ethnic or cultural minority individuals operate in relation to their ethnicity and to the dominant Western culture, because this is another within-group variation that should be considered in initial attempts to establish working relationships with patients. Through assimilation, individuals may acquire the dominant culture but lose their cultural identity (Gordon, 1964). Conversely, an individual may acquire more than one cultural identity and alternate between cultural schemas and repertoires (Rogler, Cortes, & Malgady, 1991) depending on personal preferences or the demands of the context (e.g., communication between generations of differential acculturation). In the latter case, the bicultural or multicultural individual is, in a sense, more cognitively (and perhaps behaviorally) flexible, in that he or she has a wider repertoire conceptualizing and solving problems.

The use of dual or multiple cultural health schemas to manage chronic illness may have additional advantages. There has been some criticism of the Western medical model for not treating the "whole" person; use of a variety of schemas and their associated alternative healing and care recommendations may provide a needed supplement to mainstream care. As Ataudo (1985) explained,

> traditional medicine is regarded by patients who have faith in its healing power as a "psychological opium" that helps to alleviate pain and suffering by re-creating a sense of belongingness and awareness of self in the midst of fear and death. In this way the sufferer has gained his/her sense of touch with realities in the brotherhood of relatives and friends, traditional medical doctors, and the community at large who are wholeheartedly involved in the life-and-death crusade. (p. 1346)

Relabeling and Reevaluation

Subsequent to obtaining help or advice from significant others or those who may be perceived as sources of help (which may or may not mean entering the mainstream health care system), an individual has the opportunity to either integrate or dismiss his or her newly acquired information and advice. Also, in an important sense, relabeling and reevaluation take place during every stage of an illness. The social feedback that an individual receives about whether he or she is healthy is shaped by cultural norms reflected in culturally based schemas. Because cultures differ in their definitions of what is healthy, the outcome of a reevaluation becomes partially determined by culturally defined functional criteria. For example, in many Western European cultures, mental health entails the absence of subjective distress. By contrast, in East Asian cultures, mental health is defined as one's ability to carry out a productive social role in the community (T. Murase & Johnson, 1974). Consequently, culture has a fundamental influence on all stages of the illness experience.

Implications for Research and Health Practice With Culturally Diverse Populations

The model presented in this chapter is meant to serve as a heuristic framework or guide for both researchers and practitioners. It is an attempt to incorporate both research and clinical reports from several different disciplines on the illness experiences of ethnically and culturally diverse populations into a process model. As we stated at the outset, researchers and providers alike need to be aware of the heterogeneity of ethnic populations and to avoid ethnic or cultural stereotyping. To facilitate this process, the model does not include cultural characteristics of each major ethnic group but, instead, provides generic ethnocultural dimensions. Along these dimensions, the extent that the individual's beliefs conform or are in variance with the ethnic and cultural community can be assessed.[4]

From a research perspective, it is clear that in their empirical efforts, researchers must carefully conceptualize what processes they are examining. Often, health care research may be descriptive of use and outcomes. However, what is not made clear is how cultural differences actually result in outcome and use differences. The causal mechanism is missing. As suggested by the illness experience model, different cultural factors operate at various stages. This model provides a framework for looking systematically at how culture affects the illness process. Researchers sometimes assume, depending on training or discipline, that if they find ethnic differences they are caused by a certain class of variables. For example, when psychologists found that Asian Americans underused the mental health care system, they attributed this to shame or stigma—both of which are psychological constructs. Yet there are competing culturally based hypotheses. Lack of use might be due to shame or stigma or, alternatively, to the structure of social networks (a sociological perspective) or the conceptualization of mental health problems because of underlying explanatory models (an anthropological approach). The convergence of such approaches points to the need for the interdisciplinary study of culture and health care. Often variables are tied to, or have a history within, specific disciplines. A strong interdisciplinary approach is needed to obtain a comprehensive view of how culture affects the experience of illness.

For practitioners, the model of ethnocultural influences on the illness process can highlight specific areas where these factors significantly affect the illness experiences of ethnically and culturally diverse patient populations. Within the illness process, a number of areas appear to be relatively more important in practice. The factors described in the earlier stages of the model might inform prevention programs

[4] However, for the reader interested in developing cultural competence or in working with particular groups, there are many resources available that provide guidance for working with various cultural groups. (See, e.g., Lefley & Pedersen, 1986; Lynch & Hanson, 1994; McGoldrick, Pearce, & Giordano, 1982; Tyler, Brome, & Williams, 1991.)

targeting diverse populations, but because a patient must first seek help from the health system, practitioners are not usually privy to the initial stages of the illness presented in the model. However, patients' interpretations of their state of discontinuity, their response to the illness state, and their response to health care interventions are critical processes for the practicing health care provider to keep in mind when encountering diverse patient populations.

Recent biological investigations of ethnic differences in pharmacological responsivity may be a critical consideration for practitioners, because medications are often the major treatment of choice for certain chronic illnesses. Other factors that might be of particular importance are related to the working relationship between the patient and care provider. Frequently in practice, the patient–provider relationship focuses on medical practices and procedures. Yet an ethnocultural analysis suggests that treatment compliance may be largely affected by cultural variables. For example, practitioners sometimes assume that patients will accept the practitioner's conception, or diagnosis, of the problem as well as endorse the method prescribed to remediate the problem. The biopsychosocial model predicts that cultural differences in these areas will reduce credibility, thereby reducing practitioner efficacy in implementing treatment. If a provider does not meet the patient's expectations, he or she may not be viewed as credible. If the patient does not think the recommended treatment is appropriate or is likely to help, then treatment compliance will undoubtedly be affected.

Practitioners should consider how patients interpret new health-related information in the context of acquiring a new schema. That is, if an individual already has a preexisting mainstream health schema, then the health-care provider may not need to provide the amount, detail, and justification of the information and recommendations that would be necessary for someone who has an entirely different health schema. In the latter case, the provider should think in terms of providing not only advice and information but an entire schema (health system of beliefs) to that individual so that isolated bits of information (or recommendations) can be understood in a broader context. In addition to serving in this educational capacity, the health care provider also has the role of providing a context in which the newly acquired schema can be maintained or elaborated. This contextual approach might lead to supplemental social interventions, in addition to medical care, such as community health care centers.

Likewise, the practitioner should assess the impact of an individual's social network: Is this individual's social network sufficiently tied to the health care system? How might this affect whether he or she will comply or continue with treatment? Taking into consideration ethnocultural factors may enable the practitioner to distinguish between an individual's impairment, or loss of physiological functioning, and the likelihood of disability, or the consequences of the impairment. Impairment does not necessarily lead to disability; it depends on the social and cultural environment. Does the patient's environment enable or hinder functioning? A historical example would be the binding of the feet of wealthy Chinese women: Bound feet clearly resulted in some impairment, but because these women usually had servants and were not required to walk (they could be carried from place to place), they could still move around, maintain power over their households, and participate in everyday functions. Thus, a practitioner would be informed to weigh how a patient's ethnocultural environment might minimize or worsen the consequences of an objective impairment.

It is apparent that cultural variables can affect all aspects of the illness process. Thus, it is incumbent on both researchers and health providers to acquire training in this area. We believe that it would be most helpful if health care research and training programs could systematically examine cultural factors within a heuristic framework and generate other models that can directly account for cultural variability. Furthermore, we have argued elsewhere that it is insufficient for training programs to simply provide information about different cultures; acquiring an appropriate cultural knowledge base is merely a necessary first step to developing cultural competence. We recommend experiential training, such as that developed by Pedersen (1986) or Lefley (1985), be implemented to provide health care providers with situations in which they have to work with others who may have different health schemas or symptom expressions. It has been our experience that, as ethnocultural knowledge and cognitive, affective, and role competence are developed in practitioners, they become better able to recognize when culture may be influencing clinical processes.

We have not provided a tried-and-true formula for practitioners to follow in achieving cultural competence. This is because cultural competence is too multidimensional a construct, and the illness process too dynamic, for the development of a single formula useful for all practitioners. However, the biopsychosocial model does provide an organized guide outlining those areas in which practitioners can attempt to develop both the cultural knowledge and culturally specific interpersonal awareness that form the foundations of cultural competence.

REFERENCES

Abramowitz, S. I., & Murray, J. (1983). Race effects in psychotherapy. In J. Murray & P. Abramson (Eds.), *Bias in psychotherapy* (pp. 215–255). New York: Praeger.

Agarwal, D. P., & Goedde, H. W. (1990). *Alcohol metabolism, alcohol intolerance and alcoholism*. Berlin: Springer-Verlag.

Anderson, K. E., Conney, A. H., & Kappas, A. (1982). Nutritional influences on chemical biotransformations in humans. *Nutrition Review, 40,* 161–169.

Anderson, N. B. (1989). Ethnic differences in resting and stress-induced cardiovascular and humoral activity: An overview. In N. Schneiderman, S. B. Weiss, & P. G. Kaufman (Eds.), *Handbook of research methods in cardiovascular behavioral medicine* (pp. 433–452). New York: Plenum Press.

Anderson, N. B., McNeilly, M., & Myers, H. F. (1991). Autonomic reactivity and hypertension in Blacks: A review and proposed model. *Ethnicity and Disease, 1,* 154–170.

Angel, R., & Cleary, P. D. (1984). The effects of social structure and culture on reported health. *Social Science Quarterly, 65,* 814–828.

Angel, R., & Thoits, P. (1987). The impact of culture on the cognitive structure of illness. *Culture, Medicine, and Psychiatry, 11,* 465–494.

Association of American Medical Colleges. (1989). *Minority students in medical education: Facts and figures.* Washington, DC: Author.

Ataudo, E. S. (1985). Traditional medicine and biopsychosocial fulfillment in African health. *Social Science and Medicine, 21,* 1345–1347.

Barondess, J. (1979). Disease and illness—A crucial distinction. *American Journal of Medicine, 66,* 375–376.

Betancourt, H., & Lopez, S. R. (1993). The study of culture, ethnicity, and race in American psychology. *American Psychologist, 48,* 629–637.

Blackwell, B. (1967). Upper middle class adult expectations about entering the sick role for physical and psychiatric dysfunctions. *Journal of Health and Social Behavior, 8,* 83–95.

Blackwell, B., & Gutmann, M. (1986). Management of chronic illness behavior. In S. Hugh & T. M. Vallis (Eds.), *Illness behavior: A multidisciplinary model* (pp. 401–408). New York: Plenum Press.

Brislin, R. W., Lonner, W. J., & Thorndike, R. W. (1973). *Cross-cultural research methods.* New York: Wiley.

Bureau of Health Professions. (1984). *An in-depth examination of the 1980 decennial census employment data for health occupations: Comprehensive report.* Rockville, MD: Author.

Carver, C. S., & Scheier, M. F. (1981). *Attention and self-regulation: A control-theory approach to human behavior.* New York: Springer-Verlag.

Castro, F. G., & Miranda, M. R. (1985). Stress and illness: A multivariate analysis of perceived relationships among Mexican American and Anglo-American junior college students. In W. A. Vega & M. R. Miranda (Eds.), *Stress and Hispanic mental health: Relating research to service delivery* (pp. 219–238). Rockville, MD: National Institute of Mental Health.

Chavez, L. R. (1984). Doctors, *curanderos,* and *brujas*: Health care delivery and Mexican immigrants in San Diego. *Medical Anthropology Quarterly, 15,* 31–37.

Chew, T. (1983). Sodium values of Chinese condiments and their use in sodium-restricted diets. *Journal of the American Diet Association, 82,* 397–401.

Craig, K. D. (1987). Presidential address: Consequences of caring—Pain in the human context. *Canadian Psychology, 28,* 311–321.

Cruikshank, J. K., & Beevers, D. G. (1989). *Ethnic factors in health and disease.* London: Wright.

Desai, N. K., Sheth, U. K., Mucklow, J. C., Fraser, H. S., Bulpitt, C. J., Jones, S. W., & Dollery, C. T. (1980). Antipyrine clearance in Indian villagers. *British Journal of Clinical Pharmacology, 9,* 387–394.

Dollery, C. T., Fraser, H. S., Mucklow, J. C., & Bulpitt, C. J. (1979). Contribution of environmental factors to variability in human drug metabolism. *Drug Metabolism Review, 9,* 207–220.

Draguns, J. G. (1989). Dilemmas and choices in cross-cultural counseling: The universal versus the culturally distinctive. In P. B. Pedersen, J. G. Draguns, W. J. Lonner, & J. E. Trimble (Eds.), *Counseling across cultures* (pp. 3–21). Honolulu: University of Hawaii Press.

Dutton, D. (1986). Social class, health, and illness. In L. Aiken & D. Mechanic (Eds.), *Applications of social science to clinical medicine and health policy* (pp. 31–62). New Brunswick, NJ: Rutgers University Press.

Eisenberg, D. M., Kessler, R. C., Foster, C., Norlock, F. E., Calkins, D. R., & Delbanco, T. L. (1993). Unconventional medicine in the United States: Prevalence, costs, and patterns of use. *New England Journal of Medicine, 328,* 246–252.

Eisenberg, L. (1977). Disease and illness: Distinction between professional and popular ideas of sickness. *Culture, Medicine, and Psychiatry, 1,* 9–23.

Ekman, P. (1993). Facial expression and emotion. *American Psychologist, 48,* 384–392.

Fabrega, H. (1974). *Disease and social behavior: An interdisciplinary perspective.* Cambridge, MA: MIT Press.

Flaskerud, J. H., & Hu, L. (1992a). Racial/ethnic identity and amount and type of psychiatric treatment. *American Journal of Psychiatry, 149,* 379–384.

Flaskerud, J. H., & Hu, L. (1992b). Relationship of ethnicity to psychiatric diagnosis. *Journal of Nervous and Mental Disease, 181*, 296–303.

Folkman, S., & Lazarus, R. S. (1980). An analysis of coping in a middle-aged community sample. *Journal of Health and Social Behavior, 21*, 219–239.

Foster, G. M. (1981). Relationships between Spanish and Spanish American folk medicine. In G. Henderson & M. Primeaux (Eds.), *Transcultural health care* (pp. 115–135). Reading, MA: Addison-Wesley.

Frank, J. D. (1961). *Persuasion and healing.* Baltimore: Johns Hopkins University Press.

Freeman, H. E., Blendon, R. J., Aiken, L. H., Sudman, S., Mullinix, C. F., & Corey, C. R. (1987). Americans report on their access to health care. *Health Affairs, 6*, 6–18.

Frerichs, R. R., Chapman, J. M., & Maes, E. F. (1984). Mortality due to all causes and to cardiovascular diseases among seven race–ethnic populations in Los Angeles County, 1980. *International Journal of Epidemiology, 13*, 291–298.

Freund, P. E. S., & McGuire, M. B. (1991). *Health, illness and the social body: A critical sociology.* Englewood Cliffs, NJ: Prentice Hall.

Goffman, E. (1963). *Stigma: Notes on the management of spoiled identity.* Englewood Cliffs, NJ: Prentice Hall.

Goodwin, P. J., & Boyd, N. F. (1987). Critical appraisal of the evidence that dietary fat intake is related to breast cancer in humans. *Journal of the National Cancer Institute, 79*, 473.

Gordon, M. M. (1964). *Assimilation in American life.* New York: Oxford University Press.

Grim, C. E., & Wilson, T. W. (1989). The worldwide epidemiology of hypertension in Blacks with a note on a new theory for the greater prevalence of hypertension in Western Hemisphere Blacks. In C. O. Enuonwee (Ed.), *Hypertension in Blacks and other minorities: 1988 conference proceedings of the Second Annual Nutrition Workshop* (pp. 57–73). Nashville, TN: Meharry Medical College.

Gruman, J. C., & Sloan, R. P. (1983). Disease as justice: Perceptions of the victims of physical illness. *Basic and Applied Social Psychology, 4*, 39–46.

Guarnaccia, P. J., DeLaCancela, V., & Carrillo, E. (1989). The multiple meanings of *ataques de nervios* in the Latino community. *Medical Anthropology Quarterly, 11*, 47–62.

Hann, R. S. (1994). Parasitic infestations. In N. W. S. Zane, D. T. Takeuchi, & K. Young (Eds.), *Confronting critical health issues of Asian and Pacific Islander Americans* (pp. 302–315). Newbury Park, CA: Sage.

Harburg, E., Erfurt, J. C., Haunstein, L., Chape, C., Schull, W., & Schork, M. A. (1973). Socio-ecological stress, suppressed hostility, skin color, and Black–White male blood pressure, Detroit. *Psychosomatic Medicine, 35*, 276–296.

Harwood, A. (Ed.) (1981). *Ethnicity and medical care.* Cambridge, MA: Harvard University Press.

Healy, M. (1994, February 2). "Environmental justice" for U.S. minorities is ordered. *Los Angeles Times*, p. A15.

Heggenhougen, H. K., & Shore, L. (1986). Cultural components of behavioral epidemiology: Implications for primary health care. *Social Science and Medicine, 22,* 1235–1245.

Hoang, G. N., & Erickson, R. V. (1985). Cultural barriers to effective medical care among Indochinese patients. *Annual Review of Medicine, 36,* 229–239.

Howson, C. P., Hiyama, T., & Wynder, E. L. (1986). Decline of gastric cancer: Epidemiology of an unplanned triumph. *Epidemiology Review, 8,* 1–27.

Hugh, S., & Vallis, T. M. (1986). *Illness behavior: A multidisciplinary model.* New York: Plenum Press.

Jackson, F. L. (1991). An evolutionary perspective on salt, hypertension, and human genetic variability. *Hypertension, 17*(Suppl. 1), 129–132.

Jones, E. E., Farina, A., Hastorf, A. H., Markus, H., Miller, D. T., & Scott, R. A. (1984). *Social stigma: The psychology of marked relationships.* New York: Freeman.

Kalow, W. (1989). Race and therapeutic drug response. *New England Journal of Medicine, 320,* 588–589.

Kalow, W. (1991). Interethnic variation of drug metabolism. *Trends in Pharmacological Science, 12,* 102–107.

Kalow, W., Goedde, H. W., & Agarwal, D. P. (Eds.). (1986). *Ethnic differences in reactions to drugs and xenobiotics.* New York: Alan R. Liss.

Kazdin, A. E., & Wilcoxon, L. A. (1976). Systematic desensitization and nonspecific treatment effects: A methodological evaluation. *Psychological Bulletin, 83,* 729-758.

Kinzie, J. D. (1985). Overview of clinical issues in the treatment of Southeast Asian refugees. In T. C. Owan (Ed.), *Southeast Asian mental health: Treatment, prevention, services, training, and research* (pp. 113–136). Washington, DC: U.S. Government Printing Office.

Kinzie, J. D., Boehnlein, J. K., Leung, P. K., Moore, L. J., Riley, C., & Smith, D. (1990). The prevalence of posttraumatic stress disorder and its clinical significance among Southeast Asian refugees. *American Journal of Psychiatry, 147,* 913–917.

Kleinman, A. (1980). *Patients and healers in the context of culture.* Berkeley: University of California Press.

Kleinman, A. M. (1988). *Rethinking psychiatry.* New York: Free Press.

Kleinman, A., & Kleinman, J. (1991). Suffering and its professional transformation: Toward an ethnography of interpersonal experience. *Culture, Medicine, and Psychiatry, 15,* 275–301.

Kolonel, L. N. (1988). Variability in diet and its relation to risk in ethnic and migrant groups. In A. D. Woodhead, M. A. Bender, & R. C. Leonard (Eds.), *Phenotypic variations in populations: Relevance to risk assessment* (pp. 129–135). New York: Plenum.

Kosko, D. A., & Flaskerud, J. H. (1987). Mexican American, nurse practitioner, and lay control group beliefs about the cause and treatment of chest pain. *Nursing Research, 36,* 226–231.

Koss, J. D. (1990). Somatization and somatic complaint syndromes among Hispanics: Overview and ethnopsychological perspectives. *Transcultural Psychiatric Research Review, 27,* 5–29.

Kroll, J., Habenicht, M., Mackenzie, T., Yee, M., Chan, S., Vang, T., Nguyen, T., Ly, M., Phommasouvanh, B., Nguyen, H., Vang, Y., Souvannasoth, L., & Cabugao, R. (1989). Depression and posttraumatic stress disorder in Southeast Asian refugees. *American Journal of Psychiatry, 146,* 1592–1597.

Landrine, H., & Klonoff, E. A. (1992). Culture and health-related schemas: A review and proposal for interdisciplinary integration. *Health Psychology, 11,* 267–276.

Lazarus, R. S., & Folkman, S. (1984). *Stress, appraisal, and coping.* New York: Springer.

Lefley, H. P. (1985). Mental health training across cultures. In P. Pedersen (Ed.), *Handbook of cross-cultural counseling and therapy* (pp. 259–266). Westport, CT: Greenwood Press.

Lefley, H. P., & Pedersen, P. B. (Eds.). (1986). *Cross-cultural training for mental health professionals.* Springfield, IL: Charles C Thomas.

Leslie, C. M. (1977). Pluralism and integration in the Indian and Chinese medical systems. In D. Landry (Ed.), *Culture, disease, and healing* (pp. 511–517). New York: Macmillan.

Leventhal, H., Meyer, D., & Nerenz, D. (1980). The common-sense representation of illness danger. In D. Rachman (Ed.), *Medical psychology* (pp. 7–30). Elmsford, NY: Pergamon Press.

Lin, K. M., Poland, R. E., & Nagasaki, G. (Eds.). (1993). *Psychopharmacology and psychobiology of ethnicity.* Washington, DC: American Psychiatric Press.

Lin, T., Tardiff, K., Donetz, G., & Goresky, W. (1978). Ethnicity and patterns of help seeking. *Culture, Medicine, and Psychiatry, 2,* 3–14.

Lipton, J. A., & Marbach, J. J. (1984). Ethnicity and the pain experience. *Social Science and Medicine, 19,* 1279–1298.

Lopez, S. R. (1989). Patient variable biases in clinical judgment: Conceptual overview and methodological considerations. *Psychological Bulletin, 106,* 184–203.

Lutz, C., & White, G. M. (1986). The anthropology of emotions. *Annual Review of Anthropology, 15,* 405–436.

Lynch, E. W., & Hanson, M. J. (Eds.). (1992). *Developing cross-cultural competence.* Baltimore: Paul H. Brooks.

Markus, H. R., & Kitayama, S. (1991). Culture and the self: Implications for cognition, emotion, and motivation. *Psychological Review, 98,* 224–253.

Marmot, M. G., Kogevinas, M., & Elston, M. A. (1987). Social/economic status and disease. *Annual Review of Public Health, 8,* 111–135.

Mau, W. C., & Jepson, D. A. (1990). Help-seeking perceptions and behaviors: A comparison of Chinese and American graduate students. *Journal of Multicultural Counseling and Development, 18,* 94–104.

Mayeno, L., & Hirota, S. M. (1994). Access to health care. In N. W. S. Zane, D. T. Takeuchi, & K. N. J. Young (Eds.), *Confronting critical health issues of Asian and Pacific Islander Americans* (pp. 347–375). Newbury Park, CA: Sage.

McGoldrick, M. (1982). Ethnicity and family therapy: An overview. In M. McGoldrick, J. K. Pearce, & J. Giordano (Eds.), *Ethnicity and family therapy* (pp. 3–30). New York: Guilford Press.

McGoldrick, M., Pearce, J. K., & Giordano, J. (Eds.). (1982). *Ethnicity and family therapy.* New York: Guilford Press.

McHugh, S., & Vallis, M. (1986). Illness behavior: Operationalization of the biopsychosocial model. In S. Hugh & T. M. Vallis (Eds.), *Illness behavior: A multidisiplinary model* (pp. 1–31). New York: Plenum Press.

Mechanic, D. (1978). *Medical sociology* (2nd ed.) New York: Free Press.

Mechanic, D. (1982). *Symptoms, illness behavior, and help-seeking.* New Brunswick, NJ: Rutgers University Press.

Mechanic, D. (1986). Illness behavior: An overview. In S. Hugh & T. M. Vallis (Eds.), *Illness behavior: A multidisciplinary model* (pp. 101–109). New York: Plenum Press.

Meichenbaum, D. (1976). Toward a cognitive theory of self-control. *Consciousness and Self-Regulation, 1,* 1–66.

Meinhardt, K., Tom, S., Tse, P., & Yu, C. Y. (1986). Southeast Asian refugees in the "Silicon Valley": The Asian Health Assessment Project. *Amerasia, 12,* 43–65.

Miller, L. C., Murphy, R., & Buss, A. H. (1981). Consciousness of body: Private and public. *Journal of Personality and Social Psychology, 139,* 293–296.

Mollica, R. F., Wyshak, G., & Lavelle, J. (1987). The psychosocial impact of war trauma and torture on Southeast Asian refugees. *American Journal of Psychiatry, 144,* 1567–1572.

Moser, M., & Lunn, J. (1981). Comparative effects of pindolol and hydrochlorothiazide in Black hypertensive patients. *Angiology, 32,* 561–566.

Mucklow, J. C., Caraher, M. T., Henderson, D. B., Chapman, P. H., Roberts, D. F., & Rawlins, M. D. (1982). The relationship between individual dietary constituents and antipyrine metabolism in Indo-Pakistani immigrants in Britain. *British Journal of Clinical Pharmacology, 13,* 481–486.

Mucklow, J. C., Caraher, M. T., Idle, J. R., Rawlins, M. D., Sloan, T., Smith, R. L., & Wood, P. (1980). The influences of changes in dietary fat on the clearance of antipyrine and 4-hydroxylation of debrisoquine. *British Journal of Clinical Pharmacology, 9,* 283P.

Murase, T., & Johnson, F. (1974). Naikan, Morita, and Western psychotherapy. *Archives of General Psychiatry, 31,* 121–128.

Murdock, G. P. (1980). *Theories of illness: A world survey.* Pittsburgh, PA: University of Pittsburgh Press.

Myers, H. (1993). Biopsychosocial perspective on depression in African Americans. In K. M. Lin, R. E. Poland, & G. Nagasaki (Eds.), *Psychopharmacology and psychobiology of ethnicity* (pp. 201–222). Washington, DC: American Psychiatric Association.

Neighbors, H. (1985). Seeking professional help for personal problems: Black Americans' use of health and mental health services. *Community Mental Health Journal, 21*(3), 156–166.

Neighbors, H. W., Jackson, J. S., Campbell, L., & Williams, D. (1989). The influence of racial factors on psychiatric diagnosis: A review and suggestions for research. *Community Mental Health Journal, 25,* 301–311.

O'Hare, W. P., & Felt, J. C. (1991). *Asian Americans: America's fastest growing minority group.* Washington, DC: U.S. Government Printing Office.

Palinkas, L. A. (1987). A longitudinal study of ethnicity and disease incidence. *Medical Anthropology Quarterly, 1,* 85–105.

Pantuk, E. J., Pantuk, C. B., Kappas, A., Conney, A. H., & Anderson, K. E. (1991). Effects of protein and carbohydrate content of diet on drug conjugation. *Clinical Pharmacological Therapy, 50,* 254–258.

Pedersen, P. B. (1986). Developing interculturally skilled counselors: A prototype for training. In H. P. Lefley & P. B. Pedersen (Eds.), *Cross-cultural training for mental health professionals* (pp. 73–87). Springfield, IL: Charles C Thomas.

Pennebaker, J. W. (1985). Traumatic experience and psychosomatic disease: Exploring the roles of behavioral inhibition, obsession, and confiding. *Canadian Psychology, 26,* 82–95.

Polednak, A. P. (1989). *Racial and ethnic differences in disease.* New York: Oxford University Press.

Rogler, L. H., Cortes, D. E., & Malgady, R. G. (1991). Acculturation and mental health status among Hispanics. *American Psychologist, 46,* 585–597.

Rogler, L. H., Malgady, R., & Rodriguez, T. (1989). Phase two: Help-seeking behavior. In L. H. Rogler (Ed.), *Hispanics and mental health* (pp. 45–70). Malabar, FL: Krieger.

Root, M. P. P. (Ed.). (1992). *Racially mixed people in America.* Newbury Park, CA: Sage.

Rowlison, R. H., & Felner, R. D. (1988). Major life events, hassles, and adaptation in adolescence: Confounding in the conceptualization and measurement of life stress and adjustment revisited. *Journal of Personality and Social Psychology, 55,* 432–444.

Sattler, J. M. (1977). The effects of therapist–client racial similarity. In A. S. Gurman & A. M. Razin (Eds.), *Effective psychotherapy: A handbook of research* (pp. 252–290). Elmsford, NY: Pergamon Press.

Seagall, M., & Wykle, M. (1988). The Black family's experience with dementia. *Journal of Applied Social Sciences, 13,* 170–191.

Shweder, R. A. (1990). Cultural psychology—What is it? In J. W. Stigler, R. A. Shweder, & G. Herdt (Eds.), *Cultural Psychology: Essays on comparative human development* (pp. 1–43). Cambridge, England: Cambridge University Press.

Spickard, P. R. (1992). The illogic of American racial categories. In M. P. P. Root (Ed.), *Racially mixed people in America* (pp. 12–23). Newbury Park, CA: Sage.

Steffensen, M. S., & Colker, L. (1982). Intercultural misunderstandings about health care—Recall of descriptions of illness and treatment. *Social Science and Medicine, 16,* 1949–1954.

Sue, S., Fujino, D. C., Hu, L. T., Takeuchi, D. T., & Zane, N. W. S. (1991). Community mental health services for ethnic minority groups: A test of the cultural responsiveness hypothesis. *Journal of Counseling Psychology, 59,* 533–540.

Sue, S., & Zane, N. (1987). The role of culture and cultural techniques in psychotherapy: A critique and reformulation. *American Psychologist, 82,* 37–45.

Tanaka-Matsumi, J., & Marsella, A. J. (1976). Cross-cultural variations in the phenomenological experience of depression: 1. Word association studies. *Journal of Cross-Cultural Psychology, 7,* 379–396.

Tracey, T. J., Leong, F. T. L., & Glidden, C. (1986). Help seeking and problem perception among Asian Americans. *Journal of Counseling Psychology, 33,* 331–336.

Tyler, F. B., Brome, D. R., & Williams, J. E. (1991). *Ethnic validity, ecology, and psychotherapy: A psychosocial competence model.* New York: Plenum.

U.S. Bureau of the Census. (1991). *Race and Hispanic origin.* Washington, DC: U.S. Government Printing Office.

Weisberger, J. H. (1991). Causes, relevant mechanisms, and prevention of large bowel cancer. *Seminars in Oncology, 18,* 316–336.

Weisenberg, M., Kreindler, M. L., Schachat, R., & Werboff, J. (1975). Pain: Anxiety and attitudes in Black, White, and Puerto Rican patients. *Psychosomatic Medicine, 37,* 123–135.

Wolff, P. H. (1972). Ethnic differences in alcohol sensitivity. *Science, 175,* 449–450.

Wood, A. J., & Zhou, H. H. (1991). Ethnic differences in drug disposition and responsiveness. *Clinical Pharmacokinetics, 20,* 1–24.

Yoshida, A. (1993). Genetic polymorphisms of alcohol-metabolizing enzymes related to alcohol sensitivity and alcoholic diseases. In K. M. Lin, R. E. Poland, & G. Nagasaki (Eds.), *Psychopharmacology and psychobiology of ethnicity* (pp. 169–183). Washington, DC: American Psychiatric Press.

Zane, N., & Sue, S. (1991). Culturally responsive mental health services for Asian Americans: Treatment and training issues. In H. Myers, P. Wohlford, P. Guzman, & R. Echemendia (Eds.), *Ethnic minority perspectives on clinical training and services in psychology* (pp. 48–59). Washington, DC: American Psychological Association.

Zborowski, M. (1969). *People in pain.* San Francisco: Jossey-Bass.

Zborowski, M. (1978). Cultural components in responses to pain. In M. H. Logan & E. E. Hunt (Eds.), *Health and the human condition: Perspectives on medical anthropology* (pp. 281–293). Belmont, CA: Wadsworth.

Zhou, H. H., Koshakji, R. P., Silberstein, D. J., Wilkinson, G. R., & Wood, A. J. J. (1989). Altered sensitivity to and clearance of propranolol in men of Chinese descent as compared with American Whites. *New England Journal of Medicine, 320,* 565–570.

Chapter

6

Family Assessment and Intervention

Robert D. Kerns

Across the life span, families appear to play substantial roles in the health-relevant issues of individuals. Theory and research have supported the influence of family on the development of children's concepts of health and illness and patterns of health behavior; on attempts at health behavior change; on determining responses to acute illnesses and medical interventions; on the management of chronic illness; and in issues of aging and geriatric care, terminal illness, and bereavement (Kerns, 1994; Turk & Kerns, 1985b). Personal phenomenology, clinical observation of families' interactions with health care delivery systems, theory-driven research and accumulated empirical data, and clinical intervention trials involving families all have encouraged continued attention to the role of families in health and illness issues (cf. Kerns & Weiss, 1994; Patterson & Garwick, 1994). So compelling are the arguments that Litman (1974, 1989; Litman & Venters, 1979) has offered a case for conceptualizing the family as the primary unit of health care. The development of the science and practice of family medicine is an influential example of the apparent acceptance of this perspective (Ramsey, 1989).

Theoretical and empirical contributions to the study of family influence in health and illness have historically cut across multiple fields and disciplines, including medical sociology, epidemiology and public health, psychosomatic medicine, social work, and nursing. Psychology and its several subdisciplines have also made many important contributions. Interestingly, however, the emerging specialty areas of health psychology and behavioral medicine have been relatively slow to direct attention to the family (Kerns & Turk, 1985). Turk and Kerns (1985a) have criticized these fields for largely adopting a biomedical perspective and emphasizing collaboration with investigators from the physical sciences that maintains a reductionistic focus on the individual and on disease models. Regardless of the contributors, relevant information from other disciplines and representatives of alternative theoretical perspectives on the role of families in health have largely failed to be integrated into mainstream theory and research of health psychology.

Attention to the problems posed by chronic illness continues to dominate many discussions of health care research and health care delivery. Within this domain, attention to family factors appears to be increasing as evidence mounts that the family may play a precipitating, predisposing, and contributing role in the etiology, care, and treatment of a range of chronic illnesses. Particular progress has been made in understanding family reactions to a member's chronic illness, the importance of family support, and family contributions to patient adherence to treatment regimens (Litman, 1989). It is apparent that attention to the complex interactions and transactions within the family will have important implications across the multiple challenges posed by chronic illness for the patient, the family itself, and the health care delivery system.

My goals in this chapter are threefold: (a) to review the theoretical and empirical basis for current conceptions of familial roles in chronic illness; (b) to describe in some detail the current state of clinical psychological assessment and intervention efforts involving the family; and (c) to offer some suggestions for future research and clinical development in the field. I place attention on how families influence individuals with chronic illnesses as well as on how such individuals affect the family, and, importantly, I examine their reciprocal effects. I emphasize emerging etiological and explanatory models of chronic illness; issues related to managing chronic illness, including treatment adherence; and factors associated with behavioral and psychological adjustment to chronic illness and quality of life for both the patient and family. Examples are drawn from investigations and clinical work related to a range of disorders to compare and contrast important differences related to disease characteristics and effects. Examples also cut across the life span and, therefore, attend to important developmental issues. Although this chapter is not intended as a comprehensive or exhaustive review of the issues, I hope that it informs the reader broadly about the current state of theory, research, and practice in the area of family health psychology.

Chronic Illness Perspective

Articulation of the four broad domains representing important dimensions of most chronic illnesses is helpful in any consideration of transactions between chronically ill individuals and their families. The disease process itself is one important domain. Chronic diseases vary depending on the biological system involved, their evolving versus resolving natures, their speeds of progression, and so forth. These and other factors have proven relevant in considerations of the contributions of family functioning to managing a disorder (e.g., Hanson et al., 1992; Hauser et al., 1986) and, conversely, in examinations of the impact of the disease on siblings, parents, and spouses (e.g., Kovacs et al., 1990).

A second domain relates to the clinical and symptomatic expression of the disease. Observable evidence of chronic illnesses varies greatly—from those that are largely asymptomatic (such as hypertension), to those with discrete symptomatic episodes (such as epilepsy and angina pectoris), to those in which persistent signs or symptoms are present (as with many musculoskeletal disorders). An emerging empirical literature in the area of chronic pain (e.g., Kerns et al., 1991; Romano et al., 1992; Turk, Kerns, & Rosenberg, 1992), for example, has suggested that spouses in particular may have key roles in reinforcing expressions of pain and pain behaviors (i.e., complaints of pain, guarding, or taking pain medications) and, therefore, may theoretically maintain the experience of pain in the absence of continued nociception.

Impairment and disability comprise a third important domain. For many chronic illnesses, effects on behavior are most often limited to managing the disease or its symptoms, for example, in the case of chronic skin disorders or hypertension. At the other extreme, however, are severe physical impairments or functional limitations posed by disorders affecting the central nervous system, such as cerebrovascular disease and multiple sclerosis, or by neuromuscular disorders, such as the dystrophies. Also within this domain is functional disability. Disability may or may not be associated with evidence of physical limitations. For example, chronic pain may be present in the absence of a neurological deficit limiting functioning, and it is commonly associated with functional declines in many areas of a patient's life. From this perspective, impairment and disability represent both direct and indirect behavioral effects of the underlying disease.

A final domain is the affective response of the individual. It is increasingly apparent that affective response may be a direct function of the disease—for example, in the case of brain disorders and certain endocrine and metabolic disorders. Alternatively, response may be affected by side effects of pharmacological treatment for the disorder or its symptoms. In the absence of these apparent effects, this domain represents individuals' affective adjustments to chronic illness in the broader context of their lives. Although depression and anxiety are commonly associated with chronic illness, the majority of individuals with chronic illnesses do not experience clinically significant affective distress (Banks & Kerns, in press). There is even evidence that some individuals may construct a largely positive emotional response to the challenges of chronic illness. Attention to the specific nature and intensity of the affective response as a dimension to be separated from the chronic illness experience is clearly indicated.

It is reasonable to assume significant relationships among the four domains of the chronic illness experience, but it is equally apparent that divergence among these domains is also common. Take, for example, the case of someone with chronic low-back pain: Despite a lay perspective associating severity of pain (the predominant symptom of the illness) with the extent of underlying structural pathology (the disease), empirical evidence has failed to support even a modest relationship between these variables (e.g., Boden, Davis, Dina, Patronis, & Wiesel, 1990). Among samples of chronic pain patients, there has been evidence supporting statistically significant, but surprisingly modest, relationships between the domains of pain and disability or distress (Kerns & Haythornthwaite, 1988).

Examples from the literature on coronary heart disease further emphasize the complexity of relationships among these domains. It is now apparent that a certain proportion of individuals with significant ischemic heart disease do not experience chest pain in conjunction with episodes of pronounced myocardial ischemia (Rozanski & Berman, 1987). Moreover, the association between disease severity and the presence or absence of symptoms is minimal—a conclusion that has encouraged exploration of other factors, both physiological and psychosocial, that may account for this variance in the expression of the disease (Burg, Jain, Soufer, Kerns, & Zaret, 1993). Finally, evidence has mounted in support of the efficacy of coronary artery bypass graft surgery for a subset of patients who have coronary artery disease. In over 90% of cases, patients have reported elimination or a significant reduction in symptoms of their disorder after revascularization (theoretically, a reversal of the extent of the underlying disease). Unfortunately, positive outcomes in the domains of disability and affective distress have not been as apparent (Kinchla & Weiss, 1985).

Health psychologists have relied on highly varied theories and methodologies to examine relationships among these important domains of chronic illness. Many of these approaches have emphasized the social context as a primary target for consideration. Reciprocal interactions between the individual with chronic illness and his or her family are a critically important, but relatively neglected, focus for continued attention.

A Family Perspective on Health and Illness

It is important to acknowledge the broad array of contemporary social structures to which the term *family* may apply. One particularly accommodating view was presented by Dean, Lin, and Ensel (1981): Families are groups composed of members who have mutual obligations to provide a broad range of emotional and material support. Turk and Kerns (1985a) have further suggested that discussions of health, illness, and families should consider at least seven components of families to appreciate the complexity of family transactions with health and illness. Families have (a) structure (e.g., gender, age distribution, number of members), (b) functions and assigned roles, (c) modes of interacting (e.g., with regard to decision making and problem solving, (d) resources (e.g., general health of family members, social skills, personality characteristics, or financial support), (e) a life cycle, (f) a history (e.g., sociocultural history as well as histories of coping with illness or stress), and (g) a set of individual members with unique histories.

Multiple family theories have been applied in the consideration of health and illness issues, including those posed by chronic illness. Baker and Patterson (1989) have suggested that five theories in particular are beginning to offer a framework for efforts in the family medicine arena, although none of these theoretical perspectives has found its way into the health psychology domain to any great extent. Each of these perspectives has emerged specifically from studies of family systems that were not specific attempts at considering the family's role in health and illness. Nevertheless, these models have led to the development of assessment and intervention strategies that appear directly relevant to the family health psychologist.

Beavers's Systems Model of Family Functioning

As is true of each family theory I present, Beavers's (1981, 1989) model of family functioning emerged from clinical experience and research that was largely focused on psychiatric disorders. As a systems model, Beavers's model emphasizes the importance of multiple levels of analysis and their interactions while targeting the family system specifically as critical to understanding the functioning of individuals. Family functioning is described in terms of two continuous variables: family competence and family style. *Family competence* includes adaptability or flexibility with regard to change and acceptance of individual autonomy. Competence is characterized as varying from severely dysfunctional to optimal, with three intermediate categories of competence. *Family style* is viewed as having two poles: one characterized by a "centripetal style," associated with a family belief that satisfaction comes from within the family and a tendency to draw family members in, and the other representing a "centrifugal style," consistent with a belief that satisfaction is most likely to be had in the world around the family and a resulting tendency to push family members out. "Mixed" families switch their styles depending on the circumstances and individual members' needs. Beavers (1989) emphasized that the model is consistent with other family systems theories and major clinical concepts of family functioning. Indeed, the model has served as the cornerstone for the development of an observation-based assessment scheme as well as for a self-report instrument (Beavers, 1989), although the clinical and empirical use of these is only beginning to be evaluated. A psychotherapeutic approach based on the model has also been described (Beavers, 1981).

A case of childhood epilepsy can illustrate the relevance of the model. A relatively large clinical literature has described the dilemma that families face in making decisions about the need to protect a child who has epilepsy, on the one hand, and the need to encourage independence in functioning, on the other. A high degree of overprotectiveness by some parents is presumed to have deleterious effects on the child. Within Beavers's (1981, 1989) system, such a family might be described as rigid and inflexible, in terms of family competence and demonstrating a centripetal family style that fosters unnecessary dependence. Psychotherapy would encourage family beliefs in the ultimate competence of the child to function increasingly independently.

Circumflex Model

Central to the circumflex model (Olson, 1989) are two core dimensions, labeled *cohesion* and *adaptability to change,* and one central process, communication. Cohesion and adaptability are viewed as continuous variables that range from very low to very high, with optimally functioning families lying in the midrange of both variables. For example, on the dimension of adaptability, families may be characterized by a style of functioning that ranges from a high degree of rigidity in adapting to change (i.e., a very low level of adaptability) to a chaotic (i.e., extremely changeable) style of functioning. More optimal levels of adaptability exist in families that might be characterized as either relatively "structured" or "flexible." Similarly, with regard to level of cohesion, families may be characterized as relatively disengaged, separated, connected, or enmeshed.

Olson (1989) has described how the circumflex model might apply in describing the family's process of adapting to a chronic physical illness in a member depending on the family's characteristic style of functioning. Predictable changes in family functioning might be expected in response to illness, given particular characteristics of the family's premorbid functioning. In general, "balanced" families are predicted to respond better to illness in one family member because of their ability to change the family system to cope most effectively with the stress or demands of the illness. Unfortunately, to date no empirical research has been reported that has tested this model with a sample suffering from chronic illness.

A widely used questionnaire that assesses the individual's perceived and ideal views of his or her family's functioning according to the circumflex model is the Family Adaptability and Cohesion Evaluation Scales (FACES III; Olson, Portner, & Lavee, 1985). This third version of the original scale comprises 20 items and has shown satisfactory reliability and validity estimates (Olson, 1989). An additional scale developed to be consistent with the model is the Clinical Rating Scale (CRS; Olson, 1989; Olson & Killorin, 1985). On the CRS, clinicians make 21 specific ratings as well as three global ratings of the degree of cohesion, adaptability, and communication during either interview or task performances. Reported interrater reliability estimates for the rating system have been satisfactory (Olson & Killorin, 1985). The availability of these instruments should encourage the testing of predictions about family response to chronic illness on the basis of Olson's model.

Family Adjustment and Adaptation Response Model

The family adjustment and adaptation response (FAAR) model (Patterson, 1989; Patterson & Garwick, 1994) is a relatively recent refinement of family stress theories that owe much to the work of Hill (1949) and his family crisis model. According to the traditional model, the degree of stress experienced by a family is a function of the interaction between potentially stressful events and those family resources that serve to maintain homeostasis in the face of stress. Under this model, stressors may include physiological challenges to the family system, such as physical illness. Resources are hypothesized as moderators of the response to stress by the family and include physical, psychological, and social resources and coping behaviors of the family. A third moderating factor within the model is the family's perceptions of the stressor and its interactions with family resources. This factor can be broken into situational meanings, or appraisals, regarding specific challenges and the family's capacities to cope with them, and global meanings or family schema regarding the family's views of itself and its interactions with the larger community. Reiss's (1981, 1989) description of family paradigms—that is, styles of problem solving that distinguish families—has aided the operationalization and assessment of this third factor in the FAAR model. A further description of Reiss's paradigm model of family functioning is offered below.

The FAAR model does not merely provide a framework for considering a family's characteristic patterns of interactions with the world in which the primary goal is adjustment to stress and maintenance of homeostasis. It also explicitly considers the ongoing role of the family once the family's resources are taxed beyond its capacity to maintain homeostasis or once a crisis has occurred. During this phase of family functioning, adaptation and recovery from the crisis become a central motivating factor. The FAAR model appears to have important strengths that enhance its potential utility in the health psychology field. Given the central role it attributes to the constructs of stress and coping, the model is consistent with a conceptual framework that has a primary place in the health psychology field (Friedman, 1992). Similarly, the model emphasizes the important role of family appraisal processes in much the same way that they have been conceptualized for individuals within a stress-and-coping paradigm and cognitive–social learning theory. The model is also important to the extent that it attempts to explain links between physiological and psychosocial variables. Particular to the investigation of chronic illness, the model offers a developmental and dynamic framework in which to consider the constructs of adjustment and adaptation to chronic illness and associated concerns. The model is also likely to be important because of its continued attention to individual family members in addition to the family as an integrated system.

Ultimately, the value of the FAAR model may rest in its ability to foster the development of specific instruments for measuring the variables of interest that it identifies as relevant. Many psychometrically sound measures have been developed for each of the factors outlined in the FAAR model. For example, the Family Inventory of Life Events and Changes (FILE; H. I. McCubbin, Patterson, & Wilson, 1981) is a 71-item instrument designed for completion by adult family members that offers an index of the accumulation of family-related stressors and strains over the previous year. The Family Inventory of Resources for Management (FIRM; H. McCubbin, Comeau, & Harkins, 1981) is a 98-item scale with four identified subscales: Family Strengths I, including esteem and communication; Family Strengths II, including mastery and health; extended family support, and financial well-being. A measure of family coping developed on the basis of the FAAR model is the Coping Health Inventory for Parents (CHIP; H. McCubbin et al., 1983). Three family-coping subscales have also been developed: measuring maintenance of family integration, self-esteem, and getting medical consultation. Another measure, the Family Coping Strategies (F-COPES; H. McCubbin, Larsen, & Olson, 1982), assesses five coping patterns: acquiring social and spiritual support, getting help, reframing, and passive appraisal. Multiple measures of the family's perceptions or meanings of events have also been developed and include an adaptation of the FILE, the Family Index of Cohesion (FIC; H. I. McCubbin & Patterson, 1982), and the Family Hardiness Index (FHI; M. A. McCubbin, McCubbin, & Thompson, 1987). Patterson (1989) has encouraged the use of these measures as well as many other instruments that have been derived from other family systems frameworks but that are directly applicable to tests of the FAAR model.

Challenges to the use of the FAAR model are similar to those raised for other systems-theory frameworks. Some feel that the model's scope and complexity may be too cumbersome to be practically applied in most studies. Despite the model's relative specificity, the operational definitions of its major constructs of demands, resources, coping, and so forth may be thought too general and may obscure identification of important relationships among critical and specific components or processes. Ultimately, care in the design of studies based on the model and caution in interpreting the results of such studies will be important for advancing the FAAR model and its value in health psychological research.

Family Paradigm Model

Family paradigm models (see Reiss, 1989) draw upon clinical observations of differences among family styles of interaction in the world and, particularly, in confronting challenges. Reiss (1981) has referred to these differing characteristics as rooted in distinct sets of assumptions or beliefs about the environment, the family, and their interactions. These assumptions direct the family to attend to certain aspects of the environment and to ignore others and to view certain circumstances as either threatening or benign. Just as these paradigms influence daily problem solving, they also determine the family's response to challenge, such as the physical illness of a family member.

Reiss (1981) described three relatively orthogonal dimensions of family functioning. *Configuration* refers to the belief that the environment is relatively ordered and, therefore, holds the potential to be mastered as opposed to a perception of the world as chaotic and uncontrollable. *Coordination* is the family's perception of itself as either a collection of individuals or a single unit. Families scoring high on this dimension place a greater value on the solidarity of the family group in responding to the environment in contrast with valuing the autonomous interactions of each family member. The third dimension, *closure*, refers to the family's ability to adapt to new experiences versus being dominated by past experiences.

Reiss (1989) suggested that his model has particular appeal because it adopts an ecologic approach to describing both adaptive and dysfunctional responses to challenge. In this regard, the model may be particularly relevant for describing, if not explaining, differences among families in responding to chronic illness. In particular, the model has important implications for describing how families may appear to handle one or more aspects of adjusting to chronic illness well (e.g., appearing to be cooperative with health care providers' efforts) but may perform poorly on other dimensions of the chronic illness experience (e.g., encouraging dependence of the patient through overly solicitous behavior; Reiss, Gonzalez, & Kramer, 1986). Ultimately, the paradigm model downplays assumptions about normalcy and pathology and, instead, encourages clinical assessment and intervention efforts that respond to the particular strengths and weaknesses of each family.

Oscillation Theory

Oscillation theory (Breunlin, 1989) emphasizes a developmental perspective on family functioning. Central to this model is the notion that a family gains complexity and flexibility in its adaptive functioning through a process of accommodating to the growing competence of its members over the life cycle. Consistent with most life developmental models, growth occurs largely in spurts or increments in which a family is confronted with specific developmental tasks. Periods of oscillation are hypothesized to occur during these specific episodes of growth as the family vacillates between accommodating to the increased competence of its members and promoting growth and maintaining homeostasis and stability. Families that fail to dampen the amplitude of these periods of oscillation in a reasonable time frame or to shorten their duration are prone to the emergence of physical symptoms in the family member whose increased competence is not accepted and incorporated. Thus therapeutic efforts should presumably foster this restrictive, or dampening, process, to promote family development and competence as well as competence of the symptomatic family member.

Chronic illness has not been examined specifically from within the framework of the oscillation theory of family functioning. However, it is reasonable to assume that families may become "stuck" in their efforts to accommodate to a chronically ill member and his or her efforts to manage the disease, its symptoms, and other sequelae. Although the model has not fostered the development of specific clinical assessment procedures, Breunlin (1989) has described the value of careful interviewing and observation to identify episodes of oscillation. Clinical intervention methods based on the work of structural family therapists (Haley, 1976; Minuchin & Fishman, 1981) are particularly encouraged and supported by the model.

Cognitive–Behavioral Perspective

The past 20 years have witnessed a growing dominance of behavioral and cognitive–behavioral perspectives in health psychological and behavioral medicine research and practice. These perspectives emphasize active transactions between individuals and their social environments in the maintenance of health and the treatment and management of illness. These important social interactions are hypothesized to contribute to developing and maintaining health-related cognition and health behaviors; efforts at health behavior change; decisions related to managing physical symptoms, including decisions regarding health care use; experiences during aversive medical diagnostic procedures and surgery; recovery from acute physical illness; adherence to medical and rehabilitation recommendations; and a broad range of health outcomes.

Kerns and colleagues (Kerns & Payne, in press; Kerns & Weiss, 1994; Turk & Kerns, 1985a) have specified a transactional model of family functioning that draws on the family adjustment and adaptation model (Hill, 1949; Patterson, 1989) and family paradigm model (Reiss, 1989) as well as on contemporary models of stress and coping (R. S. Lazarus & Folkman, 1984) within a cognitive–behavioral framework. The transactional model views the family and its individual members as active processors of information who

> (a) seek out information and evaluate the features and characteristics of the information or of specific sources of stress and disruption (e.g., disease); (b) evaluate resources available for responding to the threat; (c) act on the environment and after responding; (d) evaluate the adequacy of the response. (Turk & Kerns, 1985a, p. 12)

In short, the model gives a predominant role to the process of the family appraising itself (including interactions among its members), the environment, and their reciprocal interactions.

Several characteristics of families can be emphasized through the transactional model. A family, as well as its members, develops relatively stable beliefs or schemas about the world and its social interactions that are based in its history and its sociocultural context. Similarly, families develop an array of resources that can be accessed in response to perceived stress and challenge. Although perceptions of stress occur within the family system, they are importantly influenced by the individual member who experiences stress and manifests symptoms that are observable to other members of the family. As is emphasized in the oscillation model of family functioning, the family's resources are enhanced through the growth of individual family members' coping capacities and the incorporation of these additional strengths into the family's coping arsenal. The family's schema and perceptions of available resources will interact to determine its experience of stress, its efforts to respond, and the relative success of its response in eliminating or managing the stress or symptoms. Finally, structural features of the family and its stage in the life cycle each play important roles in determining the perceived nature of stress and the family's response.

The transactional nature of the cognitive–behavioral model of family functioning emphasizes that the family's responses to stress in turn shape the experience of stress, and so on in a reciprocal and dynamic manner. An example of the complicated nature of this transactional process has been documented in the chronic pain literature. Several studies have documented a positive relationship between positive spouse or significant others' responses to demonstrations of pain and patient reports of pain severity and disability (e.g., Kerns et al., 1991; Romano et al., 1992). The results have been interpreted to support an operant conditioning model of chronic pain that highlights the role of positive reinforcement for "pain behaviors" and the maintenance of the chronic pain experience. It appears likely that family members' efforts to offer support to the member in pain may inadvertently exacerbate or perpetuate the experience of pain, declines in activity, and growing disability. The resulting increases in pain may lead to further "solicitous" responding on the part of concerned others, in a manner consistent with a positive feedback loop.

Consistent with the cognitive–behavioral perspective, Kerns and his colleagues (1991) have recently suggested that future research should examine patient attributions of spousal responses to more fully understand the nature of these interactions. For example, a patient may view a spouse's efforts at "distraction" as either a supportive and selfless action or an effort to terminate the pain behavior (e.g., complaints of pain) for more selfish reasons (cf. Fincham & Bradbury, 1992). Similarly, a pain patient who perceives others as generally unsympathetic may be particularly prone to depression as an additional consequence of experiencing pain. Alternatively, a patient who experiences a generally high level of global marital satisfaction may view a spouse's "negative" response, such as an expression of irritation, as a reasonable cue for more adaptive coping. Evidence has suggested that such patients report relatively low levels of pain, disability, and distress (Kerns, Haythornthwaite, Southwick, & Giller, 1990; Turk, Kerns, & Rosenberg, 1992).

The transactional model of family functioning proposed encourages clinical assessment at the individual, dyadic, and family levels of analysis. As a model based in learning theory, it focuses on contingent relationships between environmental events and the response of the family and its members, particularly at the microlevel or behaviorally specific level of analysis. As such, attention has largely been limited to analyzing dyadic interactions within families—for example, between spouses (e.g., Romano et al., 1992) or between mother and child (e.g., Bush, Melamed, Sheras, & Greenbaum, 1986). Direct observation of such interactions is the cornerstone of the model, and researchers have been encouraged to develop reliable, structured observation systems. Most recently, Hops and his colleagues (Hops et al., 1988) have developed the Living in Family Environments (LIFE) coding system to provide real-time analysis of multiple ongoing interactions within the family. So far, application of these methods has been limited to research settings because of the time required and expense incurred in the coding process. Alternative, behaviorally specific self-report inventories and diary procedures that may have both clinical and research utility have begun to be developed. Examples include the Significant Other Response Scales from the West Haven–Yale Multidimensional Pain Inventory (Kerns, Turk, & Rudy, 1985) and the Spouse Diary (Flor, Kerns, & Turk, 1987), which are designed to assess the frequency of solicitous, distracting, and negative responses from others in the presence of a family member's expressions of pain.

In the assessment of the family's cognition regarding its transactions, specific measures grounded in cognitive theory have not been forthcoming. Recent advances in the cognitive marital therapy literature, such as the development of measures of causal attributions for spouse communication, may prove useful in assessing family cognition (Fincham & Bradbury, 1992). In addition to these efforts, it is apparent that clinical and research procedures based in other models of family functioning may be applicable, including measures designed to characterize important family schema and typical modes of appraisal, problem solving, and coping. Future research and clinical experience with these numerous measures by those wedded to a cognitive–behavioral perspective is necessary to determine their ultimate validity within this conceptual framework. See Table 1 for an overview of family models and their salient clinical features.

Role of the Family in the Development of Chronic Illness

Increasing evidence has supported the contributions of such behavioral risk factors as smoking, lack of exercise, and poor diet to the development of a number of chronic illnesses. The family's role in the initiation and maintenance of many of these pathogenic behaviors has become an important target of speculation and investigation (Burg & Seeman, 1994). For example, there is some evidence to support widely held beliefs that parents substantially influence their children's development of conceptions of health and illness and health behaviors (Mechanic, 1964; Pratt, 1976). There is also growing evidence of shared risk factors among family members (Baranowski & Nader, 1985; Barrett-Connor, Suarez, & Criqui, 1982; Deutscher, Epstein, & Kjelsberg, 1966; Smith, 1992), that families contribute to determinations of members' compliance with risk behavior change (Becker & Green, 1975), and that involvement of family members in health-risk-intervention trials can improve success (Epstein, Koeske, Wing, & Va-

Table 1

Models of Family Functioning Relevant to Considering the Role of the Family in Chronic Illness

Model	Central concepts	Assessment	Intervention
Beavers System Model (Beavers, 1981, 1989)	Family competence; Family style	Obervational system: self-report instrument (Beavers, 1989)	Psychotherapy based on the model
Circumflex Model	Two core dimensions: cohesion and adaptability and core process communication	Family Adaptability and Cohesion Evaluation Scales (FACES III; Olson, Portner, & Lavee, 1985); Clinical Rating Scale (CRS; Olson & Killorin, 1985)	None described
Family Adjustment and Adaptation Response Model (FAAR; Patterson, 1989)	Perceived stress; family resources; family paradigms	Family Inventory of Life Events and Changes (FILE; H. I. McCubbin, Patterson, & Wilson, 1981); Family Inventory of Resources for Management (FIRM; H. McCubbin, Comeau, & Harkins, 1981); Coping Health Inventory for Parents (CHIP; H. McCubbin et al., 1983); Family Coping	None described

		Strategies (F-COPES; H. McCubbin, Larsen, & Olson, 1982); Family Hardiness Index (FHI; M. A. McCubbin, McCubbin, & Thompson, 1987)	
Family Paradigm Model (Reiss, 1989)	Confirmation, coordination, and closure	As above, for FAAR Model	None described
Oscillation Theory (Breunlin, 1989)	Developmental model; complexity, flexibility, and oscillation	None specifically described	Structural family therapy to promote dampening of the oscillation process
Cognitive–behavioral perspective (Kerns & Weiss, 1994; Turk & Kerns, 1985a)	Transactional model; family appraisal, family beliefs and schema, family coping resources	Behavioral observation (LIFE; Hops et al., 1988); Significant Other Response Scales (WHYMPI; Kerns, Turk, & Rudy, 1985); Spouse Diary (Flor, Kerns, & Turk, 1987)	Cognitive–behavioral therapy

loski, 1986; Epstein, Wing, Koeske, Andrasik, & Ossip, 1981; Mermelstein, Lichtenstein, & McIntyre, 1983). In fact, spousal or partner support has been found to be the best predictor of continued abstinence from smoking (Coppotelli & Orleans, 1985; Mermelstein et al., 1983).

Social interaction, particularly among family members, has recently been hypothesized to interact with individuals' pervasive hostile beliefs about others to create a heightened state of vulnerability for cardiovascular disease (Brown & Smith, 1992; Ewart, Taylor, Kraemer, & Agras, 1984; Smith, 1992; Smith & Christensen, 1992). According to this thesis, individuals most at risk are those who not only maintain a hostile and cynical view of the world and others but also contribute to, and frequently experience, interpersonal challenges that reinforce these pathogenic beliefs and elicit heightened cardiovascular reactivity. As researchers begin to consider the synergistic effects of behavioral risk factors, the role of family interactions is likely to become a greater focus of attention (e.g., Venters, 1989). Ultimately, family or marital interventions targeting improved communication may serve to lower risks for developing chronic illness (e.g., Ewart et al., 1984).

The influence of the family in the development of chronic nonmalignant pain offers one more example of the possible effect that the family has in the development of a chronic health problem. According to operant theory, expressions of acute pain (e.g., complaining of pain, grimacing, avoidance of activity, and use of pain medication)—because they are overt and observable—may be selectively reinforced by expressions of concern from others and, over time, may come under the control of such social contingencies. Recent research has supported this model by demonstrating that spousal solicitousness in response to expressions of pain is positively associated with higher levels of reported pain, pain behavior frequency, and disability (Romano et al., 1992). The importance of these observations extends well beyond the chronic pain literature and has implications for the development and perpetuation of symptoms and disabilities associated with other chronic illnesses.

Finally, the experience of chronic stress within the family can be hypothesized to contribute to the development of chronic illness. The rapidly emerging field of psychoneuroimmunology (Ader, 1981; Borysenko, 1989), for example, encourages more specific consideration of the role of family stress and the emergence and progression of infectious disease (Schmidt & Schmidt, 1989) and cancer (Fox, 1989). Similarly, the relationship between family stress and the endocrine and cardiovascular systems deserves continued attention (Eliot, 1989). The models of family functioning already described in this chapter may be particularly useful as frameworks for considering the role of family stress in the development of biological dysfunction.

Efforts to intervene within families to reduce risk for the development of chronic illness are rarely considered by clinicians, let alone reported in the literature. In spite of this apparent neglect, several suggestions can be offered to the health psychologist. First, when assessing the risk-factor status of an individual, one should consider the possibility of shared risk within the family. In the case of such risk factors as poor diet and lack of exercise, for example, specific barriers to behavior change within the family should be considered: for example, the spouse who is primarily responsible for food purchasing and preparation may need to be drawn into the clinical assessment and intervention-planning processes. Family as well as individual beliefs about risk behavior are additional targets for assessment. Again, the family assessment strategies outlined in this chapter may be particularly helpful in this regard.

Health psychologists are increasingly involved in efforts to support individuals and their families during acute illness episodes, in preparation for aversive medical diagnostic procedures, and before and after surgery (e.g., Manne et al., 1992). Clinical engagement of families during these periods of heightened risk for the development of unnecessary disability and distress may serve a preventive purpose. In this context, assessing family functioning and identifying patterns that may undermine adaptive coping and optimal recovery may prove helpful. Specific efforts that encourage delivery of emotional and instrumental support from families to patients are particularly encouraged in light of recent empirical findings (Fontana, Kerns, Rosenberg, & Colonese, 1989; Jay & Elliott, 1990; Kulik & Mahler, 1989; Madan-Swain & Brown, 1991).

It is the promise of a science of family systems medicine to develop methods that are useful for detecting maladaptive patterns of family functioning as well as successful intervention strategies for promoting the health of the family and its members. As they move toward attaining this goal, health psychologists in a range of health care settings should attend to the contemporary models of family functioning outlined above and incorporate family assessment strategies into their routine clinical work.

Role of the Family in the Management of Chronic Illness

It has been asserted that the family of an individual with a diagnosed chronic illness may significantly determine the course of the illness with regard to each of its four primary domains: (a) the disease itself, (b) its symptomatic expression, (c) the extent of its associated disability, and (d) the extent of distress it causes. Within this multidimensional framework, transactions within the family may differentially affect each of these domains. The clinician working to promote adaptation and optimal management of an illness by involving family members should consider the different facets of the illness along with the family's specific roles with regard to each domain.

Applications of family systems theories in the health domain have generally acknowledged the inadvertent deleterious effects of the family on disease progression, symptomatic expression, and disability in the apparent service of maintaining a homeostasis and managing distress within the family and its members, including the patient. Within the cognitive–behavioral transaction model, families may maintain a high level of positive interaction that promotes general feelings of marital and family satisfaction and psychological well-being at the expense of reinforcing such illness behaviors as verbal and nonverbal expressions of the illness, dependency on others, and reduced productive activity. Empirical evidence from the chronic pain literature has offered support for this common clinical observation (Kerns et al., 1991).

Several additional functional family variables may affect the progression of disease. To the extent that other family members share such risk factors as smoking or diet, the family may actively resist or simply fail to support the patient's efforts to change his or her behavior. Cues for the risk behavior may remain present in the family environment and family members may even directly or inadvertently reinforce the risk behavior of the patient.

Family cognition may also substantially undermine efforts to change risk behaviors or manage illness. Families with a generally avoidant problem-solving style or those that lack specific skills or confidence in their ability to make decisions on behalf of the patient's illness may further interfere with optimal management. For example, the management regimen of a child with insulin-dependent diabetes mellitus is complicated and requires considerable knowledge and skill. The problem-solving style and skills of the family in this situation are likely to be critical (Hanson, Henggeler, Harris, Burghen, & Moore, 1989).

Observation of the patient following acute myocardial infarction offers another compelling example of this multidimensional perspective on chronic illness. The frequency of denial among cardiac patients has been documented in several studies. Levine et al. (1987) noted that patients who deny or minimize their reports of the severity of an acute myocardial infarction benefit by reduced experiences of distress as well as fewer complications and shorter stays in the hospital. However, denial was found to be associated with poor adherence to recommendations for behavior risk reduction and predicted increased morbidity over the following year. Families, in their efforts to be supportive and protective of the patient, may unwittingly discourage more realistic appraisal and important lifestyle changes. Therefore, positive effects of the family's response in terms of reduced affective distress and disability unfortunately may be associated with more rapid progression of chronic disease. Continued empirical examination and clinical assessment of these differential effects is indicated.

Management of the Disease Process

Some discussion of the possible roles of the family with regard to each of the four domains of chronic illness may prove helpful in emphasizing this multidimensional perspective. Similar to the role hypothesized for the family in primary prevention efforts, an important family role in efforts to arrest or reduce the progression of a chronic disease can be assumed. Drawing on this perspective, there have been increasing attempts by health care practitioners to involve family members in educating patients about risk factors and methods of behavior change. Additional efforts to involve family members in promoting adherence to medication and rehabilitation regimens and other aspects of disease management have also been increasingly documented (e.g., Radojevic, Nicassio, & Weisman, 1992). Although not yet well described, interventions to reduce the experience of stress and promote adaptive coping within the family are worth encouraging—not only because of their more apparent effects on psychological well-being but also in support of other efforts to reduce potential stress-related effects on physical functioning and disease progression.

Examples from the childhood diabetes literature represent this perspective (Hauser et al., 1986; Johnson, 1985). Educating parents about the disease itself and principles of glucose metabolism serves as the basis for collaborative efforts to promote optimal regulation. Additional family-based interventions have been encouraged that promote a generally healthy lifestyle, stress reduction, adherence to a complicated behavioral regimen, and, ultimately, shifting responsibility for management from the parents to the maturing child or adolescent. An ongoing relationship between the health care provider and the family of a child with diabetes is critical to maximize disease control and reduce the devastating effects of its progression. Involvement of a family health psychologist as part of an interdisciplinary effort in this regard is increasingly common.

Symptom Management

It is increasingly apparent that the family's response to the observable manifestations of the disease itself plays an important, if not central, role in determining the frequency, severity, and impact of these symptoms. The hypothesis that chronic illness behaviors—that is, the "sick role"—may develop largely as a function of solicitous responding by others has a long history and is a widely held belief among health care providers. Increasingly apparent, however, is the likelihood that the responses of others (particularly family members) may have effects across the illness spectrum and may serve to minimize symptom expression as well as encourage it. Examples from the clinical and research literatures across the human life span support these notions. There has been evidence that a family's style of interacting may influence seizure frequency among children with epilepsy (Hauck, 1972) and diabetic control among children (Johnson, 1980), complaints of pain and pain intensity among adult chronic-pain patients (e.g., Flor et al., 1987) and those with rheumatoid arthritis and fibromyalgia syndrome (Nicassio & Radojevic, 1993), and increased symptoms among elderly patients with Alzheimer's disease (Blumenthal, 1979).

Clinical health psychologists are called on in health care settings to evaluate patients who, in the opinion of their physicians, are experiencing symptoms at a frequency or intensity beyond that explained by the severity of physical findings. Assessment of these patients should routinely consider the social and, particularly, the family context in which they live. Beliefs of patients and family members about a disease and its symptomatic expression are important targets for assessment, as are observations and reports of family patterns of response to patients' symptoms.

Almost invariably, when patterns of solicitousness or overprotectiveness are observed, family members also express heightened concern for the patient as well as a pervasive sense of helplessness about how to help him or her cope more effectively or manage his or her level of symptoms and associated distress. Most often, family members acknowledge that their efforts at providing support are ineffective. Likewise, patients are often able to acknowledge their sense of burden on their families. Family systems models offer varying concepts to describe or even explain this frequently observed constellation of family cognition and behavior. Generally, the pattern appears to reflect an inflexibility within the family to meet the particular challenges of the illness, efforts to manage distress at virtually all costs, and a willingness to compromise the individual family member's autonomy on behalf of the "sick" family.

As an important first step in the therapeutic process, the transactional cognitive–behavioral perspective encourages relatively direct feedback to the family about its characteristic patterns of communicating about a member's illness. Patterns of communication are described in learning terms that encourage perceptions of hopefulness about the possibility for change rather than frameworks implying relatively rigid and inflexible patterns of family functioning. Similarly, rather than criticizing the family for "causing" the symptoms, the clinician should demonstrate an understanding of the adaptive function of the patterns of behavior while beginning to address some of their most obvious deleterious effects. Reflection of the family members' distress is critically important in engaging the patient and family members in future efforts to change.

While acknowledging the family's perceptions of helplessness, the clinician can offer suggestions about alternative ways of communicating support and concern. He or she should emphasize collaborative problem solving that moves toward identifying responses that encourage more adaptive behavioral coping on the part of the patient. Cognitive and behavioral barriers to these responses should also be identified and discussed. The patient and family members are ultimately encouraged to negotiate alternative means of communicating about the illness, but more general styles of communicating about other domains of family activities and functions are emphasized. Clinicians routinely assign family members "homework" in the form of planned communication exercises and pleasurable family activities.

Disability Management

Closely linked to the patient's symptomatic manifestations of an illness are behaviors that leave him or her functionally disabled. In the case of many musculoskeletal and neurological disorders, for example, primary symptoms such as fatigue, distorted ambulation, or complaints of pain are relatively directly associated with avoidance of or declines in productive activity. Family transactions that support symptom expression may serve as primary contributors to the development and perpetuation of these functional declines.

In the case of primarily asymptomatic chronic illnesses such as hypertension, illness-related cognition may play a greater role in perpetuation of the disability. Family schema that encourage overprotection of the patient and reduction of roles within and outside the family could specifically contribute to progressive declines in activity. The clinician should consider using cognitive assessment and focused interventions within a cognitive–behavioral framework with these families. To date, however, there have been no empirical efforts to evaluate the efficacy of a family-focused intervention of this type.

Promotion of a Positive Affective Response

Considerable attention has been paid by psychologists to the family's influence on the ill family member's psychological adaptation to the illness. Generally speaking, clinical observation and empirical evidence have documented that chronically ill individuals as a group suffer from increased psychological distress and diminished quality of life. However, it is equally apparent that only a subset of chronically ill individuals suffer from significant psychopathology and that many report a high level of life satisfaction (Banks & Kerns, in press). In addition to the characteristics of the disease itself and the individual's premorbid coping resources, the role of the family as a determinant of the psychological adaptation of the chronically ill individual remains an important question. In general, it appears that a family viewed as supportive is associated with lower levels of distress (e.g., Kerns & Turk, 1984). However, more specific aspects of an illness and its interactions within the family deserve focused attention.

A cognitive–behavioral mediational model of depression secondary to chronic pain, with relevance to chronic illness more generally, has been proposed (Rudy, Kerns, & Turk, 1988). According to the model, declines in instrumental activity and perceptions of self-control that are frequently associated with chronic pain are important mediators of the development of depression. Spousal support has been further hypothesized to mediate the relationship between the experience of pain and declines in activity and self-control (Turk, Kerns, & Rudy, 1984). To the extent that spouses' responding to patients' expressions of pain serves to promote disability, dependence, and declines in perceptions of control, patients may be more likely to experience depressive symptoms. Alternatively, G. M. Goldberg, Kerns, & Rosenberg (1993) found that pain-relevant spouse support could be an important buffer from depression in the context of a general decline in activity. These results suggest a level of complexity beyond the realm of examination of main effects or even simple interactions.

Certainly the most frequent reason for referring a chronically ill patient to a clinical health psychologist is the presence of significant affective distress, most frequently manifested as either depression or anxiety. In virtually every case, it is critical to consider the patient's social and, in particular, familial, context. Assessment should target global family satisfaction as well as more specific transactions focused on the illness itself and efforts to manage it, family members' responses to symptoms and behavioral disability, and their responses to displays of distress. Knowledge related to patient and family members' attributions about these transactions may prove particularly useful. Interventions designed to promote constructive communication among family members, to encourage continued productive and pleasurable activity within and outside the family, and to enhance perceptions of self-control and mastery related to the illness appear to have the strongest theoretical and empirical support (Kerns & Weiss, 1994).

Impact of Chronic Illness on the Family

Until recently, disproportionate attention has been placed on observing and evaluating how chronic illness affects the family, as opposed to considering how the family might influence the chronically ill individual. The basis for this discrepancy almost certainly lies in the dominant biomedical perspective that generally fails to consider the importance of psychosocial variables. Similarly, inspection of the literature on the impact of chronic illness on the family shows that the family has only recently begun to be considered as playing an active and dynamic role in determining the illness experience. Historically, a significant negative impact on others in a patients' environment has been presumed, and optimal adaptation has frequently been considered an anomaly.

There can be no doubt that chronic illness in a family member, regardless of the developmental phase of the family unit, poses a tremendous series of challenges to the family and its members. Nevertheless, theory, clinical observation, and research have begun to appreciate the complexity of the determinants of family adaptation to such illness (e.g., Croog & Fitzgerald, 1978; Fife, Norton, & Groom, 1987; Kazak, 1989; Madan-Swain & Brown, 1991; Magni, Carli, De Leo, Tshilolo, & Zanesco, 1986; Revenson & Majerovitz, 1991; Tompkins, Schulz, & Rau, 1988; Turk, Flor, & Rudy, 1987). Outcomes of interest include the physical and social well-being of other family members, in addition to the more limited historical concern focused on identifying psychological distress and psychiatric disorder among them. Longitudinal observation has replaced cross-sectional investigation as the state of the art in research design, allowing for examination of the dynamic interplay of important determinants of adaptation over time (e.g., Fife et al., 1987; Fontana et al., 1989; Kovacs et al., 1990; Magni et al., 1986; Tompkins et al., 1988). Clinical efforts in this domain are understandably broader in scope and better informed by research. An exciting development is the recent effort to identify early predictors of later distress among family members, which promises to lead to increased efficiency in service delivery (e.g., Kovacs et al., 1990).

Variables of Influence

The perspective on the domains of chronic illness outlined in this chapter may be helpful in considerations of how chronic illness affects the family. For example, it is clear that aspects of the disease itself significantly determine the challenges placed on the family. Disease variables that influence the impact on the family include the age of onset (and, therefore, the developmental stage of the family), the prognosis (i.e., life threatening, uncertain, or clearly benign), the evolving versus resolving nature (e.g., of cancer vs. stroke) of the disorder, and the level of complexity of the medical management regimen, among others. Similarly, symptom severity and degree of impairment and disability have important implications both for the family's developing beliefs about the disorder and for family functioning. Finally, the patient's degree of adaptation to the disorder—including his or her affective response—can be expected to affect the family's response.

Significant interactions among these domains can also be considered. For example, childhood disorders that require heightened parental vigilance and child dependence, although certainly challenging, may be less threatening to the established parenting roles of the caregivers than a similarly disabling disorder in a spouse that requires dramatic shifts in familial roles and responsibilities. Equally complex are situations in which the family member with a life-threatening disorder or severe cognitive and physical impairment fails to display a true appreciation of the disorder and prognosis, minimizes symptoms, and shows affective indifference. This example stands in contrast to the family member with a relatively benign disorder who demonstrates continuous and pronounced symptoms, disability, and affective distress. From these examples, it is easy to appreciate the differential contributions of aspects of chronic illness in attempts to understand the family's response.

Trends and Recommendations for Assessment and Intervention

Despite an extensive literature that helps to describe the varied effects of chronic illness on the family, explanatory models are in their infancy, and little empirical information is available to guide clinical efforts on behalf of families. Nevertheless, a few general principles can be offered.

Careful clinical assessment of how chronic illness affects the family should certainly include those involved most closely with the patient (e.g., a parent or spouse), but others in the immediate or even extended family network should be considered as well. There has been growing evidence that reliance on a single family member for information about the family may be misleading (Litman, 1989). Specifically, two studies have revealed that siblings of children with chronic illnesses may develop perceptions of relative neglect by their parents or may feel pressure to compensate for the perceived deficiencies of their sibling (Carr-Gregg & White, 1987; Long & Moore, 1979). A similar situation may develop among children whose parents serve primary caregiver roles for an elderly family member. Assessment of families should target members' attitudes about the illness and its impact (e.g., Willer, Allen, Liss, & Zicht, 1991), perceived changes in familial and extrafamilial roles and responsibilities (e.g., Allaire, Meenan, & Anderson, 1991), perceptions of burden and the broader emotional response of family members (Brooks & McKinlay, 1983), and perceptions of support within the family and from those outside the family (Hobfoll & Lerman, 1989; Revenson & Majerovitz, 1991). Critically important are family members' reports on the availability of information about the illness and their perceptions of their access to health care providers (e.g., Oddy, Humphrey, & Uttley, 1978).

A wide variety of family interventions have been encouraged and described as valuable components of comprehensive care for those who are chronically ill. Group interventions for members of multiple families have particularly been encouraged because of the perceived importance of sharing concerns, problem solving with others in similar situations, and delivering emotional and informational support. Self-help as well as professionally led group programs for family members of chronically ill patients have increasingly become available (Levy, 1976). Over the past several years, there have been increasing efforts to develop and evaluate the efficacy of specific group intervention programs for family members, which may or may not include patients (R. J. Goldberg, Wool, Tull, & Boor, 1984; L. W. Lazarus, Stafford, Cooper, Cohler, & Dysken, 1981). Future efforts to provide families with professional support through group therapy will benefit from attention to the specific goals of intervention, the theoretical and clinical basis for selecting the intervention process and its components, and efforts to evaluate their efficacy.

Intervention with the family of a chronically ill individual should follow a careful multidimensional assessment. The transactional framework I described earlier encourages a process that leads to identifying specific areas of concern or stress as well as to evaluating the family's available resources for managing challenges posed by the illness. The therapist should develop an overarching conceptualization of the reciprocal interactions between the family and identified patient that informs the development of a detailed and goal-directed treatment plan. The specific strategies used will depend on the problems identified and the illness and family variables that are hypothesized to contribute to the problems. Several specific targets for intervention are frequently identified through this process of assessment and treatment planning.

Complaints of a lack of information and limits on the accessibility of physicians are a common concern among families of chronically ill patients. Clinicians may serve as a patient and family advocate in some situations and intervene directly on their behalf to facilitate communication. More commonly, family cognition that interferes with assertiveness and, in some cases, family members' assertiveness skill deficits, are important targets for intervention.

Patients and families often report problems of communication within the family with regard to the illness and its sequelae (Kerns & Curley, 1985). Patients report a range of concerns: feelings of burden, guilt, and discomfort with growing dependence, on the one hand, or anger that family members do not appreciate the extent of the illness and expect too much, on the other hand. Families similarly report a range of concerns about the patient's response to the illness, their own behaviors on behalf of the patient, and his or her efforts to manage the illness and adapt to its presence. Clinicians may generally serve an important role by encouraging open sharing and discussion of beliefs and feelings, may attempt to interpret patterns of communication and offer feedback about its adaptive versus maladaptive nature, and may intervene directly to alter patterns of communication.

Related concerns are issues of shifting roles and responsibilities within the family. Clinicians may facilitate discussions about these concerns and intervene to help families renegotiate or clarify these changes. Specific problem-solving discussions are often indicated. Particular challenges for families about the fine line between fostering dependency versus realistic appraisal of the patients' deficits are important areas for discussion (Blumenthal, 1979).

A particular challenge for many families is the need to maintain a reasonable frequency of pleasurable activity in the face of illness—both as a family or, for parents of a chronically ill child or adult caregivers of an elderly family member, activities as a couple. Specific attention from clinicians to this concern is frequently indicated. In addition, family members often benefit from clinicians' encouragement for independent activities away from the home. Discussion of the beliefs that interfere with planning for activities as well as use of goal setting and social contracting can be helpful to many families.

In families of a terminally ill or severely cognitively impaired family member, feelings of loss, grief, and guilt are important targets for intervention. Clinician–family discussions focusing on acknowledging and exploring these and associated feelings are encouraged. When appropriate, discussions that move toward a consideration of a future without the family member can also be helpful. However, timing of such discussions is a difficult decision that warrants specific thought and planning.

Encouragement and assistance to the family with regard to specific planning around finances and advanced directives for medical care (LaPuma, Orentlicher, & Moss, 1991) are increasingly roles that may involve the family health psychologist (see Zisook, Peterkin, Shuchter, & Bardone, chap. 10, this book). Other issues, such as decisions regarding institutionalization, also fall within this realm (Blumenthal, 1979). Helping the family articulate its concerns and discuss alternatives is important. Referral to others who can more explicitly assist the family and patient with these problems is an additionally valuable service.

The empirical literature increasingly documents the value of social support for the family coping with a chronically ill member in moderating or buffering the experience of stress (e.g., Revenson & Majerovitz, 1991). Explicit discussions with the family members that define their current level of support and their beliefs and efforts regarding the engagement of others as support are recommended as routine components of family intervention. Attention can be focused on family efforts to support one another within the family and to engage friends and extended family members in obtaining emotional support. Family members can also be encouraged to identify their needs for assistance in the care of the chronically ill patient on an ongoing or intermittent basis. Specific assistance in arranging for additional care or even respite may be reasonably offered by the health psychologist, or referrals to more appropriate providers can be made.

The question of when to offer clinical services to the family of a chronically ill individual remains open. Increasingly, psychologists serve as part of interdisciplinary teams and offer, at a minimum, brief consultations to families on a relatively routine basis. Even more extensive assessment and treatment of the family is now common in many clinical settings, such as programs for the management of chronic pain, cardiac rehabilitation programs, comprehensive cancer centers, and renal dialysis centers. Ongoing and intensive involvement of families in the care of children or adolescents who have chronic illnesses is almost universal.

In clinical settings not involving interdisciplinary team functioning, evaluation of the family context is most often initiated in one of two common scenarios. In the first, psychologists may be consulted to assess a family that is noted to be experiencing an unusually high level of distress. Most often, open discussions of the family's concerns and efforts to "normalize" concerns, provide information, or provide minimal feedback about alternative perspectives on concerns may be sufficient. In some situations, however, more formal assessment and intervention planning may be indicated. In these cases it is not uncommon for family members to be quite accepting of professional support.

Patient nonadherence and the clinician's assessment that the family may play a key role in soliciting nonadherence is a second common reason for psychological consultation. In these cases, careful interviewing, observation of interaction patterns among family members, and, occasionally, the use of standardized questionnaires and inventories are important for developing and testing hypotheses about family influence on a patient's overall adaptation to the illness and adherence to medical and other recommendations. Clinicians must provide direct feedback to the family and patient regarding the results of this assessment in terms that the family can understand to set the stage for more extensive interventions. Brief family therapy that targets concrete behavioral change and, rarely, more substantial involvement that targets family schema and communication, can prove helpful in improving outcomes. Pending further systematic investigations, the alternative conceptual frameworks described earlier in this chapter may be equally effective to clinicians undertaking this more substantial work with families. Future clinical trials evaluating the comparative efficacy of these frameworks with specific chronic illness populations will document their use for the practitioner.

Summary

I have provided a broad overview of the various issues relevant to considering the families of chronically ill individuals. The breadth of this domain is represented by considerations of the multidimensional aspects of chronic illness and family functioning, as well as their interaction. The importance and magnitude of this area are also exemplified by the several models of family functioning, clinical assessment and intervention, and research that have been highlighted in this chapter. The role of the family in chronic illness brings into focus numerous salient issues illustrated by the biopsychosocial model. Attention to the multidimensional and transactional nature of the issues faced by families of chronically ill patients is critical to advances in theory, research, and practice in this area.

REFERENCES

Ader, R. (1981). *Psychoneuroimmunology.* San Diego, CA: Academic Press.

Allaire, S. H., Meenan, R. F., & Anderson, J. J. (1991). The impact of rheumatoid arthritis on the household work performance of women. *Arthritis and Rheumatism, 34,* 669–678.

Baker, L. C., & Patterson, J. M. (1989). Introduction to family theory. In C. N. Ramsey, Jr. (Ed.), *Family systems in medicine* (pp. 57–61). New York: Guilford Press.

Banks, S., & Kerns, R. D. (in press). Explaining high rates of depression in chronic pain: A diathesis-stress framework. *Psychological Bulletin.*

Baranowski, T., & Nader, P. R. (1985). Family health behavior. In D. C. Turk & R. D. Kerns (Eds.), *Families, health and illness: A life-span perspective* (pp. 51–80). New York: Wiley Interscience.

Barrett-Connor, E., Suarez, L., & Criqui, M. H. (1982). A spouse concordance of plasma cholesterol and triglyceride. *Journal of Chronic Diseases, 35,* 333–340.

Beavers, W. R. (1981). A systems model of family for family therapists. *Journal of Marital and Family Therapy, 203,* 299–307.

Beavers, W. R. (1989). Beavers systems model. In C. N. Ramsey, Jr. (Ed.), *Family systems in medicine* (pp. 62–74). New York: Guilford Press.

Becker, M. H., & Green, L. W. (1975). A family approach to compliance with medical treatment: A selective review of the literature. *International Journal of Health Education, 18,* 2–11.

Blumenthal, M. D. (1979). Psychosocial factors in reversible and irreversible brain damage. *Journal of Clinical and Experimental Gerontology, 1,* 39–55.

Boden, S. D., Davis, D. O., Dina, T. S., Patronis, N. J., & Wiesel, S. W. (1990). Abnormal magnetic-resonance scans of the lumbar spine in asymptomatic subjects. *Journal of Bone and Joint Surgery, 72-A,* 403–408.

Borysenko, J. (1989). Psychoneuroimmunology. In C. N. Ramsey, Jr. (Ed.), *Family systems in medicine* (pp. 243–256). New York: Guilford Press.

Breunlin, D. C. (1989). Clinical implications of oscillation theory: Family development and the process of change. In C. N. Ramsey (Ed.), *Family systems in medicine* (pp. 135–149). New York: Guilford Press.

Brooks, D. N., & McKinlay, W. (1983). Personality and behavioral change after severe blunt head injury—A relative's view. *Journal of Neurology, Neurosurgery, and Psychiatry, 46,* 336–344.

Brown, P. C., & Smith, T. W. (1992). Social influence, marriage, and the heart: Cardiovascular consequences of interpersonal control in husbands and wives. *Health Psychology, 11,* 88–96.

Burg, M. M., Jain, D., Soufer, R., Kerns, R. D., & Zaret, B. L. (1993). Role of behavioral and psychological factors in mental-stress-induced silent left ventricular dysfunction in coronary artery disease. *Journal of the American College of Cardiology, 22,* 440–448.

Burg, M. M., & Seeman, T. E. (1994). Families and health: The negative side of social ties. *Annals of Behavioral Medicine, 16,* 109–115.

Bush, J. P., Melamed, B. G., Sheras, P. L., & Greenbaum, P. E. (1986). Mother–child patterns of coping with anticipatory medical stress. *Health Psychology, 5,* 137–157.

Carr-Gregg, M., & White, L. (1987). Siblings of pediatric cancer patients: A population at risk. *Medical and Pediatric Oncology, 15,* 62–68.

Coppotelli, H. C., & Orleans, C. T. (1985). Partner support and other determinants of smoking cessation maintenance among women. *Journal of Consulting and Clinical Psychology, 53,* 455–460.

Croog, S. H., & Fitzgerald, E. F. (1978). Subjective stress and serious illness of a spouse: Wives of heart patients. *Journal of Health and Social Behavior, 19,* 166–178.

Dean, A., Lin, N., & Ensel, W. M. (1981). The epidemiological significance of social support systems in depression. In R. G. Simmons (Ed.), *Research in community mental health: Vol. 2. A research annual* (pp. 77–109). Greenwich, CT: JAI Press.

Deutscher, S., Epstein, F. H., & Kjelsberg, M. O. (1966). Familial aggregation of factors associated with coronary heart disease. *Circulation, 33,* 911–924.

Eliot, R. S. (1989). Family systems, stress, the endocrine system, and the heart. In C. N. Ramsey, Jr. (Ed.), *Family systems in medicine* (pp. 283–293). New York: Guilford Press.

Epstein, L. H., Koeske, R., Wing, R. R., & Valoski, A. (1986). The effect of family variables on child weight change. *Health Psychology, 5,* 1–12.

Epstein, L. H., Wing, R. R., Koeske, R., Andrasik, F., & Ossip, D. J. (1981). Child and parent weight loss in family-based behavior modification programs. *Journal of Consulting and Clinical Psychology, 49,* 674–685.

Ewart, C. K., Taylor, C. B., Kraemer, H. C., & Agras, W. S. (1984). Reducing blood pressure reactivity during interpersonal conflict: Effects of marital communication training. *Behavior Therapy, 15,* 473–484.

Fife, B., Norton, J., & Groom, G. (1987). The family's adaptation to childhood leukemia. *Social Science and Medicine, 24,* 159–168.

Fincham, F. D., & Bradbury, T. N. (1992). Assessing attributions in marriage: The relationship attribution measure. *Journal of Personality and Social Psychology, 62,* 457–468.

Flor, H., Kerns, R. D., & Turk, D. C. (1987). The role of spouse reinforcement, perceived pain, and activity levels of chronic pain patients. *Journal of Psychosomatic Research, 31,* 251–259.

Fontana, A. F., Kerns, R. D., Rosenberg, R. L., & Colonese, K. L. (1989). Support, stress, and recovery from coronary heart disease: A longitudinal causal model. *Health Psychology, 8,* 175–194.

Fox, B. H. (1989). Cancer survival and the family. In C. N. Ramsey, Jr. (Ed.), *Family systems in medicine* (pp. 273–280). New York: Guilford Press.

Friedman, H. (1992). *Hostility, coping and health.* Washington, DC: American Psychological Association.

Goldberg, G. M., Kerns, R. D., & Rosenberg, R. (1993). Pain relevant support as a buffer from depression among chronic pain patients low in instrumental activity. *Clinical Journal of Pain, 9,* 34–40.

Goldberg, R. J., Wool, M., Tull, R., & Boor, M. (1984). Teaching brief psychotherapy for spouses of cancer patients: Use of a codable supervision format. *Psychotherapy and Psychosomatics, 41,* 12–19.

Haley, J. (1976). *Problem-solving therapy.* San Francisco: Jossey-Bass.

Hanson, C. L., Henggeler, S. W., Harris, M. A., Burghen, G. A., & Moore, M. (1989). Family system variables and the health status of adolescents with insulin-dependent diabetes mellitus. *Health Psychology, 8,* 239–254.

Hanson, C. L., Henggeler, S. W., Harris, M. A., Cigrang, J. A., Schinkel, A. M., Rodrigue, J. R., & Klesges, R. C. (1992). Contributions of sibling relations to the adaptation of youth with insulin-dependent diabetes mellitus. *Journal of Consulting and Clinical Psychology, 60,* 104–112.

Hauck, G. (1972). Sociological aspects of epilepsy research. *Epilepsia, 13,* 79–85.

Hauser, S. T., Jacobson, A. M., Wertlieb, D., Weiss-Perry, B., Follansbee, D., Wolfsdorf, J. I., Herskowitz, R. D., Houlihan, J., & Rajapark, D. C. (1986). Children with recently diagnosed diabetes: Interactions with their families. *Health Psychology, 5,* 273–296.

Hill, R. (1949). *Families under stress.* New York: Harper and Row.

Hobfoll, S. E., & Lerman, M. (1989). Predicting receipt of social support: A longitudinal study of parents' reactions to their child's illness. *Health Psychology, 8,* 61–78.

Hops, H., Biglan, A., Arthur, J., Warner, P., Holcomb, C., Sherman, L., Oosternink, N., Osteen, V., & Tolman, A. (1988). *Living in Family Environments (LIFE) coding system.* Eugene: Oregon Research Institute.

Jay, S. M., & Elliott, C. H. (1990). A stress inoculation program for parents whose children are undergoing painful medical procedures. *Journal of Consulting and Clinical Psychology, 58,* 799–804.

Johnson, S. B. (1980). Psychosocial factors in juvenile onset diabetes: A review. *Journal of Behavioral Medicine, 3,* 95–116.

Johnson, S. B. (1985). The family and the child with chronic illness. In D. C. Turk & R. D. Kerns (Eds.), *Health, illness, and families: A life-span perspective* (pp. 220–254). New York: Wiley Interscience.

Kazak, A. E. (1989). Families of chronically ill children: A systems and social–ecological model of adaptation and challenge. *Journal of Consulting and Clinical Psychology, 57,* 25–30.

Kerns, R. D. (1994). Introduction: Families and chronic illness. *Annals of Behavioral Medicine, 16,* 107–108.

Kerns, R. D., & Curley, A. (1985). A biopsychosocial approach to illness and the family: Neurological diseases across the life-span. In D. C. Turk & R. D. Kerns (Eds.), *Health, illness, and families: A life-span perspective* (pp. 146–182). New York: Wiley.

Kerns, R. D., & Haythornthwaite, J. (1988). Depression among chronic pain patients: Cognitive–behavioral analysis and effect on rehabilitation outcome. *Journal of Consulting and Clinical Psychology, 56,* 870–876.

Kerns, R. D., Haythornthwaite, J., Southwick, S., & Giller, E. L. (1990). The role of marital interaction in chronic pain and depressive symptom severity. *Journal of Psychosomatic Research, 34,* 401–408.

Kerns, R. D., & Payne, A. (in press). Treating families of chronic pain patients. In R. J. Gatchel & D. C. Turk (Eds.), *Psychological treatments for pain: A practitioner's handbook.* New York: Guilford Press.

Kerns, R. D., Southwick, S., Giller, E. L., Haythornthwaite, J. A., Jacob, M. C., & Rosenberg, R. (1991). The relationship between reports of pain-relevant social interactions and expressions of pain and affective distress. *Behavior Therapy, 22,* 101–111.

Kerns, R. D., & Turk, D. C. (1984). Depression and chronic pain: The mediating role of the spouse. *Journal of Marriage and the Family, 46,* 845–852.

Kerns, R. D., & Turk, D. C. (1985). Behavioral medicine and the family: Historical perspectives and future directions. In D. C. Turk & R. D. Kerns (Eds.), *Health, illness and families: A life-span perspective* (pp. 338–354). New York: Wiley Interscience.

Kerns, R. D., Turk, D. C., & Rudy, T. E. (1985). The West Haven–Yale Multidimensional Pain Inventory. *Pain, 23,* 345–356.

Kerns, R. D., & Weiss, L. (1994). Family influences on the course of chronic illness: A cognitive–behavioral transactional model. *Annals of Behavioral Medicine, 16,* 116–121.

Kinchla, J., & Weiss, T. (1985). Psychologic and social outcomes following coronary artery bypass surgery. *Journal of Cardiopulmonary Rehabilitation, 5,* 274–283.

Kovacs, M., Iyengar, S., Goldston, D., Obrosky, D. S., Stewart, J., & March, J. (1990). Psychological functioning among mothers of children with insulin-dependent diabetes mellitus: A longitudinal study. *Journal of Consulting and Clinical Psychology, 58,* 189–196.

Kulik, J. A., & Mahler, H. I. M. (1989). Social support and recovery from surgery. *Health Psychology, 8,* 221–238.

LaPuma, J., Orentlicher, D., & Moss, R. J. (1991). Advanced directives on admission: Clinical implications and analysis of the Patient Self-Determination Act of 1990. *Journal of the American Medical Association, 266,* 402–405.

Lazarus, L. W., Stafford, B., Cooper, K., Cohler, B., & Dysken, M. (1981). A pilot study of an Alzheimer patient's relatives discussion group. *Gerontologist, 21,* 353–358.

Lazarus, R. S., & Folkman, S. (1984). *Stress, appraisal, and coping.* New York: Springer.

Levine, J., Warrenburg, S., Kerns, R. D., Schwartz, G., Delaney, R. C., Fontana, A., Gradman, A., Smith, S., Allen, S., & Cascione, R. (1987). The role of denial in recovery from coronary heart disease. *Psychosomatic Medicine, 49,* 109–117.

Levy, L. H. (1976). Self-help groups: Types and psychological processes. *Journal of Applied Behavioral Science, 12,* 310–322.

Litman, T. J. (1974). The family as a basic unit in health and medical care: A social–behavioral overview. *Social Science and Medicine, 8,* 495–519.

Litman, T. J. (1989). Some methodological problems and issues in family health research. In C. N. Ramsey, Jr. (Ed.), *Family systems in medicine* (pp. 167–180). New York: Guilford Press.

Litman, T. J., & Venters, M. (1979). Research on health care and the family: A methodological review. *Social Science and Medicine, 13A,* 379–385.

Long, C. G., & Moore, J. R. (1979). Parental expectations for their epileptic children. *Journal of Child Psychology and Psychiatry, 24,* 299–312.

Madan-Swain, A., & Brown, R. T. (1991). Cognitive and psychosocial sequelae for children with acute lymphocytic leukemia and their families. *Clinical Psychology Review, 11,* 267–294.

Magni, G., Carli, M., De Leo, D., Tshilolo, M., & Zanesco, L. (1986). Longitudinal evaluations of psychological distress in parents of children with malignancies. *Acta Psychiatrica Scandinavia, 75,* 283–288.

Manne, S. L., Bakeman, R., Jacobsen, P. B., Gorfinkle, K., Bernstein, D., & Redd, W. H. (1992). Adult–child interaction during invasive medical procedures. *Health Psychology, 11,* 241–249.

McCubbin, H., Comeau, J., & Harkins, J. (1981). *FIRM—Family Inventory for Resources for Management (research instrument).* St. Paul: Department of Family Social Science, University of Minnesota.

McCubbin, H., Larsen, A., & Olson, D. (1982). *F-COPES—Family Crisis-Oriented Personal Evaluation Scales (research instrument).* St. Paul: Department of Family Social Science, University of Minnesota.

McCubbin, H., McCubbin, M., Patterson, J., Cauble, A., Wilson, L., & Warwick, D. (1983). CHIP—Coping Health Inventory for Parents: An assessment of parental coping patterns in the care of the chronically ill child. *Journal of Marriage and the Family, 45,* 359–370.

McCubbin, H. I., & Patterson, J. M. (1982). *FIC—Family Index of Coherence (research instrument).* St. Paul: Department of Family Social Science, University of Minnesota.

McCubbin, H. I., Patterson, J. M., & Wilson, L. (1981). *FILE—Family Inventory of Life Events and Changes (research instrument).* St. Paul: Department of Family Social Science, University of Minnesota.

McCubbin, M. A., McCubbin, H. I., & Thompson, A. I. (1987). FHI—Family Hardiness Index. In H. I. McCubbin & A. I. Thompson (Eds.), *Family assessment inventories for research and practice* (pp. 125–132). Madison: University of Wisconsin.

Mechanic, D. (1964). The influence of mothers on their children's health attitudes and behaviors. *Pediatrics, 33,* 444–453.

Mermelstein, R., Lichtenstein, E., & McIntyre, K. O. (1983). Partner support and relapse in smoking cessation programs. *Journal of Consulting and Clinical Psychology, 51,* 464–466.

Minuchin, S., & Fishman, C. (1981). *Family therapy techniques.* Cambridge, MA: Harvard University Press.

Nicassio, P., & Radojevic, V. (1993). Models of family functioning and their contribution to patient outcomes in chronic pain. *Motivation and Emotion, 17,* 295–316.

Oddy, M., Humphrey, M., & Uttley, D. (1978). Stress upon the relatives of head injured patients. *British Journal of Psychiatry, 133,* 507–513.

Olson, D. H. (1989). Circumflex model and family health. In C. N. Ramsey (Ed.), *Family systems in medicine* (pp. 75–94). New York: Guilford Press.

Olson, D. H., & Killorin, E. (1985). *Clinical rating scale for circumflex model.* St. Paul: Department of Family Social Science, University of Minnesota.

Olson, D. H., Portner, J., & Lavee, Y. (1985). FACES III—Family Adaptability and Cohesion Evaluation Scales. St. Paul: Department of Family Social Sciences, University of Minnesota.

Patterson, J. M. (1989). A family stress model: The family adjustment and adaptation response. In C. N. Ramsey (Ed.), *Family systems in medicine* (pp. 95–118). New York: Guilford Press.

Patterson, J. M., & Garwick, A. W. (1994). The impact of chronic illness on the family: A family systems perspective. *Annals of Behavioral Medicine, 16,* 131–142.

Pratt, L. (1976). *Family structure and effective health behavior. The energized family.* Boston: Houghton-Mifflin.

Radojevic, V., Nicassio, P. M., & Weisman, M. H. (1992). Behavioral intervention with and without family support for rheumatoid arthritis. *Behavior Therapy, 23,* 13–30.

Ramsey, C. N., Jr. (1989). *Family systems in medicine.* New York: Guilford Press.

Reiss, D. (1981). *The family's construction of reality.* Cambridge, MA: Harvard University Press.

Reiss, D. (1989). Families and their paradigms: An ecologic approach to understanding the family and its social world. In C. N. Ramsey (Ed.), *Family systems in medicine* (pp. 119–134). New York: Guilford Press.

Reiss, D., Gonzalez, S., & Kramer, N. (1986). Family process, chronic illness and death: On the weakness of strong bonds. *Archives of General Psychiatry, 43,* 795–804.

Revenson, T. A., & Majerovitz, S. D. (1991). The effects of chronic illness on the spouse: Social resources as stress buffers. *Arthritis Care and Research, 4,* 63–72.

Romano, J. M., Turner, J. A., Friedman, L. S., Bulcroft, R. A., Jensen, M. P., Hops, H., & Wright, S. F. (1992). Sequential analysis of chronic pain behaviors and spouse responses. *Journal of Consulting and Clinical Psychology, 60,* 777–782.

Rozanski, A., & Berman, D. S. (1987). Silent myocardial ischemia: I. Pathophysiology, frequency of occurrence, and approaches toward detection. *American Heart Journal, 114,* 615–626.

Rudy, T. E., Kerns, R. D., & Turk, D. C. (1988). Chronic pain and depression: Toward a cognitive–behavioral mediation model. *Pain, 35,* 129–140.

Schmidt, D. D., & Schmidt, P. M. (1989). Family systems, stress, and infectious diseases. In C. N. Ramsey, Jr. (Ed.), *Family systems in medicine* (pp. 263–272). New York: Guilford Press.

Smith, T. W. (1992). Hostility and health: Current status of a psychosomatic hypothesis. *Health Psychology, 11,* 139–150.

Smith, T. W., & Christensen, A. (1992). Hostility, health and social contexts. In H. S. Friedman (Ed.), *Hostility, coping and health* (pp. 33–48). Washington, DC: American Psychological Association.

Tompkins, C. A., Schulz, R., & Rau, M. T. (1988). Poststroke depression in primary support persons: Predicting those at risk. *Journal of Consulting and Clinical Psychology, 56,* 502–508.

Turk, D. C., Flor, H., & Rudy, T. E. (1987). Pain and families: I. Etiology, maintenance and psychological impact. *Pain, 30,* 3–28.

Turk, D. C., & Kerns, R. D. (1985a). The family in health and illness. In D. C. Turk & R. D. Kerns (Eds.), *Health, illness and families: A life-span perspective* (pp. 1–22). New York: Wiley Interscience.

Turk, D. C., & Kerns, R. D. (1985b). *Health, illness and families: A life-span perspective.* New York: Wiley Interscience.

Turk, D. C., Kerns, R. D., & Rosenberg, R. 1992). Effects of marital interaction on chronic pain and disability: Examining the down-side of social support. *Rehabilitation Psychology, 37,* 259–274.

Turk, D. C., Kerns, R. D., & Rudy, T. E. (1984, August). *Identifying the links between chronic illness and depression.* Paper presented at the 92nd Annual Convention of the American Psychological Association, Toronto, Ontario, Canada.

Venters, M. (1989). Chronic illness and the family: The example of cardiovascular disease. In C. N. Ramsey (Ed.), *Family systems in medicine* (pp. 307–320). New York: Guilford Press.

Willer, B. S., Allen, K. M., Liss, M., & Zicht, M. S. (1991). Problems and coping strategies of individuals with traumatic brain injury and their spouses. *Archives of Physical Medicine and Rehabilitation, 72,* 460–464.

Chapter

7

Cognitive–Behavioral Treatment of Illness Behavior

Dennis C. Turk and Peter Salovey

All chronic diseases represent assaults on multiple areas of functioning, not just on the person's body (Cohen & Lazarus, 1979; Turk, 1979). People with chronic disease and physical impairments may face separation from family, friends, and other sources of gratification; loss of key roles; disruption of plans for the future; assault on self-image and self-esteem; loss of autonomy and control; uncertain and unpredictable futures; distressing emotions such as anxiety, depression, resentment, and helplessness; and such disease-related factors as permanent changes in physical appearance or bodily function. On the basis of such an extensive array of adjustive demands, one might expect that chronic illness inevitably results in significant emotional difficulties for individuals and the breakdown of integrated functioning. Nevertheless, a substantial proportion of individuals make satisfactory and even heroic adjustments—keeping distress within manageable limits, establishing a sense of self-worth, and maintaining relations with significant others (e.g., Visotsky, Hamburg, Goss, & Lebovits, 1961; Weisman, 1976). Yet, other individuals with the same objective degrees of physical impairment evidence much less satisfactory adaptation to their predicaments. For these people, impairments in primary roles (e.g., vocational, social, or familial) may exceed the limitations imposed by their physical condition. Furthermore, they may experience emotional distress that inhibits optimal adjustment to the realities imposed by the disease or physical impairments. It is this population that is in need of psychological consultation and intervention.

In this chapter, we examine some of the factors that may contribute to discrepant responses by people who are suffering from the same chronic illness—in particular, focusing on idiosyncratic illness schema or representations (Leventhal, 1983; Turk, Rudy, & Salovey, 1986) and illness behavior (Mechanic, 1962). We contrast this cognitive-information-processing approach with traditional psychiatric and behavioral speculations regarding "abnormal illness behavior" (Pilowsky, 1978; Wooley, Blackwell, & Winget, 1978). Next, we present a cognitive–behavioral perspective as a background against which to conceptualize interventions useful with chronic illness sufferers. We then take a practical focus—discussing such important clinical issues as how to prepare people with chronic illnesses for referral for psychological consultation and a comprehensive approach to assessment and treatment that is based on a cognitive–behavioral formulation.

Illness Behavior

It appears that people tend to notice bodily sensations when these feelings depart from more ordinary ones. Because not all available information can be processed, some form of selective filtering is required. People experiencing changes in their feeling states and physical functioning attempt to make sense of what is happening by examining different intuitive hypotheses about the seriousness of their problems and the need for attention (Leventhal, 1983). Individuals appraise new bodily perceptions against prior experiences and their anticipations according to some preexisting model or schema (i.e., an organized set of beliefs and expectations stored in memory). These representations of illness, or *illness schemas,* are based on the experiences of others and on general knowledge (Turk et al., 1986). It is through a matching process of current state to established illness representations that people identify and evaluate symptoms, interpret their causes and implications, and decide what types of help to seek.

Mechanic (1962) has referred to the manner in which people monitor their bodies, respond to symptoms, and decide on a remedial course of action as "illness behavior." The concept of illness behavior brings together all the psychological, social, and cultural influences on illness and the entire range of psychological and social consequences of being ill. Illness behavior can be distinguished from the sociological construct of the "sick role," which describes society's explicit norms and expectations regarding appropriate behavior among individuals designated as sick (Parsons, 1951). Parsons regarded the sick role as a partially and conditionally legitimized state that individuals may be granted, provided they accept that it is undesirable and recognize their obligation to cooperate with others for the purpose of achieving health as soon as possible. Furthermore, sick individuals are expected to show clear evidence of having recognized their obligation by consulting those whom society regards as competent to diagnose and treat illness.

The concept of illness behavior has been used in many different ways. It is sometimes synonymous with sick role, and in the psychiatric literature it is frequently seen with the modifier "inappropriate" or "abnormal" (Pilowsky, 1978). The phrase *abnormal illness behavior* incorporates a rather arbitrary definition of abnormality with an emphasis on disability that is "disproportionate" to the disease, a lifestyle that revolves around the illness role, and a perpetual search for additional medical care (Wooley et al., 1978). The definition of *abnormal illness behavior* has been expanded in psychiatry to incorporate (a) a syndrome of mental disorder (e.g., hypochondriasis or somatoform disorders), (b) a symptom, (c) a dimension of behavior ranging from denial to abnormal that is orthogonal to a second dimension of extent of physical disability, and (d) a social explanation for maladaptive behavior (Mayou, 1989). The diagnosis of abnormal illness behavior is made on the basis of a perceived discrepancy between the nature of the somatic pathology observed and the patient's reaction to it. This diagnostic process assumes that the physician's opinion is accurate, that examination and laboratory diagnostic procedures are capable of identifying all sources of pathology and symptoms, and that there are objective criteria against which to contrast an individual's response. None of these assumptions are warranted in all instances, however.

In considering treatment for people with chronic diseases and physical impairments, we take a somewhat different tack than usual for abnormal illness behavior and the psychiatric diagnoses that often accompany it. We suggest that subjective interpretations and appraisal of symptoms as well as social reinforcement contingencies affect physical and psychological functioning based on an individual's unique illness schema. Thus, for all patients with a chronic condition, one must attend to individuals' own conceptualizations of their symptoms, disease, and the responses from significant people in their environment because all of this may affect physical and psychological responses. Such responses in turn influence physical and psychological functioning as well as response to treatment and rehabilitation. In contrast to some, we do not refer to "abnormal" illness behavior, which, by definition, assumes that we know what normal and abnormal responses to illness should be. We focus our discussion primarily on psychologically healthy people confronted with physical impairments and chronic diseases.

The health care system often encourages patterns of illness behavior in people with chronic illness that limit personal responsibility and their sense of control over their fate. When chronically ill people are having trouble coping and adjusting and thus are referred to a psychologist, they need help in accommodating to their restrictions or limitations while retaining a sense of activity, participation, and personal efficacy. In addition to focusing on the individual with the chronic illness, the psychologist needs to target sources of social support, because these support systems may provide positive reinforcement contingent on adaptive behaviors or, alternatively, problematic, unhelpful, and even negative support that may promote disability and other dysfunctional responses (Turk, Kerns, & Rosenberg, 1992).

A Cognitive–Behavioral Perspective

Rationale

The cognitive–behavioral perspective suggests that behavior and emotions are influenced by interpretations of events, rather than solely by objective characteristics of an event itself. Instead of focusing on cognitive and affective contributions to the perception of a set of symptoms in a static fashion or exclusively examining behavioral responses and environmental reinforcement contingencies (as in the operant conditioning model), cognitive–behavioralists use a transactional view to emphasize the ongoing reciprocal relationships among physical, cognitive, affective, social, and behavioral factors.

According to the cognitive–behavioral model, each patient's perspective—based on his or her idiosyncratic attitudes, beliefs, and unique schemas—filters and interacts reciprocally with emotional factors, social influences, behavioral responses, and sensory phenomena. Moreover, patients' behaviors elicit responses from significant others that can reinforce both adaptive and maladaptive modes of thinking, feeling, and behaving. Thus, a transactional, reciprocal, and synergistic model of chronic illness is indicated.

Assumptions of Treatment

Five central assumptions characterize the cognitive–behavioral perspective on treatment (Turk & Meichenbaum, 1994). The first is that all individuals are active processors of information rather than passive reactors to environmental contingencies. Individuals attempt to make sense of the stimuli that impinge on them from the external environment by filtering information through organizing schema derived from their prior learning histories and by using general strategies that guide the processing of information (e.g., Nisbett & Ross, 1980; Taylor & Crocker, 1981). Individuals' responses (overt as well as covert) are based on these appraisals and subsequent expectations and so are not totally contingent on the actual consequences of their behaviors (i.e., positive and negative reinforcements and punishments). From this perspective, anticipated consequences are as important in governing behavior as actual consequences.

A second assumption of the cognitive–behavioral perspective is that one's thoughts (e.g., appraisals, attributions, or expectancies) can elicit or modulate affect and physiological arousal—either of which may serve as an impetus for behavior. Conversely, affect, physiology, and behavior can instigate or influence one's thinking processes. Thus, the causal priority depends on where in the cycle one chooses to begin. Causal priority may be less of a concern than the view of a transactional process that extends over time with the interaction of thoughts, feelings, physiological activity, and behavior (Lazarus & Folkman, 1984).

Unlike more behavioral models emphasizing environmental influences on behavior, the cognitive–behavioral perspective focuses on the reciprocal effects of the individual on the environment as well as on how the environment influences behavior (Bandura, 1986). Individuals not only passively respond to their environment but also elicit environmental responses by their behavior. In a very real sense, individuals create their environments. Therefore, someone who becomes aware of a physical perturbation and decides that the symptom requires attention from a health care provider initiates a set of circumstances different from an individual with the same symptom who chooses to self-medicate. The third assumption of the cognitive–behavioral perspective, therefore, is that behavior is reciprocally determined by the environment and the individual (Bandura, 1978, 1986).

According to the fourth cognitive–behavioral assumption, if individuals have learned maladaptive ways of thinking, feeling, and responding, then successful interventions designed to alter behavior should target each of these thoughts, feelings, physiology, and behaviors and not one to the exclusion of the others. In other words, there is no expectancy (faith) that changing thoughts, feelings, or behaviors exclusively will necessarily result in the other two following suit.

The final assumption of the cognitive–behavioral perspective posits that, in the same way that individuals are instrumental in developing and maintaining maladaptive thoughts, feelings, and behaviors, they can, are, and should be considered active agents of change for their maladaptive modes of responding. Patients with chronic diseases and physical impairments, no matter how severe and despite their common beliefs to the contrary, are not helpless pawns of fate. They can and should become instrumental in learning and carrying out more effective modes of responding to their environment and their plight.

Preparing Individuals for Psychological Referral

Before reviewing techniques used to treat people with various chronic illness or physical impairments, it is important that we consider how to prepare individuals for referral to a psychologist or other mental health professional (DeGood, 1983; Turk, Meichenbaum, & Genest,

1983). Patients with chronic illnesses or physical impairments are not typically receptive to referrals to psychologists. Such actions may be interpreted to imply that the individual is weak, incompetent, or emotionally disturbed; that his or her symptoms are psychologically induced, or that he or she is exaggerating (if not faking) symptoms.

Many chronic illness sufferers fear that a referral for psychological intervention implies that they can no longer be helped by the traditional health care systems and that they are being abandoned as "hopeless cases." They may view the referral as a requirement that they prove that they do have legitimate reasons for reporting symptoms. These individuals usually believe that psychological assessment is not relevant to their problems, when they have a known physical basis for their symptoms. They may believe that cure of the disease or elimination of the symptoms or physical limitations is all that is required. Conversely, if an individual is significantly convinced that there is an undiagnosed medical disorder responsible for his or her symptoms that has not been adequately addressed, then he or she will reject any implication that psychological factors may be contributing to (causing) the symptoms or exacerbating the symptoms.

For these reasons, chronic illness sufferers and physically impaired individuals may be particularly defensive when referral to a psychologist is raised. Their defensiveness may be expressed in the form of reticence, hostility, or an overly positive presentation (with the intent of projecting an image of psychological well-being by denying even minimal psychological distress or difficulties). Even if patients do not raise concerns, the health care provider making the referral should assume the potential for a problem and inform them why a psychological referral is being made, the specific nature of the referral question, how the results of the consultation will be used, and who will have access to information discussed with the psychologist.

It is helpful for health care providers recommending psychological referral to acknowledge the devastating effects that chronic illnesses and physical impairments can have on patients' lives (other than their physical status), such as disruption of vocational, familial, and social functioning. Observance of these difficulties can provide an additional rationale for further consultation. Patients are usually willing to acknowledge that their impairments and symptoms have caused and continue to cause disruption across a number of areas of their functioning, both physical and psychological. Such a discussion may alleviate some of the resistance, defensiveness, and hostility that the individual feels and that may undermine the psychological consultation and subsequent intervention.

It is important for health care providers and psychologists to be familiar with each other and to acknowledge what is expected of each in the treatment of the patient. Vague referrals without clear requests and expectancies or inadequate communication can lead to treatment failure and dissatisfaction of both psychologist and health care provider.

When discussing psychological referrals, the health care provider should describe the psychologist as a part of the clinical team who has specialized training in helping people with chronic diseases and physical impairments. Specifically, it should be noted that the psychologist can teach techniques to help reduce the suffering created by a disease or its subsequent physical limitations. In addition, the health care provider can acknowledge that having chronic physical problems can create psychological distress and affect self-esteem and emotional well-being for those who must cope with the restrictions in physical capacities, alterations in roles, and changes in lifestyle created by chronic illness or impairment. The health care provider can indicate that psychologists can be especially useful in helping patients with these issues.

It should also be made clear that while the psychologist will help with the areas noted above, the health care provider will attend to physical aspects of the patient's condition. It is important for the health care provider to note that he or she and the psychologist will share information to ensure that each is aware of the other's treatment.

The first task of the psychologist is to ask the patient about his or her reactions to the referral, to correct misconceptions, and to allow the patient to ask questions. An example of an initial interaction between psychologist and patient is presented in transcript form in Exhibit 1.

Several points should be noted about the narrative in Exhibit 1. First, the description of what will take place during therapy sessions is made within a positive framework with an expectancy of success. As we have noted, most people with troubling physical symptoms and physical limitations are defensive and demoralized; thus, they have little belief that such a nonphysical approach will succeed. Although each individual may feel that he or she is a unique case—that he or she cannot be helped—it is important that the psychologist ex-

Exhibit 1

Sample Initial Interaction

> My name is Dr. ______________. You were referred to this clinic by Dr. ______________. I would like to begin by asking you to tell me what your understanding is of why Dr. ______________ referred you to me: What do you think about his [her] explanation [rationale]? What concerns do you have about seeing a psychologist?
>
> What I would like to do today is to learn about the symptoms, especially how they affect your life. Your doctor has referred you to me [this clinic] because he [she] has determined that there is nothing medically or surgically that he [she] can offer to eliminate your symptoms [alter your physical impairments].
>
> Some patients who come here are worried that their doctors do not think that their symptoms are real—that they are overreacting, faking, or have psychological problems. You might not have had this concern, but let me tell you that there is no question that the physical symptoms you experience are real and there is no question that you are suffering. If I did not believe that your symptoms [physical limitations] were real, I would not consider treating you. Let me explain what we know about your condition and your symptoms and relate this to current understandings.
>
> Dr. ______________ referred you here because I [this clinic] have had [has had] experience helping people like you, that is, people who have long-term physical problems that affect their lives greatly. This is not the same thing as saying your symptoms are caused by emotional problems. Rather, it suggests that living with long-term physical problems can cause you to feel upset, angry, frustrated, and depressed. These are normal reactions.
>
> You may be surprised to learn that you are not alone. There are many millions of people who suffer with similar problems that you have experienced. Referral to a psychologist is not intended to imply that your symptoms are not real, that nothing can be done to help you, or that your symptoms are not causing you distress.

Many patients have unspoken fears about the progression of their condition and injuring themselves by performing certain activities or that they will be told they will just have to learn to live with their symptoms [physical limitations] and that nothing can be done. Many patients are reluctant to or perhaps cannot even articulate these concerns. The psychologist may initiate a discussion of them by stating the following:

> I am not sure if this is a concern for you, however, some people that I have seen with problems similar to yours have been worried that there was nothing that could be done to help them. Let me assure you that there is a great deal that you can do to help yourself and that I can be of assistance to you.

Of course, the message will vary depending on which concern the psychologist chooses to address. The important point is to anticipate such concerns by bringing them up even if the person does not spontane-

Exhibit continues

Exhibit 1 (contd.)

ously mention them. In the case of the concern about there being nothing to be done for symptoms, the psychologist might proceed in the following manner:

> What I will attempt to do is to work with you and teach you more effective ways to deal with some of the problems created by your physical symptoms [disease], to reduce distress, and to cope more effectively with the discomfort created by your physical condition. I will teach you a number of self-control strategies, and you may be surprised to learn just how much of your symptoms, as well as their effect on your life, you can learn to control.
>
> Some people are skeptical when I tell them this. They think that I don't believe their symptoms are real, that I don't understand how disabled they have become, or that the approach I have mentioned can be helpful for some, but not for them. To the contrary, I know your symptoms and suffering are real, and I have confidence that the procedures that I will teach you will be of help to you, if you accept some responsibility and are willing to actively try. I am not asking you to believe me on faith, but, rather, I encourage you to work with me. We will be a team, working together. I will be something of a coach to you, teaching you some new skills that you will need to learn and use.
>
> If you are willing to give it a try, I believe that you will be surprised to learn how much you can do to help yourself. Do you have any questions? Do you have any reservations?
>
> What I need to do is to begin by learning more about you, your circumstances, and the problems that your symptoms [disease or impairments] have created for you. If you have any questions or concerns at any time, please bring them up. If we hope to succeed, we must learn to work together and to trust one another.
>
> All of our discussion will remain confidential, and I will only release information with your consent and to those who are most likely to need this information, such as your referring physician. But even in the case of the referring physician, I will release no information unless you agree to this.

press that the psychologically oriented treatment to be undertaken has been proven successful with other people who have similar problems.

It is critical that the psychologist solicit questions and comments from patients and significant others. Many patients tend to be nonassertive in the office of their health care professional. For patients who do not ask questions, it is worthwhile to say something such as "Although it may not have occurred to you, many people with problems similar to yours are concerned about. . . . This is quite natural." These concerns may focus on the belief that because the interviewer is a psychologist, he or she can only help people who have psychological problems, not physical ones. It is imperative that the therapist address such concerns and fears. It is likely that the patient is thinking about such issues; and, if not addressed, these fears and concerns may inhibit their participation in the treatment.

Preliminary Formulation of Treatment Goals

The therapist and patient must cooperate in establishing treatment goals that will return the patient to optimal functioning in light of any physical impairments and that are consistent with the patient's wishes. From our perspective, this collaboration is essential because it helps patients to assume responsibility for what occurs throughout treatment and for its outcomes. Often useful for generating specific goals is information obtained from interviews—through such questions as "How would your life be different if your symptoms (physical impairments) could be relieved?" Above all, goals for patients should be specific and measurable. For example, the goal to simply "feel better" is inadequate; the patient needs to specify concretely what he or she will do that would indicate such improvement. Treatment goals typically include symptom reduction, reduced emotional distress, increased or improved functioning (in physical, recreational, or vocational activities), and reduction in the inappropriate use of the health care system.

Cognitive–Behavioral Assessment

Dimensions

A critical assumption in the psychosocial evaluation of patients with chronic illness is that biomedical disease status, symptoms, and disability compose three important and distinct dimensions of adjustment. In some instances, patients with the most severe physical pathology may also report high symptoms and extensive disability. In other instances, however, there may not be strong concordance between levels of dysfunction in these three areas. As an illustration of such potential disparity, Fordyce (1988), in an analysis of chronic pain, noted that a fundamental distinction can be made between the *input system* (the experience of pain and the factors that cause pain) and the *output system* (the emotional and behavioral reactions of the patient). This framework recognizes that the variables affecting the experience of pain may be very distinct from those affecting emotional responses or disability. Environmental factors—such as the reactions of others, for example—may significantly affect expressions of pain behavior independently of the factors (e.g., tissue damage) that are causing pain. Similarly, patients with chronic illness may exhibit different patterns of dysfunction within biomedical, symptom, and behavioral domains because the factors controlling each domain may be functionally separate from one another. It is a major challenge for the health psychologist to assess the level of dysfunction in these areas, to identify the variables affecting such dysfunction, and to use this information in rational treatment planning for the patient.

From the cognitive–behavioral perspective, assessing a patient with a chronic disease or physical limitation requires a comprehensive strategy of examining a range of psychosocial and behavioral factors in addition to the pathophysiology, subjective report of symptoms, and observable illness behaviors (e.g., grimacing or distorted ambulation or postures). Turk and his colleagues (Turk & Meichenbaum, 1994; Turk & Rudy, 1987) have suggested that two central questions guide assessment:

1. What is the extent of the patient's disease or injury (physical impairment)?
2. Is the illness behavior appropriate to the disease or injury, or is there evidence of amplification of symptoms for any of a variety of psychological or social reasons or purposes?

Turk and Rudy (1987) proposed a model of assessment, labeled the *Multiaxial Assessment of Patients* (MAP), to address the questions above. Although the MAP model was specifically designed to assess people who have chronic pain, the approach has been applied to other populations with chronic diseases or physical impairments, namely, diabetic individuals (Turk & Rudy, 1986a), end-stage renal disease patients (McRae, 1987), and patients with spinal cord injuries (Summers, Rapoff, Varghese, Porter, & Palmer, 1991). The MAP postulates that three axes are essential for assessing the patient: biomedical, psychosocial, and behavioral. From this perspective, each of these three general domains must be assessed and the results combined into a meaningful taxonomy or classification system that guides decision making and treatment planning. Turk and Rudy suggested that operationalizations of these axes should include the following: (a) biomedical—quantification of laboratory and other diagnostic procedures as well as a physical examination; (b) psychosocial—evaluation of patients' perceptions of their symptoms, impairments, disease, affective distress, perceived control over their lives, and interference with social, vocational, marital, recreational, and physical domains; and (c) behavioral—measurement of observable communication of symptoms, distress, and suffering; symptomatic use of the health care system; medication use; activity levels; and responses of significant others.

Under the MAP model, patients receive a dual diagnosis—one medical and one psychosocial (Turk, 1990). Turk and Rudy (1986b, 1987) demonstrated that chronic pain patients could be classified into one of three psychosocial diagnoses on the basis of their responses to questions about how they perceived their symptoms, the impact of their symptoms on diverse domains of their lives, mood, perceptions of control, how significant others responded to them, and restrictions in common daily activities due to their symptoms or physical limitations. One subgroup of patients was characterized by high symptom severity, impact on activities, affective distress, and low levels of activity; this type of response was labeled *dysfunctional.* A second group was characterized by feelings of reduced support from significant others and labeled *interpersonally distressed.* The third group consisted of a set of patients who appeared to be coping and functioning quite well despite the presence of symptoms; these patients were labeled *adaptive copers.* According to the dual-diagnostic, MAP approach, two patients may each receive the same medical diagnosis—for example, insulin dependent diabetes mellitus—but could have quite different psychosocial–behavioral diagnoses.

To examine whether patients with similar physical symptoms might be classified within the category system identified and described above, Turk and Rudy (1990) examined patients who had very different physical symptoms (i.e., oral–facial pain and dysfunction, headaches, and low back pain). They confirmed that, despite the diverse symptoms, patients with each of these symptoms could be classified into the subgroups described above. They concluded that some patients with different physical symptoms were, according to their psychosocial–behavioral characteristics, more similar to each other than they were to some patients with the same physical symptoms.

A number of assessment instruments and procedures are available to measure each of the three MAP axes. A detailed examination of the range of assessment procedures is beyond the scope of this chapter, and so we do not review them here (see Karoly, 1985; Turk & Melzack, 1992). We do, however, note several tactics that have been used to assess the psychosocial and behavioral axes.

Interview

When conducting an interview from the cognitive–behavioral perspective, the psychologist should focus on patients' and significant others' illness schemas and on specific thoughts and feelings as well as observe specific behaviors. Exhibit 2 shows screening questions that may be used to cover these areas. Depending on the patient's response to each question, the clinician may want to follow these up with more in-depth probing.

During an interview, it is important for the clinician to adopt the patient's perspective. Patients' beliefs about the cause of symptoms, their trajectory, and beneficial treatments appear to have important influences on emotional adjustment and compliance with therapeutic interventions (Meichenbaum & Turk, 1987). A habitual pattern of maladaptive thoughts may contribute to a sense of hopelessness, dysphoria, and unwillingness to engage in activity. The psychologist should determine both the patient's and, if applicable, a significant other's expectancies and goals for treatment.

Attention should focus on the patient's reports of specific thoughts, behaviors, emotions, and physiological responses that precede, accompany, and follow target behaviors, as well as on the environmental conditions and consequences associated with the response. During the interview, the psychologist should attend to how these cognitive, affective, and behavioral events are associated in time; their specificity versus generality across situations; the frequency of their occurrence; and so forth—to elucidate the topography of the target behaviors, including the controlling variables. The interviewer seeks information that will assist in the development of potential alternative behaviors, appropriate goals for the patient, and possible reinforcers for these alternatives.

Self-monitoring prior to or following the initial interview is a useful strategy that is not as reliant on recall. It also introduces the patient

Exhibit 2

Screening Questions

- □ When did the symptoms start?
- □ Why did you seek treatment now?
- □ Do you have any fears about your problem [symptoms or diagnosis]?
- □ What do you think is causing or caused the symptoms?
- □ What do you think is happening to your body [mind]?
- □ What do you think the symptoms are a sign of [What do you think is wrong with you]?
- □ What have others told you they think is wrong?
- □ What have you tried to do to alleviate the symptoms?
- □ What was the effect?
- □ Have you had similar symptoms in the past or other symptoms and diseases that have caused you distress?
- □ Does anyone in your family or anyone you know suffer from similar symptoms? If yes, what was their diagnosis, how were they treated, and what was the result of the treatment?
- □ What was going on in life at the time of symptom onset [i.e., recent changes, conflicts, or problems of a financial, occupational, social, marital, or familial nature]?
- □ How upset [anxious, depressed, frustrated, irritable, or angry] have you been about your symptoms?
- □ Do you have any concerns [complaints] about treatment by other health care providers?

to the active role they will be required to play in treatment. A sample self-monitoring form is shown in Table 1.

In addition to interviews, psychologists have developed a number of assessment instruments designed to evaluate patients' attitudes, beliefs, and expectancies about themselves, their symptoms, and the health care system. Standardized assessment instruments have advantages over semistructured and unstructured interviews. Specifically, they are easy to administer, less time-consuming (for the psychologist), and most important, they can be subjected to analyses that permit determination of their reliability and validity. These standardized instruments should not be viewed as alternatives to interviews but, rather, as measures that suggest issues to be addressed in more depth

Table 1

Sample Record of Symptoms, Feelings, Thoughts, and Actions

Name: ______

Date & time	Symptoms (How bad, 0–10?) Situation (What were you doing or thinking?)	How did you feel? (How bad, 0–10?)	What were you thinking?	What did you do? With what result?

during the interview. Space does not permit a detailed examination of all relevant instruments; several books contain examinations of these instruments in more detail (e.g., Karoly, 1985; Turk & Melzack, 1992).

Assessment of Illness Behaviors

Pilowksy (1978) defined *abnormal illness behavior* as the persistence of an inappropriate or maladaptive mode of perceiving, evaluating, and acting in relation to one's own state of health. This inappropriate stance develops despite the fact that a doctor (or other appropriate social agent) has offered a reasonably lucid explanation of the nature of the illness and the appropriate course of management to be followed, on the basis of a thorough examination and assessment of all parameters of functioning in which the individual's sociocultural background has been taken into account. He developed an instrument to specifically measure abnormal illness behavior: the Illness Behavior Questionnaire (Pilowsky & Spence, 1975). The Illness Behavior Questionnaire is a 62-item self-report instrument that includes subscales labeled *General Hypochondriasis, Disease Conviction, Psychological Focus, Affective Inhibition,* and *Denial.* This instrument has received significant support, although some investigators have challenged its psychometric properties (Main & Waddell, 1987; Stretton, Salovey, & Mayer, 1992).

From a very different perspective, Fordyce (1976) has described the importance of the observable behaviors of people who have chronic diseases and physical limitations. The emphasis here is on observable manifestations of pain, distress, and suffering. Fordyce suggested that these behaviors are particularly important because they are subject to contingencies of reinforcement and might be controlled, at least to some extent, by operant conditioning.

The most systematic approach to quantifying the behavior of one large population of people with chronic illnesses—chronic pain sufferers—was designed by Keefe and colleagues. Keefe and Block (1982) developed a coding system for observing five pain behaviors in back-pain patients (grimacing, rubbing, bracing, guarded movement, and sighing) that occur under static and dynamic movement conditions. The frequency of pain behaviors emitted during the specified activities is aggregated for each of the five categories under both conditions to create a total pain behavior score. Their approach to behavioral observation has been extended to work with such populations as arthritis sufferers (McDaniel et al., 1986) and cancer patients (Keefe, Brantley, Manuel, & Crisson, 1985).

A caveat is in order, however. There has been evidence that frequency of pain behaviors during physical examinations is positively correlated with the presence of organic pathology in patients presenting for neurosurgical evaluation; thus, considerable caution needs to be exercised in interpreting pain behaviors solely as a response to reinforcement contingencies (Turk & Flor, 1987; Turk & Matyas, 1992). Moreover, patients may believe that they need to convince a health care provider that pain is real and, thus, may exaggerate symptoms. As a result, the frequency of pain behaviors observed during an interview may not be related to the presence of these behaviors in the patient's usual environment.

Cognitive–Behavioral Treatment

With the background provided above, some specific components of cognitive–behavioral interventions can be considered. It should be emphasized that appropriate treatment of patients with chronic illnesses requires communication, cooperation, and the active involvement of all health care professionals who provide specialized treatments (e.g., referring physicians, physical therapists, and occupational therapists) in addition to psychologists (Turk & Stieg, 1987).

To comprehend the cognitive–behavioral approach to treating patients with chronic diseases or physical impairments, it is important to understand that the techniques used are viewed as less important than the more general cognitive–behavioral conceptualizations and orientation described earlier. These factors—often somewhat dismissively described as "nonspecifics" of treatment—may in reality be the most important components of successful treatment (see Frank, 1963/1974). Although technical details of the tactics used are important, they will contribute to treatment efficacy only if they are embedded in a more strategic treatment framework (Turk & Holzman, 1986; Turk, Holzman, & Kerns, 1986).

Strategic Overview

When patients with chronic diseases and physical impairments come to psychologists, they have received multiple evaluations and a range of treatments provided by a host of health care professionals. A common feature across all patients despite their medical diagnoses is that the array of interventions has not adequately ameliorated their suffering. Figure 1 shows the downward course that characterizes the experience of some patients with chronic diseases and physical impairments. It is important to note that this downward course does not occur for all people, not even, in fact, for the majority. But it does describe the experience of many who are referred to psychologists. Thus, it is not surprising that when such a patient sees a psychologist, he or she may be demoralized and frustrated—feeling that the situation is hopeless, yet continuing to seek "the" cure for his or her suffering. This is the background against which psychologists must view any therapeutic regimens that will be offered.

Cognitive–behavioral therapy is designed to help patients identify, evaluate, and correct maladaptive conceptualizations and dysfunctional beliefs about themselves and their predicament. Additionally, patients are taught to recognize the connections linking cognition, affect, and behavior along with their joint consequences. Patients are encouraged to become aware of and to monitor the impact that negative symptom-engendering or exacerbating thoughts and feelings may play in maintaining and exacerbating maladaptive behaviors.

The cognitive–behavioral therapist is concerned not only with the role that patients' thoughts play in contributing to disability and to

Awareness and Interpretation of Symptoms
↓
Help Seeking
↓
Diagnostic Uncertainty and Lack of Cure
↓
Frustration
↓
Doctor Shopping
↓
Multiple Costly Diagnostic Tests
↓
Suggestion of Psychological Causation or Emotional Distress
↓
Increased Symptom Reporting, Illness Behavior, and Help Seeking
↓
Increased Psychological Distress

Figure 1. The natural history of chronic illnesses.

maintaining and exacerbating symptoms but also with the nature and adequacy of each patient's behavioral repertoire. The strategic plan of a cognitive–behavioral intervention, then, is to help patients reconceptualize how they view their plight. Patients initially believe that their illness is exclusively a medical problem. They thus view their symptoms as overwhelming and beyond their own personal control.

The cognitive–behavioral approach is designed to be optimistic—emphasizing both the effectiveness of the intervention and patients' abilities to alleviate much of their suffering, even if they cannot exert total control over their disease and physical limitations. An important proviso is that the patient must be willing to work with the psychologist and other members of the rehabilitation team.

Throughout the rehabilitation process, symptoms are reconceptualized so that patients come to view their situations as amenable to change through a combination of psychologically and physically based approaches. Thus, there is an attempt to change the patient's illness schema. The treatment program is designed to teach patients a range of cognitive and behavioral skills and to assist them in dealing with maladaptive thoughts and feelings, as well as with noxious sensations that may precede, accompany, and follow the experience of symptoms or symptom exacerbation, and thereby escalate emotional suffering.

Many behavioral (reinforcement and exposure) and cognitive techniques (e.g., cognitive restructuring, problem-solving training, and coping-skills training) are used. However, in the cognitive–behavioral approach, techniques based on these models (e.g., biofeedback, extinction of inappropriate illness behaviors, or reinforcement of activity) represent feedback trials that provide an opportunity for the patient to question, reappraise, and acquire self-control over maladaptive thoughts, feelings, behaviors (including avoidance behaviors), and physiological responses, as well as adaptive skills.

We view the cognitive–behavioral approach as very much a collaborative endeavor that attempts to foster an increased sense of self-efficacy and intrinsic motivation. Even the most ideal treatment plan has little likelihood of success if the patient does not continue to engage in the prescribed behaviors once discharged from the treatment program.

The cognitive–behavioral perspective described above can be a basis for some physical as well as psychological interventions. When physical therapists or nurses work with disabled individuals, they can make use of the same principles that we have discussed. The emphasis is on helping the patient reconceptualize his or her situation and personal role in improving physical functioning and positively adapting to and accommodating limitations imposed by physical impairments.

Objectives and Components of Cognitive–Behavioral Intervention

Having described the cognitive–behavioral perspective, we can now consider what the implications of this perspective are for developing interventions for people with diverse chronic diseases and physical impairments. The four general aims of cognitive–behavioral treatment are (a) to reduce stress, (b) to reduce disability and improve physical functioning, (c) to reduce symptoms, and (d) to limit inappropriate use of medical care (Sharpe, Peveler, & Mayou, 1992). Each component of the treatment should be directed toward accomplishing these four objectives.

The cognitive–behavioral perspective will differ markedly from what patients have come to view as appropriate treatment for their symptoms or impairment (medical problems). The therapist must therefore be prepared to discuss the discrepancy between patients' conceptualizations of their problems and expectancies for treatment (i.e., illness schema) and the specific rationale for cognitive–behavioral treatment. Even if not acknowledged, there is no doubt that patients will harbor some misconceptions and reservations about what appears to be a radical departure from conventional, physically based treatments, and if these are not addressed by the therapist, the treatment is destined to fail because the patient will not be motivated to become actively engaged. We now consider some of the specific components of intervention. Treatment comprises four interrelated components: reconceptualization, skills acquisition, skills consolidation, and generalization and maintenance.

Reconceptualization. The crucial element in successful treatment is bringing about a shift in the patient's repertoire—from well-established, habitual, and automatic but ineffective responses, toward systematic problem solving and planning, control of affect, behavioral persistence, or disengagement (when appropriate). The reconceptualization process serves several essential functions. First, it translates patients' symptoms into difficulties that can be pinpointed as specific, addressable problems. Second, it recasts problems in forms amenable to solutions and, thus, can foster hope, positive anticipation, and expectations of success. Finally, reconceptualization creates positive expectations that the treatment offered is appropriate for the problem.

Reconceptualization goes on throughout treatment. Initially, it involves reorienting the patient from his or her belief that symptoms or physical impairments are an overwhelming, all-encompassing sensory experience resulting solely from tissue pathology and that he or she is helpless to do anything about them. Next, a concept of symptoms and impairments as experiences that can be differentiated and systematically modified and controlled by the sufferers themselves is introduced. Again, it is the patient's illness schema, not his or her objective functional limitations, that is of primary concern. Reconceptualizing the patient's maladaptive view of physical symptoms (limitations) is the framework of cognitive–behavioral treatment that provides validity and incentive for the development of proficiency with various coping skills used in symptom control.

Throughout treatment, it is important that psychologists permit and even urge patients to express their concerns, fears, frustrations, and anger directed toward the health care system, insurance companies, employers, social system, family, fate, and perhaps, themselves. Failure to address these issues will inhibit success. This educational component of treatment consists of presenting the cognitive–behavioral perspective on physical and emotional symptoms and their control (i.e., role of cognitions, affect, behavior, environmental factors, and physical factors). At the outset of treatment and throughout, one should attempt to discuss symptoms (physical limitations) and their impact on the sufferers' lives as well as how others' lives may be affected by problems created by the presence of symptoms (limitations). That is, the therapist conveys to patients that he or she will work with the patient to achieve the best possible outcome (given the constraints imposed by any physical limitations), but that he or she will not do anything to them. It is preferable to have this discussion with significant others present so that any misinformation and concerns and fears can be identified and addressed simultaneously.

During the reconceptualization process, symptoms are evaluated briefly through a simplified explanation of how stress affects physical functioning (for an extended discussion, see chap. 8 of this book). Often, health care providers have been inattentive to or dismissive of the patient's concerns, and an expression of genuine interest will help engagement. Great caution should be exercised in suggesting that psychological factors or psychiatric illness play a causal role in symptoms. For many patients, such suggestions imply that they are imagining or exaggerating symptoms, are at fault for being ill, or are going insane. Common ground can be established by discussing the role of stress in medical conditions (Sharpe et al., 1992). Consider the following example of a discussion with a patient who has chronic musculoskeletal pain:

> When people get upset, there is an unconscious tendency to tense their muscles. Muscle tension can create symptoms such as those that you experience. You have noted that you have been under a lot of pressure on your job lately. It is quite possible that the heavy demands of your job at this time are promoting the symptoms that you have been experiencing. There are a number of ways that you can affect your symptoms. We can consider some alternatives and see whether the symptoms are alleviated or improved. Does this make sense to you?

The last question is crucial; the patient is not likely to be motivated to participate in a treatment that is not consistent with his or her conceptualization of the cause of symptoms. To reduce defensiveness, we have also found it useful at times to provide additional explanation:

> When we have explained the relationship between stress, muscle tension, autonomic arousal, and symptoms to some people, they have been skeptical. What we have told them is that when we become upset, there is a tendency for our muscles to increase the level of tension, to become tight, and for stress hormones to increase—making us feel more aroused and anxious. Have you ever noticed this happening to you?

If the patient says no, then the psychologist might note that stress often happens without people being aware of it. He or she might even use biofeedback to demonstrate the effect of stress on muscle tension. Offering examples from everyday life can also be helpful: For example, how does one feel and what does one experience after a near miss in an automobile accident? The psychologist would then proceed to note that tense muscle and stress hormones can affect people's emotional states as well as exacerbate symptoms.

For patients with other diseases and physical impairments, stress may have a less direct effect on their physical symptoms but will be related to emotional distress. In these cases, the psychologist would present somewhat different explanations. In either case, the psychologist can note that a great deal can be done by individuals to control their levels of arousal and emotional distress once it is identified as a problem. Control should be presented not as a complex scientific theory but to demonstrate to the patient the multidimensional aspect of physical symptoms. Psychologists should present this in a way that the patient can understand by using personally relevant examples. Symptoms and physical disability should be described as a multidimensional experience having physiological, cognitive, affective, and behavioral features.

Patients are encouraged to review recent stressful episodes or circumstances and to examine the course their symptoms followed at that time. For example, a recent conflict with a spouse might be examined to determine whether the patient's getting upset had any effect on the physical and psychological symptoms experienced.

Imaginal presentation or recall of previous symptomatic exacerbations can be especially useful at this juncture. Patients can be asked to recall not only the situation but also their accompanying thoughts and feelings. With the help of the therapist, they can then discover the impact of thoughts and feelings on the experience of symptoms. In this manner, the therapist engages patients in a dialogue, using the patient's maladaptive thoughts and feelings to illustrate how such thinking may influence inappropriate behavior and exacerbate the problem.

In summary the reconceptualization process serves at least five important functions:

1. It provides a more benign view of the problem than the patient's original view.
2. It translates patients' physical and psychological symptoms into difficulties that can be pinpointed as specific, addressable problems rather than problems that are vague, undifferentiated, overwhelming, and uncontrollable.
3. It recasts problems in forms that are amenable to solutions and, thus, should foster hope, positive anticipation, and expectancy for success.
4. It prepares patients for interventions contained within the treatment regimen that are directly linked to the conceptualization proposed.
5. It creates a positive expectancy that the treatment being offered is appropriate for the patient's problems.

Skills acquisition. In all cases, it is essential for patients to understand the rationale for the specific skills being taught and the tasks they are being asked to perform. If patients do not understand the rationale for treatment components and have opportunities to raise issues and sources of confusion about them, they are less likely to persevere in the face of obstacles, to benefit from therapy, or to maintain therapeutic gains. In rehabilitation, this is true both for physical and psychological interventions. For example, physical therapists should explain the rationale for specific physical exercises; explain concepts of pacing so that patients will not "overdo" exercises—to reserve strength and avoid exacerbating symptoms; discuss the differences between hurt or fatigue and harm; and review the possibility of flare-ups and relapse and how these might be addressed. In this manner, physical therapists can adopt a cognitive–behavioral perspective rather than the more conventional physical–mechanistic approach that they have been taught. Psychologists can serve as consultants to other health care providers—assisting them in taking a broader perspective that focuses on the individual and not exclusively on the symptom or physical diagnosis.

Cognitive–behavioral treatment makes use of a whole range of techniques and procedures designed to bring about alterations in patients' perceptions of their situation, their mood, and their behavior and abilities to modify these psychological processes. Techniques such as progressive relaxation training, problem-solving training, distraction skills training, and communication skills training—to name only a few—have all been incorporated within the general cognitive–behavioral framework. Specific techniques have been described in some detail in several publications, and the interested readers might want to consult them (e.g., see Bernstein & Borkovec, 1973; Kanfer & Goldstein, 1986; Turk et al., 1983).

A number of specific skills have been reported useful for helping patients cope with symptoms. At this point, research does not permit selecting among them. We believe that more important than pinpointing useful, specific tactics is accomplishing the strategic goals of enhancing self-control and intrinsic motivation. That is, the manner in which the various skills are described, taught, and practiced may be more important than the skills per se.

Again, it is essential for therapists to keep in mind the patients' perspective and how they perceive each skill and assignment. The therapist's skills and the therapist–patient relationship grease the gears of treatment; without a satisfactory therapeutic alliance, treatment will grind to a halt (Turk, Holzman, & Kerns, 1986). Treatment should thus not be viewed as a rigid process with fixed techniques. There is a need to individualize the treatment program for each patient; however, the cognitive–behavioral rationale described above remains constant (Turk, 1990).

Relaxation. The skills-training phase of treatment should begin with relaxation exercises. These techniques are particularly useful early in treatment because they can be readily learned by almost all patients. The teaching and practice of relaxation is designed not only to help patients learn a response that is incompatible with muscle tension but also to help patients develop a behavioral-coping skill to be used in any situation in which adaptive coping is required. The practice of relaxation strengthens patients' beliefs that they can exert some control during periods of stress and symptoms and thus are not helpless or impotent.

The therapist can discuss with patients how to identify bodily signs of physical tenseness, the stress–tension cycle, how occupying one's attention can short-circuit stress, how relaxation can reduce anxiety by enabling one to exert control, how relaxation and tension are incompatible states, and, finally, how unwinding after stressful experiences can be therapeutic.

Relaxation can be used for its direct effects on specific muscles, for reduction of generalized arousal, for its cognitive effects (i.e., as a distraction or attention-diversion strategy), and for its value in increasing the patient's sense of control and self-efficacy, which may enhance independent functioning and reduce disability. Relaxation skills are generic, and there is a wide range of different techniques (e.g., biofeedback, autogenic training, or imagery) geared toward helping patients learn how to deal with stress and, in particular, how to reduce site-specific muscular hyperarousal. Moreover, relaxation also includes active efforts—such as aerobic exercise, walking, and engaging in a range of pleasurable activities consistent with interests and physical limitations.

The rationale that is presented to patients should follow the same principles as the presentation of the original treatment rationale. The goal is to develop and enhance motivation and participation. The manner in which the rationale is presented depends on the patient's particular way of thinking about his or her physical problem and life situation. Essentially, it should be presented within a framework that sets high expectations for success and indicates that the treatment is both clinically indicated and within the patient's own competencies to achieve.

Furthermore, the relaxation procedure should be used to demonstrate to patients their ability to control their muscles (both increases and decreases in symptom intensity—biofeedback may be used to reinforce this point). We initially use a muscle-tension-reduction procedure (Bernstein & Borkovec, 1973) because (a) it has face validity; (b) it is a concrete procedure and, thus, is easy to recall and practice at home; and (c) it is less prone than passive-relaxation techniques to failure due to distraction by symptoms or cognitive intrusions. Slight symptomatic exacerbations that often accompany muscle tensing clearly demonstrate to the patient the role of muscle activity in symptom perception and possibly exacerbation. If muscle tension results in increased symptoms, then one can reason that the converse—muscle relaxation—leads to symptom reduction. Also, the results of even the first relaxation training session are often inherently reinforcing in reducing generalized arousal. The therapist can build on this to predict the potential beneficial treatment effects with extended practice.

Throughout the practice of relaxation, the therapist should continue to take the collaborator's role. This is very important for developing the conceptualization of relaxation as a self-management skill, thereby facilitating self-control of psychological and, at times, physical symptoms. The therapist also should assume a role that fosters the patient's perception of success. Failure during the initial stages of treatment can seriously undermine the patient's confidence and motivation. The patient should be frequently encouraged with statements about his or her progress. Similarly, all possible indications and reports of success by the patient should be reinforced.

At the end of each session, therapists should provide specific homework assignments for patients to perform, self-monitor, and record. At the beginning of each subsequent session, the therapist would then review the self-monitored practice charts with the patient to identify problems and reinforce effort as well as success.

After the patients have become proficient in relaxation, it is helpful to have them first imagine themselves in various stress or conflict situations and then visualize themselves using relaxation skills in those situations. The therapist may describe coping versus mastery examples derived from other patients, that is, how others have reported trying to relax, having problems, and then overcoming them. In this way, patients become aware that problems might arise, that when they do have difficulties they can overcome them, and that they are not the only ones who have difficulties. Essentially, patients should be made aware that relaxation is a skill and that, like any skill, it requires a good deal of practice.

In subsequent sessions, the therapist teaches the patient that one can relax not only by tensing and releasing muscle groups (as in progressive relaxation or by means of some passive activities such as meditation and controlled breathing) but also by becoming absorbed in such activities as exercising (e.g., walking or swimming) or hobbies (knitting or gardening). All too often, therapists fail to understand that relaxation is a state of mind as well as a state of the body: Mental relaxation may be just as important as physical relaxation.

Cognitive restructuring. As we have noted several times, the cognitive–behavioral perspective assumes that the way individuals perceive their circumstances determines their mood, perceptions of symptom intensity, and subsequent behavior, including whether they seek medical attention (e.g., Flor & Turk, 1988). Cognitive restructuring focuses on identifying anxiety engendering and other maladaptive appraisals and expectations and subsequently considering more appropriate alternative modes of interpretation. Common cognitive restructuring procedures include (a) evaluating the validity and viability of thoughts and beliefs; (b) eliciting and evaluating predictions; (c) exploring alternative explanations; (d) retraining attributions from helplessness and hopelessness to resourcefulness and competence; and (d) altering an absolutist, catastrophic thinking style. The therapist encourages the patient to test the adaptiveness (not the so-called rationality) of his or her thoughts, beliefs, expectations, and predictions.

Cognitive restructuring is designed to make patients aware of the role that thoughts and emotions play in potentiating and maintaining stress and physical symptoms. The therapist elicits the patient's thoughts, feelings, and interpretations of events; gathers evidence for or against such interpretations; identifies habitual self-statements, images, and appraisals that occur; tests the validity of these interpretations, identifies automatic thoughts that set up an escalating stream of negative, catastrophizing ideation; and helps examine how such habitual thoughts exacerbate stress and interfere with performance of adaptive coping responses.

The therapist can make use of imagery recall to assist in the process of cognitive restructuring. For example, a patient may be asked to relive one or more recent experiences of stress as if a movie were running in slow motion in his or her mind, eliciting thoughts and feelings around specific events and responses. The therapist can then perform a cognitive–functional analysis with the patient to identify common themes. In this way, the therapist helps the patient to discriminate between functional symptoms (e.g., hyperventilation-induced chest pain) and disease-based symptoms (e.g., angina on effort) and to respond appropriately to each.

By using self-monitoring, the therapist helps patients identify when they are becoming stressed, helps them to become aware of low-intensity cues, and then examines the contribution of their thoughts—all in an effort to deautomatize the connection between events and arousal or distress. The therapist may ask patients to monitor symptoms but not to overreact by assuming that all unusual or noxious sensations are attributable to worsening of disease. As noted, therapy is viewed as a collaborative process by which the therapist carefully elicits the troublesome thoughts and concerns of a patient, acknowledges their bothersome nature, and then constructs an atmosphere in which the patient can critically challenge the validity of his or her own beliefs. Rather than suggesting alternative thoughts, the therapist attempts to elicit competing thoughts from the patient and then reinforces the adaptive nature of these alternatives. Patients have well learned and frequently rehearsed thoughts about their conditions. Only after repetitions and practice in cuing competent interpretations and evaluations will patients come to change their conceptualizations. Contact with significant others may be important because they may contribute unwittingly to undermining patients' changing conceptualizations.

Attention diversion. Attention is a major factor in perception and, therefore, is of concern in examining and changing behavior. Attention-diverting coping tactics have probably been used for as long as humans have experienced aversive symptoms. A great deal of research based on attentional focus has been conducted with regard to the relative efficacy of various cognitive-coping techniques (Fernandez & Turk, 1989).

Cognitive techniques consist of several different types of procedures, including cognitive distraction or attention diversion. Patients are often preoccupied with their bodily symptoms. Every new sensation is seen as an indication of deterioration or a new problem resulting from increased exercise and activity. Cognitive distraction techniques are best used during specific illness episodes in which the patient experiences an exacerbation of his or her symptom.

Before describing different coping techniques, therapists should briefly describe to patients how attention can influence perception. One can start by suggesting that people can fully focus their attention on only one thing at a time and that they can, to some extent, control what is attended to (although at times that may require a good deal of effort).

Patients might be asked to close their eyes and focus attention on some part of their body. The therapist then notes some ambient sound, such as the ventilation system, and suggests that while attending to his or her body, the patient was not aware of the sound of the air conditioning. The therapist then calls attention to the sound of ventilation and reminds the patient that he or she has stopped focusing on his or her body. The therapist also might call attention to some part of the patient's body that the patient was not attending to, such as the gentle pressure of the watch on his or her wrist. The point is that environmental (internal and external) input exists that remains out of conscious attention until it is focused on directly. The objective is to communicate to patients that people commonly use various methods to maintain some degree of control over the focus of their attention.

To date, no one category or type of cognitive coping technique has proven to be universally effective (Fernandez & Turk, 1989; Turk et al., 1983). Thus, we suggest providing patients with education and practice in the use of many different ones. The therapist should discuss a variety of cognitive coping images and attention-diverting tasks in an attempt to reveal several that might be most appealing to individual patients.

Assertiveness and communication skills training. Assertiveness training is often an important intervention that enables patients to reestablish their roles, particularly within the family, and thus to regain a sense of self-esteem and potency. Through role-playing of existing tension-producing interpersonal transactions, patient and therapist can identify and modify maladaptive thoughts, feelings, and communication deficiencies underlying nonassertiveness, while practicing more adaptive alternatives. The patient may find assertiveness training useful in addressing reactions from family members and health care providers that may oppose the patient's self-management objectives.

Problem-solving skills training. Adopting a problem-solving perspective is particularly important for patients. That is, therapists should try to help patients identify problems that may contribute to their emotional distress and suffering and suggest that if problems can be identified then they can be solved. Specifically, we recommend the following steps be taken in training for problem solving:

- Define the source of distress or stress reactions as problems to be solved.
- Set realistic goals as concretely as possible by stating the problem in behavioral terms.
- Generate a wide range of possible alternative courses of action to reach each goal.
- Imagine and consider how others might respond if asked to deal with a similar problem.
- Evaluate the pros and cons of each proposed solution, and organize solutions in rank order from least to most practical.
- Rehearse strategies and behaviors by using imagery, role reversal, or behavioral rehearsal.
- Try out the most feasible solution.
- Expect some failures, but reward self for having tried.
- Reconsider the original problem in light of the attempted solution.
- Recycle as needed.

We also recommend linking the problem-solving steps to specific questions:

- Problem identification: What is the concern?
- Goal selection: What do I want?
- Generation of alternatives: What can I do?
- Consideration of consequences: What might happen?
- Decision making: What is my decision?
- Implementation: Now do it!
- Evaluation: Did it work? If not, re-cycle.

Skills Consolidation

During the skills-consolidation phase of the cognitive–behavioral treatment, patients practice and rehearse the skills that they have learned during the skills-acquisition phase and apply them outside the clinical context. One of the techniques used is mental, or imagery, rehearsal—during which the patient imagines using the new skills in different situations. A second method involves role reversal, where the patient interacts with the therapist as if he or she was in a specific situation and needed to use specific skills (with the therapist assuming the role of patient). Specific details of these approaches are described below, and a more in-depth review has been published by Turk et al. (1983).

Imagery rehearsal. One means of providing patients with opportunities to rehearse coping skills is to use imagery rehearsal. Much like in systematic desensitization, the patient is asked, while relaxed, to imagine himself or herself in various situations in which the intensity of symptoms, disability, or stress varies. We view imagery rehearsal with the assumption that when patients are instructed to imagine scenes, they are providing themselves with a model of their behavior. The closer the imagery comes to representing real experiences, the greater the likelihood of generalization. Through imagery, patients can mentally rehearse the specific thoughts, feelings, and behaviors they will use to cope with stress, psychological, and physical symptoms.

To maximize the similarity between images and real life, patients should be encouraged to visualize coping images as well as mastery images. *Mastery images* are those in which patients view themselves as successfully handling the problem situation. *Coping imagery,* in contrast, involves patients imaging themselves becoming anxious, beginning to experience symptoms or having maladaptive thoughts, and then coping with these difficulties by using approaches that they have learned during treatment. Coping imagery also may be very useful for patients who, because of illness-related limitations, may initially feel ineffective at coping attempts but may benefit significantly from sustained coping efforts that will gradually increase self-efficacy.

Role-playing. Role-playing is another tactic used to help patients consolidate the skills learned during the skills-acquisition phase. Role-playing is useful not only for rehearsing new skills but also for identifying potential problem areas that may require special attention. Most typically, the patient is asked to identify and participate in a role-play situation that is indicative of a particular problem area.

In a variation on role-playing—role reversal—the patient is asked to role-play a situation while switching roles with the therapist. The patient is instructed that it is his or her job to assume the role of the therapist, whereas the therapist assumes the role of another individual that has a similar physical diagnosis to the patient but has not received the specific skills training. This exercise is used because it is known from research on attitude change (Kopel & Arkowitz, 1975) that when people have to improvise, such as in a role-playing situation, they generate exactly the kinds of arguments, illustrations, and motivating appeals that they regard as most salient and convincing. In this way, patients tailor the content of their roles to fit their unique motives, predispositions, and preferences. In such role-playing situations, they not only emphasize those aspects of training most convincing for them but also focus on less conflicting thoughts, doubts, and unfavorable consequences. In summary, these exercises contribute to self-persuasion while permitting the therapist to determine areas of confusion and potential difficulties.

Preparation for Generalization and Maintenance

To maximize the likelihood of maintenance and generalization of treatment gains, cognitive–behavioral therapists focus on the cognitive activity of patients as they are confronted with problems throughout treatment (e.g., failure to achieve specified goals, plateaus in progress on physical exercises, or recurrent stressors). These events are looked upon as opportunities to help patients learn how to handle setbacks and lapses, because it is probably inevitable that these will occur once treatment is terminated: Rehabilitation is not a cure.

In the final phase of treatment, discussion focuses on possible ways of predicting and avoiding, or dealing with, symptoms and symptom-related problems after treatment ends. In our practice, we have found it helpful to assist patients in anticipating future problems, stress, and symptom-exacerbating events and to plan coping and response techniques before these problems occur. Marlatt and Gordon (1985) have referred to this process as "relapse prevention."

Briefly, *relapse prevention* involves helping the patient, before he or she completes treatment, learn to identify and cope successfully with factors that may otherwise lead to relapse. Therapists help patients identify high-risk situations and the types of coping and behavioral responses that may be necessary for successful coping.

In the final stage of treatment, discussion focuses on possible ways of predicting and avoiding difficult and problematic situations in general, as well as specific ones that were identified during treatment. Discussion of relapse must unfold delicately. On the one hand, the therapist does not wish to convey an expectancy of treatment failure, but, on the other hand, the therapist wishes to anticipate problems and assist the patient in learning how to deal with potential recurrences or problematic situations that are likely (Turk & Rudy, 1991).

It is important to note that all possible problematic circumstances cannot be anticipated. Rather, the goal during this phase—as for the entire treatment strategy—is to enable patients to develop a problem-solving perspective so that they believe they have the skills and competencies within their repertoire to respond appropriately to problems as they arise. With this in mind, the therapist tries to help the patient learn to anticipate future difficulties, develop plans for adaptive responding, and adjust his or her behavior accordingly. Successful responses should further enhance patients' sense of self-efficacy and help to form a "virtuous circle"—in contrast to the "vicious circle" formerly created and fostered by inactivity, passivity, physical deconditioning, helplessness, and hopelessness that has been characteristic of people with chronic illnesses.

We have found it useful to have patients anticipate specific symptom-exacerbating events and plan how they will deal with them. For example, one patient with rheumatoid arthritis was anticipating his daughter's wedding soon after therapy termination. Using a future-oriented problem-solving approach, the patient could identify both expected and potential problematic situations (e.g., dancing at the wedding reception and dealing with poor service by the caterer). He was able to develop a plan to cope with such situations and with general, unanticipated problems and to thereby decrease the likelihood of relapse and exacerbation of symptoms.

The generalization and maintenance phase serves at least two purposes. First, it encourages the patient to anticipate and plan for the posttreatment period, and second, it focuses on the necessary conditions for long-term success. More specifically, relapse prevention gives the patient the understanding that minor setbacks are to be expected and that they do not signal total failure. Rather, patients should view these setbacks as cues to use the coping skills with which they have already become proficient. It is important that the patient not think that his or her responsibility ends with termination of treatment, but, instead, that he or she is entering a different phase of maintenance.

Therapists should emphasize the importance of adhering to recommendations on an ongoing basis.

During the final sessions, all aspects of treatment are reviewed. Patients are engaged in a discussion of what they have learned and how they have changed from the onset of treatment and in recognition of how their own efforts contributed to positive change. The therapist should also use patients' self-monitoring charts to reinforce their accomplishments. The goal is to help each patient realize that he or she has the skills and abilities within his or her repertoire to cope with circumstances without needing to contact the therapist and without becoming dependent on others. It should be emphasized that change has been achieved and can be maintained only if patients continue to accept responsibility for their lives. Patients should thus no longer view themselves as patients but as competent people who happen to have some physical symptoms and discomfort.

Closing Comments

From our perspective, patients' attitudes and beliefs have an obvious effect on motivation and behavior. We believe that environmental contingencies can influence people's thoughts, feelings, and behaviors. Thus, we suggest using both cognitive and behavioral techniques to bring about direct change in behavior provided by environmental contingencies and indirect changes following modification of cognitive factors. External reinforcement is important at the beginning of treatment; however, unless significant changes in intrinsic motivation occur, treatment efficacy will not be maintained once direct environmental reinforcement is removed (e.g., Cairns & Pasino, 1977).

We have been unable to address all the nuances of cognitive–behavioral treatments; however, we hope to have whetted the appetite of readers such that they will consider more carefully the nature of the treatment strategies and tactics they use when interacting with patients. As is obvious from even a cursory scanning of the literature, single-modality techniques imposed on passive patients with chronic illnesses seem of limited value for the complexity of problems inherent in chronic illness and physical disability.

The efficacy of a variety of cognitive–behavioral techniques has been evaluated in a number of laboratory analog and clinical studies. The clinical effectiveness of cognitive–behavioral interventions has been demonstrated with a wide range of chronic illness and disabilities, including headaches (e.g., Holroyd, Nash, Pingel, Cordingley, & Jerome, 1991; Martin, Nathan, Milech, & van Keppel, 1989), arthritis (Bradley et al., 1987; O'Leary, Shoor, Lorig, & Holman, 1988; Parker et al., 1988), temporomandibular disorders (Olson & Malow, 1987), low back pain (Hazard et al., 1989; Nicholas, Wilson, & Goyen, 1992), spinal-cord injuries (Summers et al., 1991), atypical chest pain (Klimes, Mayou, Pearce, Coles, & Fagg, 1990), functional somatic symptoms (Salkovskis, 1989; Sharpe et al., 1992), and cancer (Warner & Swensen, 1991). These approaches have been used with patients across the age span, from adolescents (Lascelles, Cunningham, McGrath, & Sullivan, 1989) to geriatric patients (Puder, 1988).

In this chapter, we have emphasized the strategy and some tactics of cognitive–behavioral therapy. According to Turk and Holzman (1986), durable change can only be expected if the following conditions are met:

- There is a fit between patients' conceptualizations of their problems and the rationale for the treatment being offered.
- The expected value of more adaptive behaviors for patients is emphasized rather than the worth of these behaviors to the health care provider.
- Patients have or can be provided with the necessary skills to carry out more adaptive responding.
- Patients believe that the treatment components will effectively alleviate their problems.
- Patients believe that they are competent to carry out the skills learned beyond the therapeutic context.
- There is sufficient intrinsic and extrinsic reinforcement for the maintenance and generalization of skills incorporated during the treatment regimen following termination.

All of these goals are incorporated within the cognitive–behavioral treatment we have described. It is important to note in closing that, at this point, methodologically adequate process research has yet to identify the necessary or sufficient components of effectively treated people who have persistent symptoms and physical disabilities. Consequently, the treatment strategy and tactics that we have elaborated in this chapter are based as much on clinical experience as on the empirical literature.

REFERENCES

Bandura, A. (1978). The self-system in reciprocal determinism. *American Psychologist, 33,* 344–359.

Bandura, A. (1986). *Social foundations of thought and action: A social cognitive theory.* Englewood Cliffs, NJ: Prentice Hall.

Bernstein, D. A., & Borkovec, T. D. (1973). *Progressive relaxation training.* Champaign, IL: Research Press.

Bradley, L. A., Young, L. D., Anderson, K. O., Turner, R. A., Agudelo, C. A., & McDaniel, L. K. (1987). Effects of psychological therapy on pain behavior of rheumatoid arthritis patients. Treatment outcome and six-month follow-up. *Arthritis and Rheumatism, 30,* 1105–1114.

Cairns, D., & Pasino, J. A. (1977). Comparison of verbal reinforcement and feedback in operant treatment of disability due to low back pain. *Behavior Therapy, 8,* 621–630.

Cohen, F., & Lazarus, R. S. (1979). Coping with the stresses of illness. In G. C. Stone, F. Cohen, & N. E. Adler (Eds.), *Health psychology* (pp. 217–254). San Francisco: Jossey-Bass.

DeGood, D. E. (1983). Reducing medical patients' reluctance to participate in psychological therapies: The initial session. *Professional Psychology, 14,* 570–579.

Fernandez, E., & Turk, D. C. (1989). The utility of cognitive coping strategies for altering pain perception: A meta-analysis. *Pain, 38,* 124–135.

Flor, H., & Turk, D. C. (1988). Chronic back pain and rheumatoid arthritis: Predicting pain and disability from cognitive variables. *Journal of Behavioral Medicine, 11,* 251–265.

Fordyce, W. E. (1976). *Behavioral methods for chronic pain and illness.* St. Louis, MO: C. V. Mosby.

Fordyce, W. E. (1988). Pain and suffering: A reappraisal. *American Psychologist, 43,* 276–283.

Frank, J. D. (1974). *Persuasion and healing: A comparative study of psychotherapy.* New York: Shocken Books. (Original work published 1963)

Hazard, R. G., Fenwick, J. W., Kalisch, S. M., Redmond, J., Reeves, V., Reid, S., & Frymoyer, J. M. (1989). Functional restoration with behavioral support—-A one-year prospective study of patients with chronic low-back pain. *Spine, 14,* 157–161.

Holroyd, K. A., Nash, J. M., Pingel, J. D., Cordingley, G. E., & Jerome, A. (1991). A comparison of pharmacological (amitriptyline HCl) and non-pharmacological (cognitive–behavioral) therapies for chronic tension headaches. *Journal of Consulting and Clinical Psychology, 59,* 121–133.

Kanfer, F. H., & Goldstein, A. P. (1986). *Helping people change: A textbook of methods.* Elmsford, NY: Pergamon Press.

Karoly, P. (1985). *Measurement strategies in health psychology.* New York: Wiley.

Keefe, F. J., & Block, A. R. (1982). Development of an observation method for assessing pain behavior in chronic low back pain patients. *Behavior Therapy, 13,* 365–375.

Keefe, F. J., Brantley, A., Manuel, G., & Crisson, J. E. (1985). Behavioral assessment of head and neck cancer pain. *Pain, 23,* 327–336.

Klimes, I., Mayou, R. A., Pearce, M. J., Coles, L., & Fagg, J. R. (1990). Psychological treatment for atypical noncardiac chest pain: A controlled evaluation. *Psychological Medicine, 20,* 605–611.

Kopel, S., & Arkowitz, H. (1975). The role of attribution and self-perception in behavior change. *Genetic Psychology Monographs, 92,* 175–212.

Lascelles, M. A., Cunningham, S. J., McGrath, P., & Sullivan, M. J. L. (1989). Teaching coping strategies to adolescents with migraine. *Journal of Pain and Symptom Management, 4,* 135–145.

Lazarus, R. S., & Folkman, S. (1984). *Stress, appraisal, and coping.* New York: Springer-Verlag.

Leventhal, H. (1983). Behavioral medicine: Psychology in health care. In D. Mechanic (Ed.), *Handbook of health, health care, and the health professions* (pp. 709–743). New York: Free Press.

Main, C. J., & Waddell, G. (1987). Psychometric construction and validity of the Pilowsky Illness Behavior Questionnaire in British patients with chronic low back pain. *Pain, 28,* 13–25.

Marlatt, G. A., & Gordon, J. R. (1985). *Relapse prevention: Maintenance strategies in the treatment of addictive behaviors.* New York: Guilford Press.

Martin, P. R., Nathan, P. R., Milech, D., & van Keppel, M. (1989). Cognitive therapy versus self-management training in the treatment of chronic headaches. *British Journal of Clinical Psychology, 28,* 347–361.

Mayou, R. (1989). Illness behavior and psychiatry. *General Hospital Psychiatry, 11,* 307–312.

McDaniel, L. K., Anderson, K. O., Young, L. D., Turner, R. A., Agudelo, C. A., & Keefe, F. J. (1986). Development of an observation method for assessing pain behavior in rheumatoid arthritis patients. *Pain, 24,* 165–184.

McRae, C. (1987). *Cognitive–behavioral mediators of depression in chronic illness: An investigation of the links between symptoms of disease and depression in patients on home kidney dialysis.* Unpublished doctoral dissertation, University of Iowa, Iowa City.

Mechanic, D. (1962). The concept of illness behavior. *Journal of Chronic Disease, 15,* 184–194.

Meichenbaum, D., & Turk, D. C. (1987). *Facilitating treatment adherence: A practitioner's guidebook.* New York: Plenum Press.

Nicholas, M. K., Wilson, P. H., & Goyen, J. (1992). Comparison of cognitive–behavioral group treatment and an alternative non-psychological treatment for chronic low back pain. *Pain, 48,* 339–348.

Nisbett, R., & Ross, L. (1980). *Human inference: Strategies and shortcomings of social judgment.* Englewood Cliffs, NJ: Prentice Hall.

O'Leary, A., Shoor, S., Lorig, K., & Holman, H. R. (1988). A cognitive–behavioral treatment for rheumatoid arthritis. *Health Psychology, 7,* 527–544.

Olson, R. E., & Malow, R. M. (1987). Effects of biofeedback and psychotherapy on patients with myofascial pain dysfunction who are nonresponsive to conventional treatments. *Rehabilitation Psychology, 32,* 195–204.

Parker, J. C., Frank, R. G., Beck, N. C., Smarr, K. L., Buescher, K., Phillips, L. R., Smith, E. I., Anderson, S. K., & Walker, S. E. (1988). Pain management in rheumatoid arthritis patients: A cognitive–behavioral approach. *Arthritis and Rheumatism, 31,* 593–601.

Parsons, T. (1951). *Social systems.* London: Routledge & Kegan Paul.

Pilowsky, I. (1978). A general classification of abnormal illness behaviours. *British Journal of Medical Psychology, 1,* 131–137.

Pilowsky, I., & Spence, N. D. (1975). Patterns of illness behaviour in patients with intractable pain. *Journal of Psychosomatic Research, 19,* 279–288.

Puder, R. S. (1988). Age analysis of cognitive–behavioral group therapy for chronic pain outpatients. *Psychology and Aging, 3,* 204–207.

Salkovskis, P. M. (1989). Somatic problems. In K. Hawton, P. M. Salkovskis, J. Kirk, & D. M. Clark (Eds.), *Cognitive behavior therapy for psychiatric problems* (pp. 235–276). New York: Oxford Medical Publications.

Sharpe, M., Peveler, R., & Mayou, R. (1992). The psychological treatment of patients with functional somatic symptoms: A practical guide. *Journal of Psychosomatic Research, 36,* 515–529.

Stretton, M. S., Salovey, P., & Mayer, J. D. (1992). Assessing health concerns. *Imagination, Cognition and Personality, 12,* 115–137.

Summers, J. D., Rapoff, M. A., Varghese, G., Porter, K., & Palmer, R. E. (1991). Psychosocial factors in chronic spinal cord injury pain. *Pain, 47,* 183–189.

Taylor, S. E., & Crocker, J. (1981). Schematic bases of social information processing. In E. T. Higgins, C. P. Herman, & M. P. Zanna (Eds.), *Social cognition: The Ontario symposium* (Vol. 1, pp. 13–30). Hillsdale, NJ: Erlbaum.

Turk, D. C. (1979). Factors influencing the adaptive process with chronic illness: Implications for intervention. In I. G. Sarason & C. D. Spielberger (Eds.), *Stress and anxiety* (Vol. 6, pp. 291–311). New York: Halstead Press.

Turk, D. C. (1990). Customizing treatment for chronic pain patients: Who, what, and why. *Clinical Journal of Pain, 6,* 225–270.

Turk, D. C., & Flor, H. (1987). Pain > pain behavior: Utility and limitations of the pain behavior construct. *Pain, 31,* 277–295.

Turk, D. C., & Holzman, A. D. (1986). Commonalities among psychological treatments for chronic pain: Specifying the meta-constructs. In A. D. Holzman & D. C. Turk (Eds.), *Pain management: A handbook for psychological treatment approaches* (pp. 257–268). Elmsford, NY: Pergamon Press.

Turk, D. C., Holzman, A. D., & Kerns, R. D. (1986). Chronic pain. In K. A. Holroyd & T. L. Creer (Eds.), *Self-management approaches to the prevention and treatment of chronic disease* (pp. 441–472). San Diego, CA: Academic Press.

Turk, D. C., Kerns, R. D., & Rosenberg, R. (1992). Effects of marital interaction on chronic pain and disability: Examining the down-side of social support. *Rehabilitation Psychology, 37,* 259–274.

Turk, D. C., & Matyas, T. A. (1992). Pain-related behavior > communication of pain. *American Pain Society Journal, 1,* 109–111.

Turk, D. C., & Meichenbaum, D. (1994). A cognitive–behavioural approach to pain management. In P. D. Wall & R. Melzack (Eds.), *Textbook of pain* (3rd ed., pp. 1337–1348). London: Churchill Livingstone.

Turk, D. C., Meichenbaum, D., & Genest, M. (1983). *Pain and behavioral medicine: A cognitive–behavioral perspective.* New York: Guilford Press.

Turk, D. C., & Melzack, R. (1992). *Handbook of pain assessment.* New York: Guilford Press.

Turk, D. C., & Rudy, T. E. (1986a). Living with chronic disease: The importance of cognitive appraisal. In S. McHugh & T. M. Vallis (Eds.), *Illness behavior: A multidisciplinary model* (pp. 309–320). New York: Plenum Press.

Turk, D. C., & Rudy, T. E. (1986b). Toward an empirically derived taxonomy of chronic pain patients: Integration of psychological assessment data. *Journal of Consulting and Clinical Psychology, 56,* 233–238.

Turk, D. C., & Rudy, T. E. (1987). Toward the comprehensive assessment of chronic pain patients. *Behaviour Research and Therapy, 25,* 237–249.

Turk, D. C., & Rudy, T. E. (1990). Robustness of an empirically derived taxonomy of chronic pain patients. *Pain, 43,* 27–36.

Turk, D. C., & Rudy, T. E. (1991). Neglected factors in chronic pain treatment outcome studies—Relapse, noncompliance, and adherence enhancement. *Pain, 44,* 5–28.

Turk, D. C., Rudy, T. E., & Salovey, P. (1986). Implicit models of illness. *Journal of Behavioral Medicine, 9,* 453–474.

Turk, D. C., & Stieg, R. L. (1987). Chronic pain: The necessity of interdisciplinary communication. *Clinical Journal of Pain, 3,* 163–167.

Visotsky, H. M., Hamburg, D. A., Goss, M. F., & Lebovits, B. Z. (1961). Coping behavior under extreme stress. *Archives of General Psychiatry, 5,* 423–448.

Warner, J. E., & Swensen, C. H. (1991, May). *The effectiveness of stress inoculation training for cancer pain patients.* Paper presented at the meeting of the Midwest Psychological Association, Chicago, Illinois.

Weisman, A. D. (1976). Early diagnosis of vulnerability in cancer patients. *American Journal of the Medical Sciences, 271,* 187–196.

Wooley, S. C., Blackwell, B., & Winget, C. (1978). A learning theory model of chronic illness behavior: Theory, treatment, and research. *Psychosomatic Medicine, 40,* 379–401.

Chapter

8

Stress Management

Jerry C. Parker

Stress is a universal phenomenon of everyday life, but especially so for those with chronic illness. Approximately 20 million Americans experience chronic, stress-induced physical illnesses (Schaffer, 1982). The frequency of medical problems directly attributable to stress has been estimated to be as high as 75% of all medical disorders (Hughes, Pearson, & Reinhart, 1984), and epidemiological data have indicated higher levels of morbidity and mortality in psychologically distressed populations (Kiecolt-Glaser & Glaser, 1988). Annual fiscal losses as a result of stress-induced physical illness are approximately $16 billion (Adams, 1978). In addition, there is a substantial literature documenting a relationship between stressful life events and the symptomatology of physical illness (Ben-Sira, 1984; Gentry, 1984; Holmes & Masuda, 1974; Leidy, Ozbolt, & Swain, 1990; Rahe, 1988).

Studies of interrelationships between psychosocial variables and illness have gradually led to an expanded view of health. Since the sixteenth century, the predominant view has been that physical illness results from abnormal body tissues (Rasmussen, 1975). For acute illnesses, this biomedical perspective has proven useful. In the case of infectious diseases, for example, a specific causal agent usually can be identified, and treatments that destroy or remove the agent typically will restore health.

In the case of most chronic illnesses, however, a single causal agent usually cannot be identified or eliminated by available treatments. Accordingly, G. L. Engel (1977) postulated a complex interaction between chronic biological illness and a person's psychological–sociological circumstances. Engel coined the term *biopsychosocial* for his model, to highlight the psychological and sociological foundations of health and illness (see Smith & Nicassio, chap. 1, this book).

One of the most compelling biopsychosocial aspects of illness involves the concept of stress. The term *stress* was originally coined by Thomas Young to refer to the forces within a physical object that serve to counterbalance externally applied forces. In this usage from the physical sciences, stress is a precise term describing a characteristic within an object. Selye (1946) adapted the term to the biological sciences as a way of describing the general "wear and tear" encountered by an organism. Subsequently, the term *stress* has been applied to health and illness in many diverse ways. In some usages, it refers to taxing events in the environment that create coping demands for the individual. In other usages, *stress* refers to biological responses within the organism that result from taxing events. Given these two divergent usages, the literature on stress and stress management can appear confusing and contradictory. In fact, some researchers have recommended that the term be avoided entirely in the context of the human organism (B. T. Engel, 1985).

For conceptual clarity, there must at a minimum be a distinction between environmental events, defined as *stressors*, and biological reactions, defined as *stress responses*. When the term *stress* is used without such specificity, its usage is inherently ambiguous. Nevertheless, stress is a term that has intuitive meaning for most people in Western society, and the stress construct is useful within the field of health psychology. For the layperson, the term creates a bridge between the environment and the person. In contrast with the global concept of mental health, the concept of stress tends to create a normalizing view that something is partially awry in the environment, not just within the individual. Therefore, *stress* is a term that can create receptivity to psychological interventions. For most patients experiencing a chronic illness, stress management is a face-valid therapeutic strategy.

Theoretical and Research Foundations

From a theoretical standpoint, the term *stressor* should be used to describe taxing environmental events. *Stress response* should be used to describe the biological reactions to stressors. For clinical purposes, the term *stress* can be used to refer to the "sum total of stressors and stress responses" operating in a given situation. When conceptual precision is needed, however, the term *stress* is best avoided.

Stress and Appraisal

An important aspect of stressors is that there is great individual variability in what constitutes a taxing environmental circumstance. Certain "biogenic" stressors are universally capable of inducing a stress response. For example, amphetamines and strenuous exercise will trigger predictable biological reactions in most individuals. Beyond the biogenic stressors, however, most stressors are of the "psychogenic" variety. That is, most induce biological responses on the basis of the psychological interpretation placed on them. For example, speaking in public is a frightful experience for some people, whereas, for others, public speaking is a positive opportunity for self-expression. In the case of psychogenic stressors (e.g., public speaking), there is nothing about the stressor itself that induces the biological stress response. Rather, the cognitive interpretation, or appraisal, is the key factor determining the stress response for a given individual.

The role of appraisal in the stress response has been described by Lazarus and Folkman (1984), who identified two subtypes of appraisal. The first, *primary appraisal,* refers to an initial judgment about whether a stressor has the potential for producing harm or inducing an undesirable loss. If the primary appraisal reveals that there is no potential for harm or loss, then the stimulus does not meet the criteria for a stressor, and a stress response is not invoked. On the other hand, if the primary appraisal signifies a potential for harm or loss, then a secondary appraisal occurs. *Secondary appraisal* refers to a judgment about whether sufficient resources exist to cope with the stressor. If the person perceives that he or she possesses the personal and environmental resources to manage the stressor, then the stress response is minimized. If, on the other hand, the person thinks that he or she does not have adequate resources for coping with the stressor, then the stress response is exacerbated. There is a need for practitioners to recognize that the psychological interpretation of potentially stressful events is the major modulator of the stress response.

Stress Response

When a stressor has been appraised as threatening, people respond in individualistic ways. At the biological level, the stress response occurs along three primary axes, as follows: (a) the neuronal axis, (b) the neuroendocrine axis, and (c) the endocrine axis. Although these general axes have characteristic effects, there is a need for practitioners to remember that stress responses are both individualistic and specific. More precisely, people manifest their own unique pattern of the stress response, and there are specific stress responses to unique situations (B. T. Engel, 1985).

One aspect of the stress response occurs along the neuronal axis. In general, the neuronal axis involves the activity of the autonomic nervous system (ANS). There are two subdivisions of the ANS: the sympathetic nervous system (SNS) and the parasympathetic nervous system (PSNS). The SNS pathway progresses from the cortex through the limbic structures (specifically, the posterior hypothalamus), through the spinal cord, through the sympathetic ganglia, and, ultimately, to the target organs. The primary neurotransmitter of the SNS is epinephrine. The PSNS pathway progresses from the cortex through the limbic structures (specifically, the anterior hypothalamus), through the spinal cord, and, ultimately, to the target organs. The primary neurotransmitter of the PSNS is acetylcholine. In general, the SNS serves to activate and energize the organism, whereas the PSNS serves to deactivate and restore the organism.

A second aspect of the stress response occurs along the neuroendocrine axis. Cannon (1914) described the "fight or flight" response, which involves the ANS acting in conjunction with an endocrine structure (the adrenal medulla). Sympathetic stimulation of the adrenal medulla results in the release of the adrenal medullary catecholamines (specifically, norepinephrine and epinephrine). Catecholamines generally play a role in the activation and mobilization of energy for the organism.

A third aspect of the stress response occurs along the endocrine axis. Specifically, the median eminence of the hypothalamus releases hormones, such as corticotropin-releasing factor (CRF), into the hypothalamic-hypophyseal portal system from where CRF descends to the pituitary gland. In the case of CRF, the pituitary is stimulated to release adrenocorticotropic hormone (ACTH) into the peripheral blood. ACTH then circulates and stimulates the adrenal cortex to release glucocorticoids, such as cortisol. The role of glucocorticoids in the stress response is primarily to counterbalance the organism's defensive reactions to stress (Munck, Guyre, & Holbrook, 1984). Other pituitary hormones operating within the endocrine axis are somatotropic hormone, thyroid-stimulating hormone, vasopressin, and oxytocin.

Although the neuronal, neuroendocrine, and endocrine axes operate in an integrated fashion, they display different temporal sequences (see Figure 1). The neuronal axis, which relies solely on neural transmission, permits an immediate response to stressors. The neuroendocrine axis, which relies on the release of catecholamines from the adrenal medulla, has intermediate effects, including a minimum 20–30 second delay. The endocrine axis is the slowest acting but has the most prolonged effects. Selye (1956) described the integrated pattern of reactions to chronic stress as the "general adaptation syndrome" (GAS). For a more in-depth discussion of the physiological aspects of the stress response, see Field, McCabe, & Schneiderman's (1985) book.

Conceptual Framework for the Stress Response

Everly (1989) has described a model of the stress response that is useful for clinicians. The model comprises six stages in the epiphenomenology of the human stress response: (a) stressor events (real or imagined), (b) cognitive appraisal and affective integration, (c) neurological triggering mechanisms (i.e., the translation of cognitive processes into neuronal events), (d) the physiological stress response, (e) target-organ activation, and (f) coping activities. There are several important features to Everly's model. First, there is acknowledgment that the six stages are interrelated and that feedback systems are operating. Second, the coping process is conceptualized to occur after physiological responses and target-organ activation. In this manner, coping actions can be viewed as cognitive or behavioral efforts to regain ho-

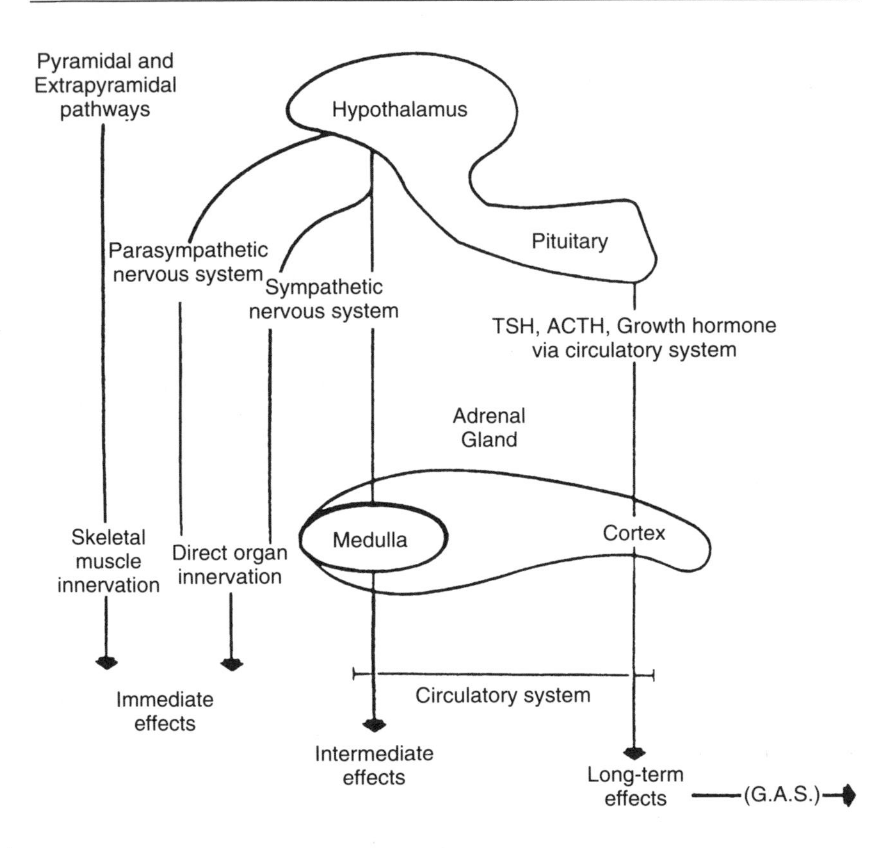

Figure 1. Temporal relationships between primary stress axes. GAS = general adaptation syndrome. From *Clinical Guide to the Treatment of the Human Stress Response* (p. 40), by G. S. Everly, 1989, New York: Plenum. Copyright 1989 by Plenum. Reprinted with permission.

meostasis. For the clinician, Everly's model provides a useful perspective for conceptualizing stress-management interventions.

Management of the Stress Response

Several stress-management strategies can be deduced from Everly's (1989) model of human stress response. One strategy is to minimize both biogenic and psychogenic stressors. In terms of biogenic stressors, this means minimizing exposure to sympathomimetics. With regard to psychogenic stressors, this means reexamining such factors as time demands and life goals. Environmental or contextual alterations can be used to alter one's exposure to biogenic and psychogenic stressors. To the extent that stressors can be minimized, target-organ activation will be reduced.

A second stress-management strategy involves modifying the cognitive–affective mediation of stressful events. Some stressful events cannot be avoided, but they can be managed more effectively at the cognitive–affective level. In terms of stress management, this may mean modifying attitudes, positively reframing events, and examining sociocultural values. Interventions at the cognitive–affective level have as their focus the restructuring of appraisals and the amelioration of emotional distress.

A third stress-management strategy involves directly reducing psychophysiological arousal through the use of progressive relaxation training, autogenic training, meditation, or biofeedback. Under the proper conditions, each of these strategies can effectively reduce psychophysiological arousal.

A fourth strategy of stress management involves constructive expression of the stress response. For individuals facing stressful events, coping may involve expression of ideas, ventilation of emotions, or the harnessing of energies to ameliorate the original stressful circumstances.

Efficacy of Stress Management

There is an extensive literature concerning the effectiveness of various forms of stress management, including relaxation training, biofeedback, and cognitive–behavioral approaches. Hyman, Feldman, Harris, Levin, and Malloy (1989) conducted a meta-analysis of the effects of relaxation training on clinical symptoms in a medical population. The meta-analyses revealed that stress-management interventions were beneficial, with the exception that the effectiveness of Benson's relaxation technique (Benson, Beary, & Carol, 1974) was questionable. Overall, the effectiveness of relaxation training was demonstrated for several chronic problems, such as hypertension, headaches, and insomnia.

Blankfield (1991) has reviewed the literature on the usefulness of suggestion, relaxation, and hypnosis as adjunctive treatments for surgical patients. Eighteen clinical trials were reviewed; 16 of these studies found that the interventions facilitated either the physical or the emotional recovery of postsurgical patients. Blankfield's review indicated that relaxation, suggestion, and hypnosis can be used to shorten postoperative stays, to promote physical recovery following surgery, and to contribute to the psychological and emotional convalescence of surgical patients.

Blenkhorn, Silove, Magarey, Krillis, and Coninet (1992) have reviewed a series of studies examining the effectiveness of several psychological interventions for enhancing immunological functioning, specifically, progressive relaxation, visual imagery, and meditation. They found preliminary evidence that immunological functioning can be altered through psychological intervention. However, the number of studies examined was small, and additional work is required to confirm these preliminary findings.

In summary, there is evidence that stress-management strategies are generally beneficial in terms of both psychological and physical functioning. Therefore, stress management can play an important role in the treatment of patients with chronic diseases.

Clinical Implementation: Rheumatoid Arthritis

Clinical implementation of a stress-management program for patients with chronic diseases can be illustrated through consideration of the case of rheumatoid arthritis (RA). There are over 110 subcategories of arthritis, ranging from relatively minor inflammations to major systemic diseases such as RA (Hollander, 1985). *Rheumatoid arthritis* is an autoimmune disease in which the immune system reacts to the patient's own tissues. The autoimmune response results in a state of chronic inflammation, particularly in the joints, which eventually leads to destruction of cartilage, erosion of bone, and loss of range of motion. RA is characterized by severe pain, chronic fatigue, and loss of functional capacities. For most patients, there is a gradual progression toward severe physical disability.

As is the case for most chronic diseases, the socioeconomic consequences of RA are profound. RA patients earn only 50% of the income predicted for them in comparison with age and education-matched control subjects (Meenan, Yelin, Nevitt, & Epstein, 1981). The divorce rate is higher for RA patients, and the remarriage rate is lower (Bradley, 1985). Nearly two thirds of RA patients experience major disruptions in their marital or family circumstances, and 85% experience major disruption in their leisure activities (Liang et al., 1984). Only

41% of RA patients are able to maintain gainful employment (Meenan et al., 1981). In the face of these severe socioeconomic stressors, a stress-management program can play an important role in the treatment of people with RA (as well as most other chronic diseases).

Preparing the Stress-Management Practitioner

Prior to embarking on a stress-management program, there are four areas in which preparation is required of the practitioner. First, there must be solid training in the area of severe psychopathology. Practitioners must be able to recognize situations in which a stress-management program is contraindicated. For a small but clinically important minority of RA patients, stress management is not appropriate as the primary therapeutic strategy. For example, Frank et al. (1988) found that 17% of RA patients met the criteria for a major depressive disorder. In the context of a major depressive disorder and other psychiatric disturbances, comprehensive mental health care is indicated, and a stress-management program, by itself, would not be expected to be effective. Therefore, stress-management practitioners should have sufficient skills in the area of psychodiagnosis to recognize cases in which stress management is not the treatment of choice.

Second, stress-management practitioners need to be well versed in the stress-management literature; that is, they need a solid foundation in the theoretical aspects of stress and coping. Practitioners should also have a basic understanding of psychophysiological responses and an in-depth mastery of stress-management modalities, such as progressive relaxation training, meditation, autogenic training, and biofeedback. Additionally, practitioners must demonstrate an appreciation for the cognitive modulators of the stress response.

Third, stress-management practitioners should be familiar with the particular chronic disease (in this example, RA) that the patient is facing. A practitioner's understanding of a disease need not extend deeply into the medical arena, but he or she must be aware of the pathogenesis, the symptomatology, the diagnostic procedures, and the conventional medical treatments. The practitioner's knowledge of these aspects of the chronic disease is critically important for gaining an awareness of the phenomenology of the patient. To orchestrate an effective stress-management program, practitioners must be sensitized to the disease-specific issues confronting the patient.

Finally, stress-management practitioners must prepare for their work by acquiring a comprehensive psychological database on each patient. The practitioner's knowledge of the patient must go beyond the specific stressors of the moment to an in-depth understanding of his or her history, background, and life circumstances. Stress management is not simply the application of specific techniques, but also the facilitation of improved adaptation. Therefore, the acquisition of a comprehensive psychological database is imperative.

Clinical Encounter

Stress management begins with the initial clinical encounter. In some instances, patients seek stress management on their own, in which case they typically present with expectations for a positive treatment outcome. In the self-referral situation, the initial clinical encounter can be directed toward educating the patient about stress management, affirming that stress management is part of a broader adaptation phenomenon, and initiating the preintervention assessment.

In other cases, the initial clinical encounter occurs as a result of referral by a physician or other health care provider. In the colleague-referred situation, there is a critical need to identify the patient's expectations. Most people with chronic diseases conceptualize their problems as being a consequence of their physical disability. In other words, the physical aspects of their illness are typically viewed as paramount, and the psychological problems are usually viewed as secondary. A patient's initial contact with a mental health professional may therefore seem dissonant, or even inappropriate, to him or her given the physical origins of the patient's difficulties. If the practitioner conveys awareness of the physical origins of the patient's problems and acknowledges that the psychological aspects are secondary to the chronic illness, then a major source of potential resistance is immediately removed. Practitioners need to take special precautions when providing psychological services to people who do not think of themselves as having mental health problems.

During the initial clinical encounter, there is a distinct advantage to beginning the interview with those topics of most immediate relevance for the patient. In chronic illnesses such as RA, immediate concerns are frequently related to pain, fatigue, sleep disturbance, daily stress, and loss of valued activities, among others. To the extent that practitioners focus on these pressing concerns, direct assistance from a mental health professional will be more consonant for the patient. For example, in the case of RA, discussions of pain or fatigue should typically occur before a discussion of depression. In general, the clinical encounter should progress from the discussion of global, disease-relevant topics to subsequent discussions of the psychological aspects of the illness. Patients should be helped to differentiate illness-related stressors from other global stressors operating in their lives.

An important objective during the initial clinical encounter is to elicit the patient's participation in a collaborative psychological assessment. To collaborate with the practitioner effectively, the patient must understand the nature of the process. In addition, the assessment must be reasonably face valid. For example, an assessment of the stressors encountered by the RA patient should include pain, because pain is a face-valid source of stress. Any unique concern of the patient should be covered in the assessment to maintain the credibility of the assessment process. When there are obvious psychiatric components to the assessment (e.g., major depression), the patient needs to understand the clinical rationale for examining these aspects. The initial encounter should be used to prepare the patient to cooperate fully during the assessment process.

Assessment Strategies

There are numerous conceptual domains that should be assessed prior to the initiation of a stress-management program. When possible, the assessment should include a clinical interview, stressor questionnaires, coping questionnaires, problem-focused questionnaires, behavioral data, psychophysiological data, and a screen for psychopathology.

Clinical interview. The clinical interview is the foundation of a stress-management assessment because it affords the opportunity to understand the phenomenology of the patient. As noted, the majority of stressors are psychogenic, so the manner in which a patient perceives a taxing event is usually the critical determinant of the degree of stress. Therefore, determining the nature of the patient's primary appraisal process is imperative. That is, to what extent does the patient perceive a threat of harm or loss? The practitioner must seek to comprehend the nature of the stressful situation from the patient's perspective. The clinical interview also provides an opportunity for the practitioner to gain an understanding of the secondary appraisal process; that is, What coping resources does the patient perceive himself or herself to possess? And are there available resources operating that the patient does not see? A thorough clinical interview (or series of interviews) permits the practitioner to gather information about the patient's primary and secondary appraisal processes.

Life-stress questionnaires. A preintervention assessment should include a review of the number and types of stressors operating in a patient's life. To some extent, assessment of stressors can occur during the clinical interview, but standardized questionnaires are also useful. For example, the Social Readjustment Rating Scale, by Holmes and Rahe (1967), is a commonly used stressor questionnaire. It contains 43 items organized so that a total life stress score can be derived. Although a practical questionnaire, with face validity, this scale does have disadvantages: It covers major life events but not minor everyday frustrations. In addition, the scale does not help one ascertain patients' cognitive appraisals of potentially stressful events.

The Life Experiences Survey is a 57-item questionnaire developed by Sarason, Johnson, and Siegel (1978). The advantage of this survey is that it asks patients to rate stressful events on a 3-point scale of severity and thus captures the patients' cognitive appraisals of stressors. Another questionnaire, the Daily Hassles Scale, is a 117-item scale that quantifies everyday pressures, irritations, and frustrations (Kanner, Coyne, Schaefer, & Lazarus, 1981). Studies have shown that the minor stressors of everyday life are more closely related to emotional state than are major life events (Monroe, 1983). In addition, the Daily Stress Inventory (Brantley, Waggoner, Jones, & Rappaport, 1987) and the Assessment of Daily Experience (Stone & Neale, 1982) are valuable life-stress questionnaires. In contrast with the Daily Hassles Scale, these measures require patients to report prospectively on the occurrence of daily stressors and have proven helpful in documenting relationships between stressors and mood disturbances and physical symptoms in individual patients.

Coping questionnaires. A standardized examination of the coping process is also important. In stress management, improved coping is the primary source of therapeutic gain, so careful examination of the coping process is required. There are several coping questionnaires from which to choose. Some questionnaires measure the coping process in a global sense; others are disease-specific coping inventories.

The Ways of Coping Scale is a 68-item questionnaire developed by Folkman and Lazarus (1980) and subsequently revised by Felton and Revenson (1984) for specific use with patients who have chronic diseases. Another coping scale—the Coping Strategies Questionnaire—was developed by Rosenstiel and Keefe (1983) to assess the ways in which patients cope with pain. This inventory comprises 10 subscales, but factor analyses have yielded the following two factors: Coping Attempts and Pain Control and Rational Thinking (Keefe et al., 1987; Parker et al., 1989). The Pain Control and Rational Thinking factor score, in particular, has proven useful for predicting the degree of psychological distress experienced by patients with RA (Parker et al., 1989).

The Arthritis Helplessness Index is a 15-item questionnaire measuring the degree of helplessness perceived by arthritis patients secondary to their chronic disease. Developed by Nicassio, Wallston, Callahan, Herbert, and Pincus (1985), it has been shown to be a reliable and valid instrument. Nicassio et al. found that high helplessness scores correlated with high levels of depression and functional impairment. Another arthritis-specific scale, the Arthritis Self-Efficacy Scale, was developed by Lorig, Chastain, Ung, Shoor, and Holman (1989). This scale is used to assess patients' degree of confidence that they can successfully manage their disease. The ability to assess self-efficacy in a disease-specific manner is a major advantage for practitioners.

Problem-focused questionnaires. During a preintervention assessment, there is potential benefit to using problem-focused questionnaires. In the case of RA, the Arthritis Impact Measurement Scales is a particularly useful measure (Meenan, Gertman, & Mason, 1980). It yields 10 subscores that cover such problems as pain, social functioning, psychological functioning, upper extremity functioning, and lower extremity functioning. In most cases, the assessment of disease-specific problems has face validity for the patient and yields valuable information for the design of a stress-management intervention. The Sickness Impact Profile, although not a disease-specific measure, is nevertheless useful for assessing functional status in the context of a wide range of chronic diseases (Bergner, Bobbitt, Pollard, Martin, & Gilson, 1976). This measure provides information about how a patient's daily life is being affected by chronic disease.

The examination of chronic pain is another important area for problem-focused assessment. For many chronically ill patients, such as those with RA, coping with pain is an everyday reality. However, pain is a particularly difficult construct to assess. In terms of self-reports, the McGill Pain Questionnaire (Melzack, 1975) is a useful measure, yielding subscores for sensory pain, affective pain, and evaluative pain, among others. This questionnaire can be easily augmented with a visual analog scale (10 cm line with endpoints of *no pain* and *pain as bad as it can be*). For diseases such as RA, a therapist's failure to assess pain may be viewed by the patient as a serious oversight. Pain is a major concern of RA patients (Kazis, Meenan, & Anderson, 1983), so a stress-management practitioner needs to assess pain carefully to understand the patient's experience.

Numerous additional questionnaires are available for assessing the concerns of people who have chronic diseases. Potential concerns include fatigue, family–marital distress, sexual dysfunction, and work-related difficulties. Fatigue can be assessed with the Piper Fatigue Scale (Piper et al., 1989), whereas family difficulties can be assessed with the Family Environment Scale (Moos & Moos, 1986) and other measures (see Kerns, chap. 6, this book). Marital difficulties can be assessed by using the Marital Adjustment Inventory (Manson & Lerner, 1962). Sexual dysfunction and work-related difficulties are typically best assessed in the context of an in-depth clinical interview.

Behavioral data. In addition to conducting clinical interviews and administering self-reports, psychologists can substantially benefit from directly observing behavior. Behavioral observations can take many forms, ranging from reviewing a patient's daily diary to objectively rate behavioral videotapes. With regard to daily diaries, time spent by patients in specific activities—such as sitting, reclining, and standing—can be recorded as recommended by Fordyce (1976). Such diary data can be averaged across time and used to monitor behavioral changes in response to a stress-management intervention.

With regard to videotaping, Keefe and Block (1982) have devised a system for objectively rating pain behaviors. These pain behavior methods were subsequently adapted by McDaniel et al. (1986) for use with RA patients. The pain behavior method involves videotaping patients during a standardized 10-minute sequence of reclining, standing, and walking. The pain behavior videotapes can subsequently be rated to yield measures of specific pain behaviors, such as grimacing, limping, and guarding. Anderson et al. (1987) have shown that videotaped pain behavior is related to RA disease activity. In general, data obtained through behavioral observations are useful for augmenting information obtained through self-reports.

Psychophysiological data. Psychophysiological monitoring is another valuable source of assessment data. The most common monitors are skin temperature, electromyographic response, and skin conductance response. One advantage of psychophysiological monitors is that the patient can be permitted to observe the recording of his or her own stress response. When a patient is able to see changes on a psychophysiological recording, one of the endpoints of stress management immediately becomes clear. Even when biofeedback will not be used as a therapeutic strategy, psychophysiological data are nevertheless helpful because they provide the patient with conceptual information. Even moderate control over psychophysiological responses can help a patient better understand the relevance of the coping process to his or her own biological reactions. A disadvantage of psychophysiological monitoring, though, is the degree of variability that typically occurs. From session to session, electrodes may not be applied in quite the same way. Similarly, background events for the patient may skew his or her psychophysiological responses for a given session. Nevertheless, baseline psychophysiological data can play an important role in helping patients grasp the conceptual aspects of a stress-management program.

Screening for psychopathology. Screening for psychopathology before starting a stress-management program is a particularly important issue. The possibility of clinically significant psychopathology in the patient's presentation must be considered. First and foremost, a practitioner bears the obligation of providing the best possible treatment for a patient's problem. In some cases, major psychopathology may dictate that stress management is inadequate for the treatment task. For example, when patients present with major depression, manic–depressive disorder, schizophrenia, or certain other psychiatric conditions, stress management, by itself, may be contraindicated. Therefore, screening for major psychopathology is imperative prior to the initiation of a stress-management program.

Screening should include a comprehensive psychological interview and a thorough family history. The interview can be used to carefully observe affective state and reality-testing capacities. In some situations, semistructured diagnostic interviews, such as the Schedule for Affective Disorders and Schizophrenia (Endicott & Spitzer, 1978), may be needed. More commonly, objective screening questionnaires—such as the Center for Epidemiologic Studies—Depression Scale (Radloff,

1977) or the Beck Depression Inventory (Beck, Steer, & Garbin, 1988)—can be used. The Symptom Checklist-90-R (Derogatis, 1983) is another useful tool for screening patients with chronic diseases (Parker et al., 1990). Although the Minnesota Multiphasic Personality Inventory can be used to screen for major psychopathology, Pincus, Callahan, Bradley, Vaughn, and Wolfe (1986) have shown that it contains items that overlap with some of the primary symptoms of RA. Therefore, this inventory should be used with great caution with patients who have chronic diseases.

The presence of major psychopathology may serve to contraindicate the implementation of a stress-management program. For some patients, alternative treatments are simply more appropriate and efficacious for the magnitude of the problem. In other cases, serious psychopathology will dictate the stress management must be conceptualized as only one component of a more comprehensive psychiatric program. If major psychopathology is not detected, then the practitioner can proceed with the confidence that a stress-management approach will have a reasonable chance of being helpful to the patient.

Stress-Management Interventions

Following the assessment, the stress-management intervention can begin. *Stress management* is a broad term that encompasses a wide range of therapeutic activities. However, most stress-management programs fall into one of the following four conceptual categories: (a) patient education programs, (b) cognitive–behavioral approaches, (c) psychophysiological interventions, and (d) psychotherapeutic strategies.

Patient education programs. With the patient education approach, the goal is to expand the patient's knowledge of the etiology, pathogenesis, symptomatology, diagnostic procedures, and treatment options for his or her disease. The expectation is that the receipt of relevant information will improve the patient's capacities for self-management and adaptation. In many cases, however, this expectation is not correct. On the basis of a comprehensive literature review, Sackett and Haynes (1976) concluded that there is minimal evidence that patient education results in improved health status for patients with medical conditions. Specifically, in the case of RA, Parker et al. (1984) found that a strictly educational approach was potentially harmful to patients with RA. This was because RA patients may have dramatically reduced their activity levels as a result of discussions of joint erosion or joint protection, and thus encountered more pain. Nevertheless, for some patients, acquiring disease-relevant information is a therapeutic process, particularly in the early stages of a chronic illness. Patient education can correct misconceptions about an illness, clarify the nature of proposed treatments, and set the stage for more in-depth strategies. In most cases, though, a stress-management program must go beyond the purely educational approach to be effective.

Cognitive–behavioral approaches. With cognitive–behavioral approaches, there is a concerted effort to move beyond patient education to the enhancement of adaptive functioning. Bandura's (1977, 1982) social learning framework is a major theoretical foundation for cognitive–behavioral programs. In these approaches, there is an emphasis on identifying specific problems of concern to the patient. Interventions are then designed to modify either the cognitive appraisals or the coping behaviors of the patient to reduce stress.

In the case of RA, several prospective outcome studies have examined the effects of cognitive–behavioral stress-management programs. Lorig, Lubeck, Kraines, Seleznick, and Holman (1985) developed the Arthritis Self-Help Program, which attempts to enhance self-efficacy as its primary treatment goal. The program is delivered by lay leaders who follow structured program guidelines. In a small-group format, participants engage in activities aimed at enhancing self-efficacy. Most trials of the Arthritis Self-Help Program have been successful (Lorig et al., 1985). In addition, trials of several other programs that have a cognitive–behavioral emphasis also have been found beneficial for patients with RA (Bradley et al., 1987; O'Leary, Shoor, Lorig, & Holman, 1988; Parker, Frank, et al., 1988).

In many respects, the stress-management program described by Parker (1992) is prototypical of the cognitive–behavioral approach. Parker and his colleagues delivered a semistructured stress-management program of 10 weeks duration to patients with RA. The patients were seen on a weekly basis for an average of 90 minutes per session. The first half of each session was devoted to enhancing active-coping and problem-solving skills in relation to disease-relevant stressors; the remainder of each session was devoted to biofeedback-assisted relaxation training. A predesigned list of frequent stressors encountered by RA patients was used to guide the active-coping and problem-solving discussions. The general approach was to address a new stressor each week, but the pace of the discussions and the specific content areas were dictated by the needs of each patient. The broad themes for the weekly stress-management sessions were as follows: (a) the rationale for stress management, (b) the sources of the stressors encountered by the patient, (c) the characteristic ways in which patients cope with the stressors associated with RA, (d) the patient's major life goals, (e) pain management, (f) the range of emotional responses that commonly occur in chronic diseases, (g) the management of the life changes that typically occur secondary to a chronic disease, (h) the manner in which chronic diseases challenge self-esteem, (i) the patient's interpersonal relationships, and (j) a general overview and consolidation of gains made during the stress-management program. There was an effort to highlight the particular themes and discussions of primary relevance for each patient. In addition, a stress-management maintenance plan was developed, and a schedule for follow-up visits was established. Recommendations for incorporating and maintaining treatment gains in everyday life were also provided.

The Parker (1992) stress-management program is only one example of a cognitive–behavioral intervention for patients with chronic diseases. Other programs also have been found effective in the context of RA (Bradley et al., 1987; O'Leary et al., 1988). Any cognitive–behavioral program should be delivered in a highly individualized manner. That is, the order and timing of the sessions should be modified to maximally meet the needs of a given patient. There also should be homework assignments between sessions to foster generalization of the stress-management program to the stressors of everyday life. In addition, the involvement of family members in the treatment process is usually indicated, and a systems perspective is highly desirable.

Psychophysiological interventions. Psychophysiological interventions focus on specific skills that can be used to directly reduce psychophysiological arousal. Psychophysiological interventions include meditation techniques, autogenic methods, progressive relaxation training, and biofeedback. These direct strategies for reducing psychophysiological arousal are rarely used in isolation. More commonly, such interventions are integrated into more comprehensive stress-management programs. However, psychophysiological interventions are sufficiently unique to warrant separate discussion.

Meditation as a stress-management strategy has been described by Benson et al. (1974), who indicated that four elements are required for the emergence of a relaxation response. These requisite elements are a comfortable position, a quiet environment, a passive attitude, and a mental or physical exercise. The rationale for meditation is that the repetition of a mental or physical exercise will, over time, successfully block anxiety-arousing thoughts. Several studies have reported psychophysiological benefits following meditation-based interventions (e.g., Parker, Gilbert, & Thoreson, 1978).

Autogenic training (Luthe, 1969) is another strategy used to directly reduce psychophysiological arousal. In this approach, comforting words, pleasant visualizations, or both are used to induce a mentally relaxed state. In the autogenic approach, audiotapes or videotapes are commonly used to stimulate feelings of peacefulness and well-being. Studies have shown that autogenic training can be useful for reducing psychophysiological arousal (Jacobs & Lubar, 1989).

Progressive relaxation training is an additional useful technique for inducing reduced psychophysiological arousal (Bernstein & Borkovec, 1973). Progressive relaxation training involves teaching a standardized sequence of "tensing and releasing" exercises that can lead to a relaxed mental and physical state. The principles of progressive relaxation training were developed by Jacobson (1938) and were subsequently used by Wolpe (1958) as a component of systematic desensitization. The literature provides convincing evidence that progressive relaxation training can result in reduced psychophysiological arousal.

Biofeedback is a final strategy for directly reducing psychophysiological activity (Schwartz, 1987). There is convincing evidence that physiological responses can be brought under voluntary control, but the role of biofeedback as a therapeutic strategy remains somewhat controversial (Roberts, 1985). Shellenberger and Green (1986) have suggested that psychophysiological instrumentation is only one component of the biofeedback phenomenon. They maintained that the cognitive and motivational capacities within the individual are the critical factors that permit control over physiological responses to be achieved. There is no doubt that people can be trained to reduce psychophysiological arousal without the use of biofeedback instrumentation (Bernstein & Borkovec, 1973). Nevertheless, biofeedback-assisted approaches are helpful to some patients as they attempt to learn relaxation techniques. In addition, biofeedback can be useful for specific disorders, such as migraine headaches and Raynaud's disease.

There are several effective psychological strategies for reducing psychophysiological arousal. These strategies can be used either singly or in combination as components of a stress-management program.

Eclectic psychotherapy. In some situations, the combination of patient education, cognitive–behavioral methods, and direct psychophysiological intervention may prove to be insufficient for enhancing a patient's stress-management capacities. In such cases, using a range of psychotherapeutic approaches may be more helpful. For example, a given patient's outlook may be such that adaptive coping and problem-solving cannot be maintained. In the extreme situation, perceptions of helplessness or loss of control may immobilize a patient and keep him or her from engaging in coping activities. In addition, psychiatric disorders or long-standing personality characteristics may interfere with the usual approaches to stress management. In these situations, a skillful practitioner can call on a range of psychotherapeutic strategies to help the patient progress to the point of being able to benefit from a stress-management program.

Adjunctive Stress-Management Care

In chronic diseases, such as RA, physicians and allied health professionals play important roles in interdisciplinary approaches to stress management. Physicians can effectively provide information to both the psychologist and the patient regarding realistic expectations for disease outcomes. Physicians also can be directly involved in the problem-solving process and enlisted as allies in patients' stress-management activities. Similarly, physical therapists, occupational therapists, and exercise physiologists, among others, can provide important adjunctive components of a stress-management program. If a patient is effectively supported by an interdisciplinary team, there can be beneficial effects on the patient's perceptions of personal control and self-efficacy. Ideally, a stress-management program should be designed to be under the direct control of the patient. In effect, the patient becomes the "director" of his or her treatment team, rather than a passive recipient of a range of professional services.

Social service professionals can also be important components of a stress-management program. The economic impact of chronic illness is often profound. Work-related activities are commonly disrupted, and income may be severely curtailed. Chronic illness typically engenders a tremendous financial burden for the patient and his or her family, so a social worker can play an important role by helping the patient to reduce or manage the numerous financial stressors. Similarly, vocational rehabilitation counselors can help by designing vocational retraining programs, identifying new occupational possibilities, arranging for transportation needs, and assisting with the process of adapting to new living environments. Effective stress-management programs for patients with chronic diseases typically require the coordinated efforts of such interdisciplinary treatment teams.

Evaluation of Treatment Efficacy

The same types of assessments that are used at the initiation of a stress-management program can also be used to evaluate treatment efficacy. Self-reports can be derived through either clinical interviews or standardized questionnaires, although the possibility that the patient may choose to give socially desirable responses cannot be completely ruled out. Nevertheless, if patients are asked to respond candidly, useful outcome information can often be obtained. Another valuable source of evaluation data is direct behavioral observation. With behavioral data, social desirability does not operate to quite the same degree. In the case of videotapes of RA pain behavior, for example, the patient does not even know which specific pain behaviors will be rated. Behavioral data from diaries or self-monitoring can also figure importantly in outcome evaluations. Lastly, psychophysiological data are useful in some situations, although improved coping does not necessarily lead to identifiable psychophysiological changes on the variables being monitored. Therefore, reduced psychophysiological values should not be the sole criterion for positive treatment outcomes. In most cases, a combination of self-reports, behavioral observations, and psychophysiological recordings will be an appropriate strategy for evaluating treatment outcome.

Future Directions

From a clinical standpoint, much remains to be learned about the delivery of effective stress-management programs. Currently, most programs use multicomponent interventions, but all components may not be equally important. Ultimately, there needs to be a better understanding of which specific components are crucial for positive clinical outcomes. There also is much to be learned about which programs work best for which patients. For some patients, the patient education approach may sufficiently stimulate coping activities. For others, cognitive–behavioral approaches or psychophysiological strategies may be required. For still others, in-depth psychotherapeutic efforts may be needed to achieve beneficial treatment outcomes. Presently, there is minimal understanding of how to best match treatment approaches to a particular patient's clinical needs. Additional research in this area is needed.

The limited availability of resource materials for stress-management practitioners is a substantial problem. In the context of chronic diseases, practitioners need to be knowledgeable about the disease itself in order to be effective. The development of stress-management handbooks for specific diseases could help practitioners respond more effectively to the unique issues involved in each chronic illness. Practitioners also would benefit from the development of computer software packages and graphics components to assist in the delivery of the didactic aspects of stress-management programs.

There is also work to be done to reduce social and cultural barriers to stress-management services. Economics is one major barrier to stress-management access: Many patients with chronic illnesses do not have the financial resources or the insurance coverage to obtain assistance from stress-management practitioners. As a result, some people with chronic diseases experience greater disability than would otherwise be necessary. The progression from health to disability is modulated by numerous psychological and sociological factors (Pope & Tarlov, 1991). Stress management can help inhibit this progression toward disability by helping chronically ill people maintain viability in their social roles. Unfortunately, limited access to stress-management services is a major problem that leads to unnecessary disablement for millions of Americans.

There also are cultural barriers to the use of stress-management programs because people from some minority groups may be disinclined to participate in traditional health care services (see Young & Zane, chap. 5, this book). For many segments of society, the traditional health care system is simply not a viable alternative. Innovative programs that can gain the confidence of minority group leaders are needed to expand the use of stress-management services. Sensitivity to gender issues should also be considered in the development of stress-management programs. In American society, women encounter unique stressors associated with societal expectations for the multiple roles of spouse, mother, and worker. For women with chronic diseases, such societal expectations are extremely difficult to meet. Specialized stress-management programs should be made available to this particular group.

From a research standpoint, exciting questions are waiting to be addressed at the interface of psychology and medicine. There is an increasing scientific appreciation for the ways in which psychological factors, such as stress, can modulate disease activity. Although associations between stress and the immune system have been established, the mechanisms and the causal relationships are not fully understood. In many chronic diseases, there is a possibility that stress may contribute to the physical symptoms of the disease itself, but carefully controlled studies in this area are not yet available. In the future, it is hoped, researchers will pursue a better understanding of the ways in which stressor events exert their effects on the coping process, target-organ activation, and disease activity in relation to specific illnesses.

In conclusion, the concept of stress is centrally important to the field of health psychology. Stressors and stress responses bridge the gap between the environment and the human organism. The term *stress* has clinical value and can serve as a foundation for effective psychological interventions for individuals with chronic diseases. When used with precise terminology, the stress concept can also facilitate important investigations at the interface of health psychology and medicine.

REFERENCES

Adams, J. D. (1978). Improving stress management. *Social Change: Ideas and Application, 8*(4), 1–11.

Anderson, K. O., Bradley, L. A., McDaniel, L. K., Young, L. D., Turner, R. A., Agudelo, C. A., Gaby, N. S., Keefe, F. J., Pisko, E. J., Snyder, R. M., & Semble, E. L. (1987). The assessment of pain in rheumatoid arthritis: Disease differentiation and temporal stability of a behavioral observation method. *Journal of Rheumatology, 14,* 700–704.

Bandura, A. (1977). Self-efficacy: Toward a unifying theory of behavioral change. *Psychological Review, 84,* 191–215.

Bandura, A. (1982). Self-efficacy mechanism in human agency. *American Psychologist, 37,* 122–145.

Beck, A. T., Steer, R. A., & Garbin, M. G. (1988). Psychometric properties of the Beck Depression Inventory: Twenty-five years of evaluation. *Clinical Psychology Review, 8,* 77–100.

Ben-Sira, Z. (1984). Chronic illness, stress and coping. *Social Science and Medicine, 18,* 725–736.

Benson, H., Beary, J. F., & Carol, M. P. (1974). The relaxation response. *Psychiatry, 37,* 37–46.

Bergner, M., Bobbitt, R. A., Pollard, W. E., Martin, D. P., & Gilson, B. S. (1976). The Sickness Impact Profile: Validation of a health status measure. *Medical Care, 14,* 57–67.

Bernstein, D. A., & Borkovec, T. D. (1973). *Progressive relaxation training: A manual for the helping professions.* Champaign, IL: Research Press.

Blankfield, R. P. (1991). Suggestion, relaxation, and hypnosis as adjuncts in the care of surgery patients: A review of the literature. *American Journal of Clinical Hypnosis, 33,* 172–186.

Blenkhorn, A., Silove, D., Magarey, C., Krillis, S., & Coninet, H. (1992). The effect of a multimodal stress management program on immune and psychological functions. In A. J. Husband (Ed.), *Behavior and immunity* (pp. 189–209). Boca Raton, FL: CRC Press.

Bradley, L. A. (1985). Psychological aspects of arthritis. *Bulletin on the Rheumatic Diseases, 35*(4), 1–12.

Bradley, L. A., Young, L. D., Anderson, K. O., Turner, R. A., Agudelo, C. A., McDaniel, L. K., Pisko, E. J., Semble, E. L., & Morgan, T. M. (1987). Effects of psychological therapy on pain behavior of rheumatoid arthritis patients: Treatment outcome and six-month followup. *Arthritis and Rheumatism, 30,* 1105–1114.

Brantley, P. J., Waggoner, C. D., Jones, G. N., & Rappaport, N. B. (1987). A Daily Stress Inventory: Development, reliability, and validity. *Journal of Behavioral Medicine, 10,* 61–74.

Cannon, W. B. (1914). The emergency function of the adrenal medulla in pain and the major emotions. *American Journal of Physiology, 33,* 356–372.

Derogatis, L. R. (1983). *SCL-90-R administration, scoring & procedures manual—II.* Towson, MD: Clinical Psychometric Research.

Endicott, J., & Spitzer, R. L. (1978). A diagnostic interview: The Schedule for Affective Disorders and Schizophrenia. *Archives of General Psychiatry, 35,* 837–844.

Engel, B. T. (1985). Stress is a noun! No, a verb! No, an adjective. In T. M. Field & P. M. McCabe (Eds.), *Stress and coping* (pp. 3–12). Hillsdale, NJ: Erlbaum.

Engel, G. L. (1977, April 18). The need for a new medical model: A challenge for biomedicine. *Science, 196,* 129–136.

Everly, G. S., Jr. (1989). *A clinical guide to the treatment of the human stress response.* New York: Plenum.

Felton, B. J., & Revenson, T. A. (1984). Coping with chronic illness: A study of illness controllability and the influence of coping strategies on psychological adjustment. *Journal of Consulting and Clinical Psychology, 52,* 343–353.

Field, T. M., McCabe, P. M., & Schneiderman, N. (1985). *Stress and coping.* Hillsdale, NJ: Erlbaum.

Folkman, S., & Lazarus, R. S. (1980). An analysis of coping in a middle-aged community sample. *Journal of Health and Social Behavior, 21,* 219–239.

Fordyce, W. E. (1976). *Behavioral methods for chronic pain and illness.* St. Louis, MO: C. V. Mosby.

Frank, R. G., Beck, N. C., Parker, J. C., Kashani, J. H., Elliott, T. R., Haut, A. E., Smith, E., Atwood, C., Brownlee-Duffeck, M., & Kay, D. R. (1988). Depression in rheumatoid arthritis. *Journal of Rheumatology, 15,* 920–925.

Gentry, W. D. (1984). Behavioral medicine: A new research paradigm. In W. D. Gentry (Ed.), *Handbook of behavioral medicine* (pp. 1–12). New York: Guilford Press.

Hollander, J. L. (1985). Introduction. In D. J. McCarty (Ed.), *Arthritis and allied conditions* (pp. 3–8). Philadelphia: Lea & Febiger.

Holmes, T., & Masuda, M. (1974). Life change and illness susceptibility. In B. S. Dohrenwend & B. P. Dohrenwend (Eds.), *Stressful life events: Their nature and effects* (pp. 45–72). New York: Wiley.

Holmes, T. H., & Rahe, R. H. (1967). The Social Readjustment Rating Scale. *Journal of Psychosomatic Research, 11,* 213–218.

Hughes, G. H., Pearson, M. A., & Reinhart, G. R. (1984). Stress: Sources, effects, and management. *Family and Community Health, 7,* 47–58.

Hyman, R. B., Feldman, H. R., Harris, R. B., Levin, R. F., & Malloy, G. B. (1989). The effects of relaxation training on clinical symptoms: A meta-analysis. *Nursing Research, 38,* 216–220.

Jacobs, G. D., & Lubar, J. F. (1989). Spectral analysis of the central nervous system effects on the relaxation response elicited by autogenic training. *Behavioral Medicine, 15,* 125–132.

Jacobson, E. (1938). *Progressive relaxation.* Chicago: University of Chicago Press.

Kanner, A. D., Coyne, J. C., Schaefer, C., & Lazarus, R. S. (1981). Comparison of two modes of stress management: Daily hassles and uplifts versus major life events. *Journal of Behavioral Medicine, 4,* 1–39.

Kazis, L. E., Meenan, R. F., & Anderson, J. J. (1983). Pain in the rheumatic diseases: Investigation of a key health status component. *Arthritis and Rheumatism, 26,* 1017–1022.

Keefe, F. J., & Block, A. R. (1982). Development of an observation method for assessing pain behavior in chronic low back pain patients. *Behavior Therapy, 13,* 363–375.

Keefe, F. J., Caldwell, D. S., Queen, K. T., Gil, K. M., Martinez, S., Crisson, J. E., Ogden, W., & Nunley, J. (1987). Pain coping strategies in osteoarthritis patients. *Journal of Consulting and Clinical Psychology, 55,* 208–212.

Kiecolt-Glaser, J. K., & Glaser, R. (1988). Psychological influences on immunity: Implications for AIDS. *American Psychologist, 43,* 892–898.

Lazarus, R. S., & Folkman, S. (1984). *Stress, appraisal, and coping.* New York: Springer.

Leidy, N. K., Ozbolt, J. G., & Swain, M. A. P. (1990). Psychophysiological processes of stress in chronic physical illness: A theoretical perspective. *Journal of Advanced Nursing, 15,* 478–486.

Liang, M. H., Rogers, M., Larson, M., Eaton, H. M., Murawski, B. J., Taylor, J. E., Swafford, J., & Schur, P. H. (1984). The psychosocial impact of systemic lupus erythematosus and rheumatoid arthritis. *Arthritis and Rheumatism, 27,* 13–19.

Lorig, K., Chastain, R. L., Ung, E., Shoor, S., & Holman, H. R. (1989). Development and evaluation of a scale to measure perceived self-efficacy in people with arthritis. *Arthritis and Rheumatism, 32,* 37–44.

Lorig, K., Lubeck, D., Kraines, R. G., Seleznick, M., & Holman, H. R. (1985). Outcomes of self-help education for patients with arthritis. *Arthritis and Rheumatism, 28,* 680–685.

Luthe, W. (1969). *Autogenic therapy.* New York: Grune & Stratton.

Manson, M. P., & Lerner, A. (1962). *Marriage Adjustment Inventory.* Los Angeles: Western Psychological Services.

McDaniel, L. K., Anderson, K. O., Bradley, L. A., Young, L. D., Turner, R. A., Agudelo, C. A., & Keefe, F. J. (1986). Development of an observation method for assessing pain behavior in rheumatoid arthritis patients. *Pain, 24,* 165–184.

Meenan, R. F., Gertman, P. M., & Mason, J. H. (1980). Measuring health status in arthritis: The Arthritis Impact Measurement Scales. *Arthritis and Rheumatism, 23,* 146–152.

Meenan, R. F., Yelin, E. H., Nevitt, M., & Epstein, W. V. (1981). The impact of chronic disease: A sociomedical profile of rheumatoid arthritis. *Arthritis and Rheumatism, 24,* 544–548.

Melzack, R. (1975). The McGill Pain Questionnaire: Major properties and scoring methods. *Pain, 1,* 277–299.

Monroe, S. M. (1983). Major and minor life events as predictors of psychological distress: Further issues and findings. *Journal of Behavioral Medicine, 6,* 189–205.

Moos, R. H., & Moos, B. S. (1986). *Family Environment Scale.* Palo Alto, CA: Consulting Psychologists Press.

Munck, A., Guyre, P. M., & Holbrook, N. J. (1984). Physiological functions of glucucorticoids in stress and their relation to pharmacological actions. *Endocrine Reviews, 5,* 25–44.

Nicassio, P. M., Wallston, K. A., Callahan, L. F., Herbert, M., & Pincus, T. (1985). The measurement of helplessness in rheumatoid arthritis: The development of the Arthritis Helplessness Index. *Journal of Rheumatology, 12,* 462–467.

O'Leary, A., Shoor, S., Lorig, K., & Holman, H. R. (1988). A cognitive–behavioral treatment for rheumatoid arthritis. *Health Psychology, 7,* 527–544.

Parker, J., Buckelew, S., Smarr, K., Buescher, K., Beck, N., Frank, R., Anderson, S., & Walker, S. (1990). Psychological screening in rheumatoid arthritis. *Journal of Rheumatology, 17,* 1016–1021.

Parker, J. C. (1992, October). *Stress, stress management, and the immune system.* Paper presented at the Annual Meeting of the Arthritis Health Professions Association, Atlanta, GA.

Parker, J. C., Frank, R. G., Beck, N. C., Smarr, K. L., Buescher, K. L., Phillips, L. R., Smith, E. I., Anderson, S. K., & Walker, S. E. (1988). Pain management in rheumatoid arthritis patients: A cognitive–behavioral approach. *Arthritis and Rheumatism, 31,* 593–601.

Parker, J. C., Gilbert, G. S., & Thoreson, R. W. (1978). Reduction of autonomic arousal in alcoholics: A comparison of relaxation and meditation techniques. *Journal of Consulting and Clinical Psychology, 46,* 879–886.

Parker, J. C., Singsen, B. H., Hewett, J. E., Walker, S. E., Hazelwood, S. E., Hall, P. J., Holsten, D. J., & Rodon, C. M. (1984). Educating patients with rheumatoid arthritis: A prospective analysis. *Archives of Physical Medicine and Rehabilitation, 65,* 771–774.

Parker, J. C., Smarr, K. L., Buescher, K. L., Phillips, L. R., Frank, R. G., Beck, N. C., Anderson, S. K., & Walker, S. E. (1989). Pain control and rational thinking: Implications for rheumatoid arthritis. *Arthritis and Rheumatism, 32,* 984–990.

Pincus, T., Callahan, L. F., Bradley, L. A., Vaughn, W. K., & Wolfe, F. (1986). Elevated MMPI scores for hypochondriasis, depression, and hysteria in patients with rheumatoid arthritis reflect disease rather than psychological status. *Arthritis and Rheumatism, 29,* 1456–1466.

Piper, B. F., Lindsey, A. M., Dodd, M. J., Ferketich, S., Paul, S. M., & Weller, S. (1989). The development of an instrument to measure the subjective dimension of fatigue. In S. G. Fund, E. M. Tornquist, M. T. Champagne, L. A. Copp, & R. A. Wiese (Eds.), *Key aspects of comfort: Management of pain, fatigue, and nausea* (pp. 199–208). New York: Springer.

Pope, A. M., & Tarlov, A. R. (1991). *Disability in America: Toward a national agenda for prevention.* Washington, DC: National Academy Press.

Radloff, L. S. (1977). The CES-D scale: A self-report depression scale for research in the general population. *Applied Psychological Measurement, 1,* 385–401.

Rahe, R. H. (1988). Anxiety and physical illness. *Journal of Clinical Psychiatry, 49,* 26–29.

Rasmussen, H. (1975). Medical education: Revolution or reaction. *Pharos of Alpha Omega Honor Medical Society, 38,* 53–59.

Roberts, A. H. (1985). Biofeedback: Research, training, and clinical roles. *American Psychologist, 40,* 938–941.

Rosenstiel, A. K., & Keefe, F. J. (1983). The use of coping strategies in chronic low back pain patients: Relationship to patient characteristics and current adjustment. *Pain, 17,* 33–44.

Sackett, D. L., & Haynes, R. B. (1976). *Compliance with therapeutic regimens.* Baltimore: Johns Hopkins University Press.

Sarason, I. G., Johnson, J. H., & Siegel, J. M. (1978). Assessing the impact of life changes: Development of the Life Experiences Survey. *Journal of Consulting and Clinical Psychology, 46,* 932–946.

Schaffer, M. (1982). *Life after stress.* New York: Plenum.

Schwartz, M. S. (1987). *Biofeedback: A practitioner's guide.* New York: Guilford Press.

Selye, H. (1946). The general adaptation syndrome and the diseases of adaptation. *Journal of Clinical Endocrinology, 6,* 117–230.

Selye, H. (1956). *The stress of life*. New York: McGraw-Hill.

Shellenberger, R., & Green, J. A. (1986). *From the ghost in the box to successful biofeedback training*. Greeley, CO: Health Psychology Publications.

Stone, A. A., & Neale, J. M. (1982). Development of a methodology for assessing daily experiences. In A. Baum & J. Singer (Eds.), Advances in environmental psychology: Environment and health (Vol. 4, pp. 49–83). Hillsdale, NJ: Erlbaum.

Wolpe, J. (1958). *Psychotherapy by reciprocal inhibition*. Stanford, CA: Stanford University Press.

Chapter

Clinical Assessment and Management of Adherence to Medical Regimens

Jacqueline Dunbar-Jacob, Lora E. Burke, and Sandra Puczynski

The magnitude of the problem of poor adherence to medical regimens for chronic disease has been well documented over the past 20 years or more. The rates have changed little over that time period (Dunbar-Jacob, Dwyer, & Dunning, 1991). Even today, up to 80% of patients will not follow their treatment program sufficiently to attain therapeutic benefit. Furthermore, the problem crosses age groups, diagnoses, and socioeconomic strata as well as various treatment regimens.

The problem of nonadherence to therapeutic regimens concerns all practitioners in the health care arena. Every patient is at risk for nonadherent episodes of varying degree. Thus, the practitioner needs to advise patients and to prescribe health behaviors in ways that support adherence. For the clinical health psychology practitioner, the problem of nonadherence has relevance beyond the direct patient–provider interchange. Health psychologists may be called on to consult with the patient or with other providers of health care on issues of poor adherence. This consultation may range from behavioral assessment to the design of systemwide programs to promote adherence. Furthermore, health psychologists may be involved in the design and conduct of efficacy or effectiveness studies, with a particular role in the design of compliance assessment and intervention strategies for such studies. Attention to these issues is also crucial to the adequate interpretation of intervention studies conducted by the health psychologist himself or herself.

This chapter is designed to provide an overview of the broad and extensive literature on adherence to medical regimens. It is intended to instruct the naive reader on the extensive problem that exists in health care and to provide the experienced reader with a reference by which to evaluate assessment strategies, develop interventions, and identify the research needed to further understanding of this important behavior. Included are data on the significance of the problem of poor adherence and on the magnitude of the problem across common health behaviors as well as a discussion of the factors that contribute to low adherence. The limited literature on intervention strategies is examined. The multiple methods of assessing adherence are discussed in some detail, as no gold standard exists. Attention is also given to issues in the clinical implementation of adherence-enhancement programs. And, lastly, a discussion of key future directions for research and intervention is included. The problem of poor adherence has considerable impact on health and health care. We hope that this chapter conveys the seriousness of this problem and stimulates the health psychologist to address nonadherence in both practice and research.

The Problem of Poor Adherence and Related Issues

Significance of the Problem

Poor adherence to long-term health care regimens necessitated by chronic disease contributes to significant cost as well as morbidity. For example, 39% of single and 31% of multiple admissions for insulin-dependent diabetes have been attributed to poor compliance (H. A. Fishbein, 1985). Among elderly people, 11% of hospitalizations have been attributed to noncompliance, with nearly 33% of those hospitalized having a history of poor adherence (Nanada, Fanale, & Kronholm, 1990). There is an excess hospitalization rate among mentally ill people as well. For example, the difference in rehospitalization rates among schizophrenics is substantial: 27% for compliant and 73% for noncompliant patients (Pietzcker, 1985). Such needless hospitalizations unquestionably contribute to unnecessary costs. In a study carried out to determine the relative cost–benefit of identifying new cases of hypertension or of remediating adherence in people currently diagnosed and under treatment, the evidence clearly supported the advantage of improving adherence in known cases (Stason & Weinstein, 1977).

Cost is not the only untoward consequence of poor adherence. Increases in morbidity may also result. One illustration is in the recently noted increasing prevalence of treatment-resistant tuberculosis. A significant cause of death in the world today is infectious disease, with tuberculosis the leading contributor (Bloom & Murray, 1992). An upswing in cases of tuberculosis has been noted and is most likely due to the emergence of drug-resistant strains of organisms (Gibbons, 1992). The emergence of these treatment-resistant organisms can be attributed to poor adherence to medication regimens (Bloom & Murray, 1992). That is, poor adherence allows organisms to survive because doses of medication are inadequate, increasing the chance of mutation and selective survival of treatment-resistant organisms. Perhaps even more startling is one report indicating that nonadherence accounts for more graft loss than does uncontrollable rejection among patients who have had organ transplants (Rovelli et al., 1989).

The consequences of nonadherence are also found in the pediatric population. Unnecessary complications of disease may result from poor adherence. For example, one of the leading causes of hospitalization for ketoacidosis among children and adolescents with diabetes is nonadherence to insulin and diet therapy (White, Kolman, Wexler, Polin, & Winter, 1984). Relapse rates among adolescents with acute lymphoblastic leukemia, a life-threatening condition, are also higher among the nonadherent (Klopovich & Trueworthy, 1985; Trueworthy, 1982). Not only do preventable complications of disease occur as a result of nonadherence, but other unnecessary disease may befall the child. One unfortunate illustration of this problem is the occurrence of 27,600 cases of measles in 1990 as a result of a failure to immunize (Mason, 1992).

The impact of nonadherence or partial adherence is felt not only in the clinical setting, but in the research arena as well. The implications of partial adherence for the evaluation of therapeutic efficacy are significant. In the study of medication efficacy, for example, the accepted statistical paradigm for analysis is the intention-to-treat model. In this model, all subjects randomized to a treatment arm are included in the outcome analysis regardless of behavior during the course of the trial. In studies where adherence is less than optimal, the efficacy of treatment may be underestimated. However, less appreciated is the fact that the occurrence of untoward effects of treatment may also be underestimated. In addition to the potential for confounding outcome, poor adherence can seriously impair study power, leading to added costs because of the need for additional subjects. The curve relating adherence to sample size is steep. E. E. Davis (1990) has noted that sample sizes increase by a factor of 1.02 when just 10% of subjects fail to adhere and by up to a factor of 4 when 50% of subjects fail to adhere.

There is no doubt that the consequences of poor adherence can be significant to the costs of health care, to patients' health, and to clinical research outcomes. Efforts need to be directed toward preventing or remediating this problem.

Relevance of the Problem

Health psychology. The development and evaluation of strategies to enhance adherence is clearly a focus within the discipline of health psychology. Health psychology is concerned with the behavior of individuals in relation to health and disease. Much of health psychology addresses hypothesis testing related to the interplay of individuals' behavior, broadly defined, and their health status or the development and evaluation of interventions to modify that behavior, with the final objective being the modification of health status. Yet neither the testing nor the application of these interventions has utility unless patients (or research subjects) actually carry out the recommendations.

Through furthering the understanding of factors that contribute to poor adherence, as well as through the development and evaluation of behavioral interventions, health psychology is uniquely prepared to contribute to the promotion of patient adherence. Such interventions should have broad applicability throughout health care fields.

Perhaps more inherently relevant is the understanding that patients who are in treatment or participating in a research study with a health psychologist are just as likely to be nonadherent as patients who are receiving medically directed treatment. Consequently, it behooves the practitioner as well as the scientist to develop a fuller understanding of the phenomenon of poor adherence and to develop a set of strategies to prevent or remediate this problem.

Health professionals. The physician, the nurse, the dietitian, and the physical therapist—indeed, all health care professionals—are affected by the problem of poor adherence on at least three fronts. The first is the ability to deliver clinical care. Unless poor adherence is recognized and addressed, it is not possible for the practitioner to make reasoned decisions about the efficacy of treatment for a given patient. The second is the identification of efficacious and acceptable therapies based on empirical study. The adherence of people participating in research influences study outcomes and may mislead investigators and clinicians about the effect of a particular intervention (Collins & Dorus, 1991). Consequently, studies of treatment efficacy must, at a minimum, measure adherence, and ideally attempt to foster high adherence to the study protocol and treatment. The third problem area is provider or investigator adherence. This is a critical but underdiscussed problem in the conduct of clinical research. Clearly, the evaluation of treatment is based not only on the patient's ability to follow the regimen, but also on the investigator's ability to follow the study protocol. However, provider adherence is also an issue when treatment is delivered under commonly held guidelines or according to a structured clinical protocol.

Patient care. In designing care, the efficacy of treatment depends on the patient's ability to follow the treatment plan. Patients who are unprepared to meet the many disruptions to adequate completion of the daily treatment routine will fail to benefit from care. Consequently, the provider needs to have the knowledge and the skills to help patients adhere to the best of their abilities.

Theoretical and Research Base

Magnitude of the Problem

Up to 80% of patients can be expected to be poorly adherent to their treatment regimen at some time. Rates of inadequate compliance vary with the characteristics of the regimen. For example, poor adherence may be greater among people on long-term regimens and on more complex regimens that include multiple components or multiple doses per day (Goodall & Halford, 1991). Although adherence to medication regimens has been most widely studied, there is some suggestion that making changes in other health-related behaviors, such as diet or exercise, is even more difficult (Anderson, 1990), though patients may prefer these nonpharmacologic therapies (Swain & Steckel, 1981). The problem of poor adherence can and does affect patients on every type of regimen. Patients' failure to adhere to prescribed medical regimens may be one of the most serious problems in health care today.

Adherence to medication. Medication has been the most widely studied regimen, with the preponderance of studies occurring in chronic disease, particularly hypertension. The rates of adherence among people with hypertension tend to average about 64% (Dunbar-Jacob et al., 1991). Even with the attention to improving these rates over the past 2 decades, little change has occurred. The data do suggest that there may be differences in adherence rates among clinical settings. The highest rates have tended to be seen in family practice sites, followed by population studies, with hospital clinics showing the smallest proportion of adherent patients (Dunbar, Dunning, Dwyer, Burke, & Snetselaar, 1991).

Adherence rates among people with other disorders are equally problematic. Approximately 40% to 60% of people with rheumatoid arthritis adhere to medication designed to reduce the inflammation that causes the deformity seen in this disease (Belcon, Haynes, & Tugwell, 1984; Deyo, Inui, & Sullivan, 1981; Hicks, 1985). Among patients with chronic obstructive pulmonary disease, more than 50% reported missing or discontinuing medication, and more than 50% reported taking extra medication periodically (Dolce et al., 1991). Adherence rates of 57% to 85% have been reported among patients receiving organ transplants (Beck et al., 1980; Cooper & Lanza, 1984; Didlake, Dreyfus, Kerman, Van Buren, & Kahn, 1988; Rovelli et al., 1989; Schweitzer et al., 1990). People with hyperlipidemia prescribed daily medication were found to adhere 82% of the time (Kruse, Schlierf, & Weber, 1989). It has also been shown that just 74% of people with major depression were found to adhere to antidepressants sufficiently to obtain therapeutic benefit (Engstrom, 1991). In another antidepressant therapy study (Myers & Branthwaite, 1992), the actual rates of compliance ranged from 30% to 82% and depended on the dosing schedule and duration of therapy. Studies have also found that from 50% to 66% of people with epilepsy take sufficient medication to receive optimal treatment (Leppik, 1991). The rates reported for other specific diseases and risk factors are similar to those cited above. Although as few as 20% and as many as 80% of people may adhere to a specific treatment within a specific sample, overall these studies suggested that one half to three fourths of patients across a broad range of diseases adhere to treatment, at least sufficiently to obtain therapeutic benefit. The rates are problematic whether the disease is symptomatic or not (e.g., rheumatoid arthritis vs. hypertension) and whether the disorder is or is not more immediately life threatening (e.g., organ transplantation vs. hyperlipidemia).

The extent of the problem of poor adherence to medication described above pertains to adults. As mentioned earlier, however, adherence is also a problem among children (Dunbar & Waszak, 1990). In the pediatric population, treatment programs are administered or supervised by parents. Most of what is known about adherence with pediatric regimens has come from studies of antibiotic regimens for otitis media and from studies with the more complex, multicomponent regimens for diabetes and asthma management (Dunbar, Dunning, & Dwyer, 1993). The rates of nonadherence are no better than those found with adults. For example, in an outpatient study that examined adherence to short-term antibiotic use, more than 50% of patients had stopped their medication by the 3rd day, 71% had stopped by the 6th day, and 82% were no longer taking the medication on the 9th day (Bergman & Werner, 1963). Thus, just 12% of patients adhered to the full 10-day duration of the prescription.

The rates of adherence in chronic pediatric disease are not much better. Estimates of adherence to asthma therapy ranged from 17% to 90% (Lemanek, 1990). Recent work with children on anticonvulsant therapy reported an adherence rate of 44%, with more adherent children having fewer seizures (Hazzard, Hutchinson, & Krawiecki, 1990). Only 55% of children with juvenile rheumatoid arthritis were reported adherent to salicylate therapy (Litt & Cuskey, 1981). Surprisingly, just

57% of children with renal transplants adhered to their life-sustaining medications (Beck et al., 1980).

Adherence to diet. Dietary interventions are also a commonly prescribed regimen for both primary prevention of disease and the management of chronic conditions. Dietary changes are a particularly important treatment for hypertension, hyperlipidemia, other cardiovascular disease, diabetes, and renal disease. Furthermore, diet may be modified to promote adequate nutrition for patients with such disorders as chronic obstructive pulmonary disease and cancer. Few studies actually report adherence to dietary interventions. Where reported, the rates tend to be relatively low. For example, adherence to dietary regimens for diabetes ranges from less than 50% to 86% (Ary, Toobert, Wilson, & Glasgow, 1986; Christensen, Terry, Wyatt, Pichert, & Lorenz, 1983; Glanz, 1980; Webb et al., 1983). Rates of adherence to diets for the management of cardiovascular disease, which emphasize fat, cholesterol, and sodium reduction or weight loss, range from 13% to 76% (Carmody, Fey, Pierce, Connor, & Matarazzo, 1982; Carmody, Matarazzo, & Istvan, 1987; Dunbar, 1985; Glanz, 1979, 1980; Kruse, 1991; McCann, Retzlaff, Dowdy, Walden, & Knopp, 1990; McCann, Retzlaff, Walden, & Knopp, 1990; Witschi, Singer, Wu-Lee, & Stare, 1978). For weight reduction diets, in terms of obesity management, long-term participation tends to be less than 50%, with fewer able to maintain weight loss (Glanz, 1980; Sohar & Sneth, 1973). These studies suggest that a significant number of people are not benefiting from dietary interventions because of their inability to stay with the food plans.

Dietary adherence also is problematic in the management of childhood conditions, especially in the management of diabetes. Dietary adherence tends to be a difficult aspect of treatment for children with diabetes; as many as 47% have reported nonadherence (Delameter, Smith, Kurtz, & White, 1988). Similarly, more than 70% of children with cystic fibrosis have been reported to be nonadherent or partially adherent to diet (Geiss, Hobbs, Hammersley-Maercklein, Kramer, & Henley, 1992; Passero, Remor, & Solomon, 1981).

Adherence to exercise. Regular physical activity and exercise is an area of major importance to health status. The physiological and psychological benefits of exercise have been well documented for such chronic illnesses as coronary heart disease, hypertension, diabetes, respiratory disease, arthritis, and end-stage renal disease (Martin & Dubbert, 1987; Minor, 1991; Powell, 1988; Williams, Stephans, McKnight,

& Dodd, 1991). Because the behavioral requirements are generally much greater than the requirements of drug taking, adherence rates for exercise programs may be even lower than those for other medical regimens for chronic illnesses (Perkins & Epstein, 1988). Studies on adherence to preventive as well as rehabilitative exercise programs of about 6 months' duration have suggested that the rate of adherence is about 50% (Dishman, 1982; Martin & Dubbert, 1987; Oldridge, 1982; Ward & Morgan, 1984). In addition, the dropout rates are high; an average of 50% drop out occurs within 6 to 12 months (Emery, Hauck, & Blumenthal, 1992; Oldridge, 1988; Pollack et al., 1992).

Very little attention has been paid to the study of exercise adherence in children. A 12-session program for children ages 8 to 15 years with hemophilia indicated that at 6 months, 81% to 90% adherence was achieved (Greenan-Fowler, Powell, & Varni, 1987). However, after 9 months the exercise behavior rate was not different from baseline.

Clearly, the problem of poor adherence crosses diseases, regimens, and age groups. Furthermore, adherence is not static over time. Drops in adherence occur and recur at any point in the patient's course of treatment. Every patient is potentially susceptible to problems in the conduct of the treatment regimen. A multiplicity of factors may contribute to those problems, many of which are potentially remediable.

Factors Contributing to Low Adherence

Patient characteristics. A multitude of factors have been associated with poor adherence. Least relevant are demographic characteristics. Age, with the exception of adolescence; gender; marital status, with the exception of dietary adherence; and socioeconomic status have not been consistently related to adherence. Although no studies have examined the specific impact of culture or ethnicity on adherence, in our own work with people who have rheumatoid arthritis no differences in adherence for African American and White patients were found within the practice sites. Interestingly, Dolce et al. (1991) reported a trend ($p = .07$) for African Americans to report better adherence on one self-report measure and no difference between African Americans and Whites on a second self-report measure.

Personality characteristics also have not correlated with adherence. There is a paucity of studies addressing the impact of specific cognitive coping strategies—such as denial, learned resourcefulness, and helplessness—on patient adherence. The results from the limited studies to date are counterintuitive. Cardiac patients who use denial have been shown to have better outcomes, although adherence itself has not been evaluated in this context (e.g., Hackett, Cassem, & Wishnie, 1968; Levenson, Kay, Monteferrante, & Herman, 1984; Levenson, Mishra, Hamer, & Hastillo, 1989). Daily stress and learned resourcefulness have been shown to affect metabolic control in diabetic patients, but this does not appear to be mediated by adherence (Aikens, Wallander, Bell, & Cole, 1992). However, selective cognitive elements have been associated with adherence. For example, Sherbourne, Hays, Ordway, DiMatteo, and Kravitz (1992) noted that avoidant coping was associated with adherence. Others, working with the Common Sense Model of Illness, have noted cognitive constructions of the illness, or the model the patient holds of his or her disease and its course, to be associated with adherence (Baumann, Cameron, Zimmerman, & Leventhal, 1989). For example, if the patient believes that the absence of symptoms signals that a disease is ameliorated, then he or she may stop taking medications for asymptomatic conditions. Or, alternatively, the patient may believe that certain symptoms are associated with a condition, even in the face of counterargument by the health care provider, and engage in treatment dependent on the presence or absence of those symptoms. For example, Meyer, Leventhal, and Gutmann (1985) found that hypertensive patients believe their disorder has specific symptoms that indicate to them when their blood pressure is up, and they then take medication to treat the elevations. Self-efficacy (e.g., Ewart, 1989) has also been associated with adherence. In this case, the patient who believes that he or she is capable of adhering under different conditions is more likely to adhere. The following patient characteristics are most relevant: (a) whether or not the patient knows what he or she is to do (e.g., Boyd, Covington, Stanaszck, & Coussons, 1974; Joyce, Capla, Mason, Reynolds, & Mathews, 1969); (b) how well the patient was able to adhere at the outset of treatment or in the past (Desharnais, Bouillon, & Godin, 1986; Dunbar, 1990; Sherbourne et al., 1992); (c) self-efficacy expectations (Desharnais et al., 1986; Ewart, 1989; McCann, Follette, Driver, Brief, & Knopp, 1988); (d) barriers to implementation of the regimen (Robertson & Keller, 1992); (e) social support, particularly for diet (McCann, Brief, Follette, Walden, & Knopp, 1987); (f) satisfaction with medical care (Nagy & Wolfe, 1984); and (g) avoidance coping (Sherbourne et al., 1992). Thus, for the most part, the patient characteristics that influence adherence are potentially modifiable, rather than fixed characteristics over which the health care provider has no influence.

Regimen characteristics. Regimen features are particularly important influences on adherence. Most important is the complexity of the regimen (Haynes, 1976). Several dimensions of the regimen are critical. First is the number of times a day that the regimen needs to be carried out. The more frequently the regimen needs to be repeated, the greater the probability of nonadherent episodes. Similarly, the greater the number of regimens—for example, diet plus drug rather than drug alone—the more likely that poor adherence will be evidenced. Regimens requiring lifestyle behavior changes appear to be more complex than simply adding a medication into the daily routine and, thus, are more likely to be difficult to follow. General recommendations are to simplify the regimen, to introduce it in steps, and to tailor it to the patient to minimize complexity, although limited numbers of controlled studies have examined the utility of these procedures.

Also of importance is the duration of the regimen. Adherence tends to decline over time (Jacobson et al., 1987; McCann et al., 1987); thus, the patient on a long-term program has an increasing likelihood of episodes of nonadherence as time progresses.

Provider and practice characteristics. Over and above their influence on the nature of the treatment regimen prescribed, the providers and their practices influence patient adherence. Their skills in communicating with the patient and their attitudes toward the patient are key factors (e.g., M. S. Davis, 1978; Korsch & Negrete, 1972). Providers who are warm and address patient concerns are more likely to have patients who adhere. Furthermore, the procedural aspects of the clinical practice, such as the minimization of waiting time, play an important role in whether or not patients return for care and follow the provider's advice (Badgley & Furnal, 1961; Bierenbaum, Green, Florin, Fleischman, & Caldwell, 1967).

Intervention Strategies

A paucity of randomized, controlled intervention research exists for examining strategies for preventing or remediating nonadherence to health care regimens. And, unfortunately, those studies that are done have been often of limited duration. Even so, a number of strategies are suggested by the literature (Southam & Dunbar, 1986).

Initiating the regimen. Efforts to promote adherence at the outset of treatment could theoretically prevent many of the problems that occur during regimen management. Indeed, the value of such strategies is strengthened by the observation that initial adherence is a major predictor of long-term adherence. In the Lipid Research Clinics—Coronary Primary Prevention Trial, initial adherence accounted for 34.5% of the variance in 1-year adherence and 24% of the variance in 7-year adherence (Dunbar, 1990). Similarly, data from the Medical Outcomes Study indicated that initial nonadherence was the strongest predictor of subsequent nonadherence after 2 years (Sherbourne et al., 1992). In spite of this, little research has addressed initiation of regimens. Indeed, just one randomized, controlled investigation was identified that examined the efficacy of a strategy to promote adherence among individuals beginning treatment. This study examined a behavioral strategy to promote adherence among newly diagnosed hypertensive patients in Soweto, South Africa (Saunders, Irwig, Gear, & Ramushu, 1991). Intervention subjects received a health education package, written appointment reminders, and a record for self-monitoring of adherence and blood pressure. At 6 months, just 28% could produce a medication record and only 40% could fill in the medication record correctly. In the intervention group, 31% took 80% or more of their medication, whereas just 15% of the control subjects did. Although this study demonstrated that intervention procedures at the inception of treatment could improve initial adherence in comparison with no intervention, the rates of adherence are still low. Interventions need to be devised that will promote initial adherence at even higher rates.

Remediating adherence problems. Few randomized controlled studies of adherence intervention strategies directed toward the poor adherer have been conducted. The majority of studies have been directed toward improving the adherence of a cross section of patients in a treatment setting or research protocol without regard to individual levels of adherence. Of the studies that have been directed toward remediating poor adherence, efficacy has varied. However, the most promising interventions to date include contracting (Dapcich-Miura & Bovell, 1979; Epstein et al., 1981; Keane, Prue, & Collins, 1981; Steckel & Swain, 1977; Wenerowicz, 1979), social support and follow-up (Kirscht, Kirscht, & Rosenstock, 1981; Morisky et al., 1983; Nessman, Carnahan, & Nugent, 1980), and multicomponent behavioral strategies (Dunbar, 1977; Haynes et al., 1976; Levine et al., 1979; Logan, Milne, Achber, Campbell, & Haynes, 1979; Nessman et al., 1980). Maintenance effects have not been demonstrated with any of these strategies.

Maintaining adherence. Limited attention has been given to studying adherence maintenance strategies. One study addressing this issue focused on medication adherence. C. A. Bond and Monson (1984) combined nurse and pharmacist education with long-term monitoring and management. Adherence was found to be significantly better in the nurse–pharmacist program than in a historical usual-care control group. Good adherence rates continued to be reported over 4 years. Similarly, patients who received nurse or pharmacist home visits, in another study, were more likely to be in treatment 2 years later than those who did not receive the visits (Dickinson et al., 1981). Taken together, these studies suggest that adherence to medication can be maintained over time with the use of continuing care provided by health professionals.

As noted, the majority of adherence-enhancing studies have been conducted without regard to initial adherence levels. Instead, efforts have been directed toward raising the average adherence of the sample, which generally includes the full range of adherence. Interventions have generally consisted of educational, modeling, behavioral, social-support, and self-efficacy strategies.

Educational interventions. Although most intervention strategies include an education component, few randomized controlled studies have examined the efficacy of educational strategies on adherence. There have been two randomized controlled studies. One study directed at medication adherence and one directed at dietary adherence revealed greater adherence in the intervention conditions over a control condition, with no difference between the educational strategies (Mojonnier et al., 1980; Morisky et al., 1983). However, the educational conditions that included family support showed greater adherence than those that did not in the medication adherence study. Educational strategies in diabetes management with both adults and children have also reportedly increased adherence (e.g., deBont et al., 1981; Epstein et al., 1981; Lucey & Wing, 1985; Rettig, Shrauger, Recker, Gallager, & Wiltse, 1986). Varying settings for delivering the education, although not directly compared, seem to be effective. Education that is home based (McCaul, Glasglow, & Schafer, 1987; Rettig et al., 1986), clinic based (Lucey & Wing, 1985; Stevens, Burgess, Kaiser, & Sheppa, 1985), or computer based have been shown to improve adherence among people with diabetes (Wheeler, Wheeler, Ours, & Swider, 1985).

Modeling strategies. Modeling has been used to improve dietary and insulin-injection adherence among adults and children with diabetes. Children receiving instruction in insulin injections by observing peers on videotape demonstrated improved adherence to self-injections (Gilbert, Johnson, Silverstein, & Rosenbloom, 1982). Adults receiving dietary instruction by videotape combined with lunchtime demonstrations also showed improved adherence (McCulloh, Mitchell, Jambler, & Tattersall, 1983). Such strategies reveal the potential for cost-effective delivery of education in skills necessary for adherence to a treatment regimen.

Behavioral strategies. The majority of the interventions evaluating adherence-enhancing strategies have been behavioral in nature. These include strategies emphasizing self-monitoring, goal setting, feedback, behavioral contracting, reinforcement, cuing, and tailoring. One of the first randomized, controlled intervention studies examined the efficacy of behavioral strategies, particularly tailoring, on subsequent adherence (Haynes et al., 1976). By instituting a surreptitious pill count in the home, researchers found that patients who received the adherence intervention were more adherent than those in a control condition.

Cuing, or reminders, has been found to be effective in promoting appointment keeping. Written reminders as well as computerized monitoring systems yielded better keep rates than usual care systems (McDowell, Newell, & Rosser, 1989; Siscovick et al., 1987; Velez, Anderson, McFall, & Magruder-Habib, 1985). The use of mailed educational materials and provider follow-up has also been shown to improve appointment keeping (Smith, Norton, Weinberger, McDonald, & Katz, 1986). Thus, it appears that provider-initiated contact through written or telephone reminders may enhance retention in treatment through continued appointment keeping.

Other strategies have been examined to a limited degree for their effect on improving adherence. Included among these are contracting (e.g., Swain & Steckel, 1981) and self-monitoring (e.g., Edmonds et al., 1985; Fleece et al., 1988). These strategies also improve adherence over usual care practice.

Social support. Social support has been shown to be effective in raising adherence over usual practices. The mobilization of both provider support and family support has been useful (Morisky et al., 1983; Kirscht et al., 1981). Church-based interventions have also been used successfully to enhance adherence through the mobilization of social support, particularly among minority populations (E. Saunders, 1985). Additionally, group interventions have been used successfully in an effort to promote adherence (Nessman et al., 1980).

Self-efficacy enhancement. Following the tenets of cognitive–social learning theory (Bandura, 1986), interventions have also been directed toward the enhancement of self-efficacy with the hope of improving adherence. This has been especially evident in the areas of exercise and dietary adherence. Self-efficacy seems to be a particularly important construct at the outset of treatment (Desharnais et al., 1986; Ewart, 1989). Efficacy enhancement may also be an important component of spousal involvement. Taylor, Bandura, Ewart, Miller, and DeBusk (1985) have noted that rehabilitation efforts may be either enhanced or reduced by the spouse's belief in the patient's efficacy.

Measurement of Adherence

Adherence is a process variable that should be evaluated in all therapeutic outcome studies and in any clinically prescribed treatment that requires a self-management component. However, one of the difficulties in evaluating intervention and treatment efficacy is assessing adherence. The utility of relief from symptoms or the achievement of therapeutic goals may suggest to the clinician that the patient is following the treatment plan. However, it is no confirmation that this is indeed the case. Multiple factors may mediate the effect of treatment on physiological outcomes. Among these factors are the adequacy of level of treatment, individual variations in the absorption and metabolism of drugs, pretreatment status, comorbid conditions, and seasonal variations in physiological parameters. Thus, therapeutic outcome is not a good measure of adherence.

Although numerous methods of assessing adherence have been reported in the literature, none are sufficiently accurate for a true standard to be identified. The errors in measurement generally are biased toward an overestimate of adherence. A number of reasons may account for this bias. Perhaps most important, adherence is assessed for a specific time period, which may not be representative of the patient's ongoing behavior. For example, in using an unobtrusive electronic monitor, Norell (1981) found that patients were more likely to improve their adherence to an eyedrop regimen just before and after a physician visit. This finding has been confirmed by other investigators examining adherence across diverse regimens (Cramer, Mattson, Prevey, Scheyer, & Ouellette, 1989; Kass, Meltzer, Gordon, Cooper, & Goldberg, 1986). Thus, self-report strategies, which may be biased by the individual's tendency to report on usual behavior based on the recall of recent events, would likely overestimate adherence over a longer period of time. Similarly, drug levels, which typically assess current and recent intake of medication because of the limited half-life of the drugs, would overestimate usual behavior. Other physiological parameters that are responsive to fairly short intervention periods would be similarly affected. An overview of specific adherence-assessment methods would further detail their utility.

Self-report measures. Multiple methods have been used to assess adherence to treatment regimens. Self-report, however, is the most commonly used method. Self-report measures are perhaps the most easily administered and the least expensive. Although such measures can assume multiple formats, the most commonly used are interviews, structured questionnaires, and daily diaries.

The majority of research studies examining medication adherence report using interview methods. Generally there are no standard procedures. Two brief interviews have been published by Morisky, Green, and Levine (1986) and by Shea, Misra, Ehrlich, Field, and Francis (1992) that assess global estimates of adherence. However, very limited psychometric data are available, and these have rarely been compared with more accurate daily estimates of adherence. Norell (1981) reported that interviews that showed a correlation of .75 with pill counts detected just 12% of patients who missed medication. Similarly, research has indicated that the interview may have a limited relationship to the more accurate and direct measure of using the electronic monitor. In a study of people with rheumatoid arthritis in outpatient settings, investigators were able to identify just 7% of people who reported less than 80% adherence to a research staff member during a telephone interview where anonymity was guaranteed. Yet, a parallel assessment using an electronic monitor with the same patients identified 54% as poorly adherent (Dunbar-Jacob et al., 1992). Confounding the problem of self-report further is that the nature of the questions used in the interview will affect reported adherence (Burke et al., 1992; Dunbar et al., 1991; Petitti, Friedman, & Kahn, 1981).

Similar issues are encountered in the study of dietary adherence. The most common methods of assessing food intake through structured interview include the 24-hour recall and diet histories. The assumption underlying these methods is that an estimate of usual intake can be made from the responses to these interviews. In the case of the 24-hour recall (an assessment of the preceding day's intake) the representativeness of the 1 day is questionable (Wylie-Rosett, Wassertheil-Smoller, & Elmer, 1990). Furthermore, inability to generalize over time is acknowledged, and so the 24-hour recall is usually confined to the study of population intake rather than the study of the individual (Dolecek et al., 1986; Gordon et al., 1986; Schwerin et al., 1981). The 24-hour recall is precise, however, and draws only upon recent memory.

Specific recalls have also been used to a lesser extent in the assessment of exercise. They have shown promise in at least one study when compared with the use of electronic monitoring for adherence. In this case, the 7-day recall showed 94% overall agreement with an electronic monitor that assessed heart rate and motion (Taylor et al., 1984).

A more general measure of adherence using interview methods is the diet history. Information is requested about patients' food intake over an extended period of time, frequently the past year, along with information on factors that influence food habits. Given a well-trained interviewer, the diet history provides a comprehensive profile of intake. The diet history, however, is difficult to validate and is subject to problems in recall. Of particular consequence is the problem frequently observed in the recall of usual behavior and noted above: the bias of long-term behavior by generalization of recent behavior.

In the pediatric arena, the self-report of adherence often becomes the parent's report of the child's adherence. However, in at least one study it was found that more than 70% of parents were unable to report on regimen-related behaviors of their children (G. G. Bond, Aiken, & Somerville, 1992). Certainly, if the report of others is to be used to assess adherence, then those others need to be aware of the occurrence of the behavior.

Questionnaires are also used in the self-report of adherence. Although none are widely used for assessing medication adherence, food frequency questionnaires and physical activity questionnaires are commonly used to assess diet and exercise (Block et al., 1986; LaPorte,

Montoye, & Caspersen, 1985; Paffenbarger, Hyde, & Wing, 1986; Schechtan, Barzilai, Rost, & Fisher, 1991; Willett et al., 1985). Both types have been validated with other methods of assessment. The food frequency questionnaires are limited by the amount and types of items listed, which particularly reduces their utility among ethnic groups (Willett, 1990). The exercise questionnaires have shown good predictive validity when compared with measures of patients' maximum oxygen uptake (Schectan et al., 1991; Siconolfi, Lasater, Snow, & Carleton, 1985), as well as body mass and HDL cholesterol (Schechtan et al., 1991).

Perhaps one of the most common methods of self-reported assessment of adherence with a variety of regimens is the use of a daily record. Such diaries tend to circumvent the reliance on recall required by the use of interviews or questionnaires. However, they do require that the patient be trained in keeping daily records. Instructions should include the need to place the diary in an accessible setting and to record as near to the time of the behavior as possible.

Although daily diaries have been used to assess medication adherence, exercise adherence, and adherence to blood glucose testing among people with diabetes, few data are available on their usefulness or acceptability to patients. Generally, investigators do not report on the proportion of people who completed the diaries, the extent to which the diaries were completed, or the findings of any validity checks. In one study of children's diaries regarding blood glucose testing, 53.8% of the entries were found to be fabricated when compared with unobtrusive electronic monitoring of blood glucose testing through the test instrument itself (Wilson & Endres, 1986).

Diaries are also commonly used in the assessment of dietary adherence. Diet diaries typically cover a 7-day period or a 3-day period in which one of the days includes a weekend or day off, if that is different. A variety of formats have been used; these are frequently constructed for a specific study or clinical practice. In a study of the comparative validity of nonlaboratory measures of dietary intake, the food record was found to be somewhat better at estimating change than the interview (Hyman et al., 1982). Diaries do have the potential to modify the patient's behavior as a function of self-monitoring. Consequently, they may not provide a view of true baseline data.

In general, self-report measures are inexpensive and permit the collection of more detailed information on the circumstances surrounding poor adherence than do other types of measures. Research suggests that these measures may perform differently for different types of regimens. Their specificity in the collection of medication adherence data is questionable, yet they appear to function satisfactorily in the assessment of exercise adherence. There are insufficient alternatives, at least in the field setting, to the collection of dietary adherence data to determine their accuracy, although they have been found to predict cholesterol lowering in the Multiple Risk Factor Intervention Trial study (Dolecek et al., 1986). Care needs to be taken to minimize the potential problems posed by reliance on memory. Consideration should also be given to the impact of varying questions on reported adherence. Furthermore, patients may need specific training to accurately report their behavior through any of the self-report methods.

Biological measures. A variety of physiological measures have been used as measures of adherence. For medication adherence, such measures as the level of the drug or its metabolites in the serum, urine, or saliva have been examined. For dietary adherence, measures such as 24-hour urine samples and urine dipsticks to assess sodium intake and direct assays of physiological outcomes, such as cholesterol level and glycosylated hemoglobin, have been used. For exercise adherence, such indicators as direct or indirect calorimetry, electronic heart-rate monitoring, muscle strength, and maximal oxygen uptake have been used. The physiological measures rarely provide an assessment of the daily variability in adherence and tend to identify those people who have been adherent within a relatively recent time period, close to the time of assessment. These measures do not identify the level of adherence, but simply classify a person as having followed or not followed some of the regimen. They tend, however, to be affected by individual differences in drug metabolism, with the potential for leading to false classifications of patients. For example, 7 of 75 patients who reported adherence showed no serum drug levels, in a classic study of digoxin adherence (Weintraub, Au, & Lasagna, 1973). Further analysis of 6 showed that although 3 had misrepresented their adherence, 3 had rapid digoxin metabolism patterns.

Electronic monitoring. Newer technologies have permitted the longitudinal assessment of proxies for adherence. Technologies are available for the electronic monitoring of heart rate and muscle movement to track exercise adherence (e.g., Iyriboz, Powers, Morrow, Ayers, & Landry, 1991; LaPorte et al., 1985; Taylor et al., 1984), electronic diaries for the self-monitoring of dietary adherence (S. Shiffman, personal communication, 1992), and electronic monitors to assess medication adherence (e.g., Cramer et al., 1989; Norell, 1981; Urquhart, 1991). Although the technology has limited availability and is expensive, it does provide a reliable assessment of the temporal patterns of adherence. Event-by-event data are captured, permitting a view of adherence that is not available through other methods. Thus, more precise estimates of adherence are available. This is an important consideration in the evaluation of both intervention strategies and therapeutic failures.

Pill counts and pharmacy refills. Pill counts and pharmacy refills are unique to the assessment of medication adherence. *Pill counts* consist of counting the number of pills remaining from a prescription over a defined time period and comparing that with the number of pills that should have remained. This difference is subtracted from the number of pills dispensed to determine the number that were taken. Dividing this number by the number prescribed in the time interval of interest and multiplying by 100 gives an adherence percentage. Pill counts tend to overestimate adherence. For example, in a comparison of pill counts with electronically monitored adherence, investigators reported a .24 correlation, with pill counts overestimating the amount of medication consumed (Rudd, Ahmed, Zachary, Barton, & Bonduelle, 1990).

Pharmacy refills perform like pill counts. In this case, the time the medication is refilled is compared with the time it should have been refilled if the patient had taken all of the medication. Adherence is estimated in a similar manner to the pill count estimate. This method assumes that patients purchase all of their medication from the same pharmacy, and access to pharmacy records is also required. It is a difficult assessment procedure in all but the most controlled dispensing situations.

Multiple methods are available for the assessment of adherence. None are perfect. Those providing the most complete picture of adherence are expensive and of limited accessibility, whereas those providing the most depth surrounding adherence events are the most subject to errors. Yet methods are improving and are sufficient to provide evidence of intervention effectiveness and to disentangle therapeutic failure from partial adherence.

Issues in Clinical Implementation

Populations to Be Targeted

The potential for poor adherence exists for any patient receiving health care, regardless of age, disease, prescribed regimen, or socioeconomic characteristics. The interventions that have been studied have crossed age groups and regimens. Unfortunately, their efficacy has not been examined in cultural subgroups. However, attention to adherence enhancement should be incorporated in the treatment of any patient receiving health care.

The Clinical Encounter

Attention to adherence enhancement should begin at the initiation of treatment, whether in the clinical setting or in the research setting. As it is the rare patient who can be fully adherent over the long term, it would be appropriate to advise the patient that many people have periodic difficulties establishing a treatment regimen or maintaining it. This sets the stage for interviewing the patient, or caretaker, about factors that are likely to interfere with regimen conduct. It further sets the stage for introducing both initial and episodic assessment of adherence. In subsequent sessions, the clinician or researcher should inquire about adherence and address any problems that may have arisen.

Methods of Assessment

The clinician should use some form of self-monitoring in the initial stages of adherence, if at all possible. The structure of the assessment tools should also be relevant to the culture of the patient. In particular, food frequencies should emphasize the foods most commonly consumed within the culture. The tools should also be in the patient's language and at his or her appropriate reading level. For people who are unable to read, it may be useful to use diaries that contain pictures and use check marks for responses. This would, of course, limit the amount of information that could be collected, but may be a better alternative than no self-monitoring at all. The clinician should also use self-monitoring to encourage good adherence and to identify circumstances in which nonadherent episodes occur. These data would be available for problem solving with the patient.

Interview methods should also be used routinely throughout the maintenance period, with episodic use of a daily diary, where possible, for additional confirmation of interview reports. For the person who is suspected of poor adherence or for whom poor adherence needs to be ruled out, the electronic monitor might provide a more precise evaluation. Monitor usage, however, might be problematic for disenfranchised people, such as the homeless or the severely addicted. Special attention would need to be given to the ability of such people to retain and use diaries. At any stage in regimen management, adherence assessment should be addressed in some manner best fitting the characteristics of the patient.

For the researcher, plans need to be made during the design of study to assess adherence and how it will be handled in data analysis. Additionally, estimates of both dropouts (total nonadherers) and partial adherers need to be addressed in the calculation of sample size. More precise estimates of adherence are required of all subjects than might be necessary in the clinical setting.

Treatment Interventions

A number of intervention techniques have been shown to be more effective than usual care in promoting adherence. Unfortunately, studies of the comparative effectiveness of these strategies have yet to be done. In the meantime, the existing data suggest that the first strategy should be to provide an adequate education regarding the regimen and any skills necessary to carry it out. This would be followed by tailoring or adapting the treatment regimen to the patient's usual routine and culture. Pairing medication taking with an existing habit, adapting existing recipes to the new diet and identifying acceptable food alternatives, or building exercise into the existing routine are likely to reduce some of the initial barriers to adopting a new regimen as well as account for the culturally determined habits of daily living. Self-monitoring at this time would provide feedback and heighten awareness of the regimen.

It is important to develop the regimen at a pace that each patient can accept. Early success is important both to increase the probability of subsequent adherence and to foster high self-efficacy regarding regimen conduct. During this time the significant others in the patient's life may be instructed in the regimen and in their roles in facilitating adherence. Before instructing significant others, however, it may be well worth asking the patient about his or her preferences for involving significant others. Our own research (Dunbar-Jacob, Kwoh, Sereika, & Burke, 1995) has indicated that a portion of patients prefer to manage their treatment and not involve others. Time spent promoting successful adoption of the regimen, including adapting it to the unique characteristics of the patient, is likely to promote longer-term adherence.

The provider of care may be better versed in the adaptation of the treatment regimen and in the role of significant others when the patient matches the provider's own characteristics. This may allow the provider to offer support, identify potential problems, and adapt the regimen more quickly and successfully than when the match is not there. The provider needs to assess the limitations and variations in resources between age groups, genders, and ethnic groups. These will be important considerations and will influence the degree and type of community referrals that may be helpful. Similarly, the provider needs to be aware of the specific influences on regimen implementation. The availability of accessible and safe sites for physical exercise, the source of such nutrients as fats within the diet, and the openness of the patient's social network to treatment—including willingness to modify cooking habits and acceptance of prescribed medications—will all influence the intervention plan.

For example, consider the case of a married African American man versus the case of a single White woman—each of whom presents with borderline hypertension and is prescribed a weight-loss, low-sodium diet and exercise regimen. The support system for each is likely to be considerably different. Assume that the man has a wife who does the food shopping and prepares all the meals, the majority of which are eaten at home. This patient is likely to benefit from instruction of the wife and the elicitation of her cooperation in carrying out the dietary aspect of the treatment regimen. Assume that the female patient with hypertension lives alone, eats out frequently, and tends to snack at home. She gives little attention to her eating behavior. She would benefit from personal instruction in the selection of diet-compatible snack foods and how to identify acceptable alternatives from her preferred restaurant menus. If one assumes that the man does no structured exercise and has a job with little physical activity and the woman is a member of a health club that she attends sporadically with friends, then different strategies to promote exercise will be important. It may be that the man's wife could be involved in a walking program with the husband. This may have to be tailored to their living arrangement and could include the neighborhood, the mall, or the local school track, depending on availability, ease of use, and safety. The female patient might be able to contract with her friends to increase regular activity at her club, where safety, accessibility, and ease are already considered. These are the more obvious considerations in adapting a regimen to the unique characteristics of a person and his or her social network.

Following the successful initiation of the regimen, attention turns to maintenance. The limited research specifically addressing adherence suggests that the health provider ought to initiate regular and ongoing contact with the patient. To date, this appears to be the strategy that is most likely to promote continuation in treatment (or in the research program). Throughout this period, adherence should be routinely assessed. If the therapeutic benefit is not obtained or is lost, then a more precise estimate of adherence might be obtained, such as through one of the electronic monitors.

Should there be indications that the patient's adherence is declining, efforts to remediate this situation ought to be put in place. Several strategies might be tried, depending on the nature of the patient's adherence problem. Such strategies include tailoring, contracting, self-monitoring, or other behavioral interventions. It should be kept in mind that with cessation of the intervention, adherence is likely to fall again. So maintenance strategies become important.

Adjunctive Care

Adequate management of adherence necessitates the provision of consistent communication from providers and consistent reinforcement of adherence to the regimen. Not only is consistency of communication important, but the prescription of multiple regimens by various providers will unnecessarily complicate the treatment program. Coordinating efforts so that the patient is not overburdened with a set of complex regimens will remove one of the barriers to good adherence. Thus, it is important early on in care to involve any other care providers that the patient may be seeing. Similarly, it is important to maintain this communication over time. Efforts to improve adherence in the partially adherent patient might exacerbate side effects or other adverse effects of treatment. Other providers need to be aware of the source of these problems and, potentially, to contribute to the adjustment of the regimen itself. Ongoing linkages with the patient's other care providers are important to the success of an adherence-enhancing program.

Evaluation of Treatment Efficacy

The evaluation of the efficacy of adherence interventions needs to be based on the patient's behavior with regard to the treatment regimen. It should not be based on the attainment (or lack thereof) of therapeutic efficacy. For research studies this requires precision in measurement and the use of randomized, controlled trials. For clinical purposes this requires an assessment of whether the desired outcome is attained and whether sufficient adherence problems exist to impair the attainment of treatment efficacy. It may also require efforts to rule out adherence problems in the face of therapeutic failure. Observational and single case methods may be satisfactory in these situations.

Future Needs

Research

Although there is a voluminous literature on adherence, there are few randomized, controlled studies of adherence-intervention efficacy and fewer still that focus on subgroups, such as the newly treated or the partially adherent. Similarly, there is little research addressing the unique needs of people from various cultures or the acceptance of specific intervention strategies by various cultural groups. Very little is known about how to successfully initiate a treatment regimen to ensure adherence. Little is also known about how to maintain adherence or to remediate adherence problems. Randomized, controlled studies using accurate measures are needed if adherence is to be improved in health care. Studies that compare the efficacy of various interventions and examine the utility of interventions across cultural and ethnic groups are necessary.

Intervention development would also be furthered by a continuing investigation of the factors that contribute to poor adherence. Although numerous studies have reported on factors associated with adherence, many of these have been empirical descriptions of clinical populations. Little attention has been given to identifying factors that predict, longitudinally, adherence in a population. Furthermore, very little effort has been put into examining those factors relevant within specific subpopulations. Not considered in these studies is the impact of measurement method on the identification of factors contributing to low adherence. In an examination of factors concurrently associated with adherence, different sets of factors were identified for self-reported adherence and for electronically monitored adherence in patients with rheumatoid arthritis (Dunbar-Jacob, Sereika, Burke, & Kwoh, 1993). Thus, it is probable that the means by which adherence is assessed influences the factors associated with the behavior. Systematic examination of the factors contributing to poor adherence, with particular attention to those factors that are likely to be modifiable, would make a significant contribution to the understanding of patient adherence and to the development of intervention strategies.

Studies are also needed to improve the accuracy of adherence assessment. This is particularly the case for inexpensive and easy-to-use assessment techniques in the clinical setting. Efforts to improve self-report methods would be particularly valuable.

The preponderance of the work in adherence has been empirically driven. Little has been theoretically based. Where theory has propelled the research, a limited number of paradigms have been used. The identification of factors contributing to adherence has been influenced by the Health Belief Model (Becker, 1974; Rosenstock, 1974), the theory of reasoned intentions (Ajzen, 1985; M. Fishbein & Ajzen, 1975), the Common Sense Model (Leventhal, Meyer, & Nerenz, 1980; Meyer et al., 1985), and decision theories. Where theory has driven intervention, cognitive–social learning theory has been most influential (Bandura, 1986). It is likely that the field would advance more rapidly with increased attention to theoretically driven investigations.

Impact on the Field

The development of intervention strategies to promote adherence to medical regimens would have significant impact on the delivery and cost of health care. The extent of the problem across population groups is substantial and contributes notably to rising health care costs.

The enhancement of the accuracy of measurement parallels the development of interventions. More accurate measures would permit the identification of partial adherence more readily and, thus, facilitate the testing of interventions. Although there has been considerable attention to adherence over the past 2 decades, rates of adherence have not improved substantially (Dunbar et al., 1991), suggesting that there is considerably more to be learned about how to alter this costly and pivotal behavior.

REFERENCES

Aikens, J. E., Wallander, J. L., Bell, D. S., & Cole, J. A. (1992). Daily stress variability, learned resourcefulness, regimen adherence, and metabolic control in type I diabetes mellitus: Evaluation of a path model. *Journal of Consulting and Clinical Psychology, 60,* 113–118.

Ajzen, I. (1985). From intentions to actions: A theory of planned behavior. In J. Kuhl & J. Beckman (Eds.), *Action control: From cognition to behavior* (pp. 11–39). New York: Springer.

Anderson, L. A. (1990). Health-care communication and selected psychosocial correlates of adherence in diabetes management. *Diabetes Care, 13*(Suppl. 2), 66–76.

Ary, D. V., Toobert, D., Wilson, W., & Glasgow, R. E. (1986). Patient perspectives on factors contributing to nonadherence to diabetes regimen. *Diabetes Care, 9,* 168–172.

Badgley, R. F., & Furnal, M. A. (1961). Appointment breaking in a pediatric clinic. *Yale Journal of Biology and Medicine, 34,* 117–123.

Bandura, A. (1986). *Social foundations of thought and action: A social cognitive theory.* Englewood Cliffs, NJ: Prentice Hall.

Baumann, L. J., Cameron, L. D., Zimmerman, R. S., & Leventhal, H. (1989). Illness representations and matching labels with symptoms. *Health Psychology, 8,* 449–469.

Beck, D. E., Fennell, R. S., Yost, R. L., Robinson, J. D., Geary, D., & Richards, G. A. (1980). Evaluation of an educational program on compliance with medication regimens in pediatric patients with renal transplants. *Journal of Pediatrics, 96,* 1094–1097.

Becker, M. H. (Ed.). (1974). The health belief model and personal health behavior. *Health Education Monographs, 2,* 324–508.

Belcon, M. C., Haynes, R. B., & Tugwell, P. (1984). A critical review of compliance studies in rheumatoid arthritis. *Arthritis and Rheumatism, 27,* 1227–1233.

Bergman, A. B., & Werner, R. J. (1963). Failure of children to receive penicillin by mouth. *New England Journal of Medicine, 268,* 1334–1338.

Bierenbaum, M. L., Green, D. P., Florin, A., Fleischman, A. I., & Caldwell, A. B. (1967). Modified-fat dietary management of the young male with coronary disease: A five year report. *Journal of the American Medical Association, 202,* 1119–1123.

Block, G., Hartman, A. M., Dresser, C. M., Carroll, M. D., Gannon, J., & Gardner, L. (1986). A data-based approach to diet questionnaire and testing. *American Journal of Epidemiology, 124,* 453–469.

Bloom, B. R., & Murray, C. J. L. (1992, August 21). Tuberculosis: Commentary on a reemergent killer. *Science, 257,* 1055–1061.

Bond, C. A., & Monson, R. (1984). Sustained improvement in drug documentation, compliance, and disease control. *Archives of Internal Medicine, 144,* 1159–1162.

Bond, G. G., Aiken, L. S., & Somerville, S. C. (1992). The health belief model and adolescents with IDDM. *Health Psychology, 11,* 190–198.

Boyd, J. R., Covington, T. R., Stanaszck, W. F., & Coussons, R. T. (1974). Drug defaulting—Part 1: Determinants of compliance. *American Journal of Hospital Pharmacy, 31,* 362–364.

Burke, L., Dunbar-Jacob, J., Glaister, G., McCall, M., Sereika, S., Dwyer, K., Kwoh, C. K., & Starz, T. W. (1992, May). *Influence of question type on self-reported medication compliance in rheumatoid arthritis patients.* Paper presented at the 1992 Sigma Theta Tau International Nursing Research Conference, Columbus, OH.

Carmody, T. P., Fey, S. G., Pierce, D. K., Connor, W. E., & Matarazzo, J. D. (1982). Behavioral treatment of hyperlipidemia: Techniques, results, future directions. *Journal of Behavioral Medicine, 5,* 911–916.

Carmody, T. P., Matarazzo, J. D., & Istvan, J. A. (1987). Promoting adherence to heart-healthy diets: A review of the literature. *Journal of Compliance in Health Care, 2,* 105–124.

Christensen, N. K., Terry, R. D., Wyatt, S., Pichert, J. W., and Lorenz, R. A. (1983). Quantitative assessment of dietary adherence in patients with insulin-dependent diabetes mellitus. *Diabetes Care, 6,* 245–250.

Collins, J. F., & Dorus, W. (1991). Patient selection bias in analyses using only compliant patients. In J. A. Cramer & B. Spilker (Eds.), *Patient compliance in medical practice and clinical trials* (pp. 335–348). New York: Raven Press.

Cooper, D. K. C., & Lanza, R. P. (1984). *Heart transplantation: The present status of orthotropic and heterotropic heart transplatation.* Boston: MTP Press.

Cramer, J. A., Mattson, R. H., Prevey, M. L., Scheyer, R. D., & Ouellette, V. L. (1989). How often is medication taken as prescribed? A novel assessment technique. *Journal of the American Medical Association, 261,* 3273–3277.

Dapcich-Miura, E., & Bovell, M. F. (1979). Contingency management of adherence to a complex medical regimen in an elderly heart patient. *Behavior Therapy, 10,* 193–201.

Davis, E. E. (1990). Prerandomization compliance screening: A statistician's view. In S. A. Shumaker, E. B. Schron, & J. K. Ockene (Eds.), *The Handbook of health behavior change* (pp. 342–347). New York: Springer.

Davis, M. S. (1978). Variations in patients' compliance with doctor's advice: An empirical analysis of patterns of communication. *American Journal of Public Health, 58,* 274–288.

deBont, A. J., Baker, I. A., St. Leger, A. S., Sweetnam, P. M., Wragg, K. G., Stephans, S. M., & Hayes, T. M. (1981). A randomized controlled trial of the effect of low fat advice on dietary response in insulin dependent diabetic women. *Diabetologia, 21,* 529–533.

Delameter, A. M., Smith, J. A., Kurtz, S. M., & White, N. H. (1988). Dietary skills and adherence in children with type I diabetes mellitus. *Diabetes Educator, 14,* 33–36.

Desharnais, R., Bouillon, J., & Godin, G. (1986). Self-efficacy and outcome expectations as determinants of exercise adherence. *Psychological Reports, 59,* 1155–1159.

Deyo, R. A., Inui, T. S., & Sullivan, B. (1981). Noncompliance with arthritis drugs: Magnitude, correlates and clinical implications. *Journal of Rheumatology, 9,* 930–936.

Dickinson, J. C., Warshaw, G. A., Gehlbach, S. H., Bobula, J. A., Muhlbaier, L. H., & Parkerson, G. R. (1981). Improving hypertension control: Impact of computer feedback and physician education. *Medical Care, 19,* 843–854.

Didlake, R. H., Dreyfus, K., Kerman, R. H., Van Buren, C. T., & Kahn, B. D. (1988). Patient noncompliance: A major cause of late graft rejection in cyclosporine-treated renal transplants. *Transplantation Proceedings, 20* (Suppl. 3), 63–69.

Dishman, R. K. (1982). Compliance/adherence in health-related exercise. *Health Psychology, 1,* 237–267.

Dolce, J. J., Crisp, C., Manzella, B., Richards, J. M., Hardin, J. M., & Bailey, W. C. (1991). Medication adherence patterns in chronic obstructive pulmonary disease. *Chest, 99,* 837–841.

Dolecek, T. A., Milas, N. C., Van Horn, L. V., Farrand, M. E., Gorder, D. D., Duchene, A. G., Dyer, J. R., Stone, P. A., & Randall, B. A. (1986). A long-term nutrition intervention experience: Lipid responses and dietary adherence patterns in the Multiple Risk Factor Intervention Trial. *Journal of the American Dietetic Association, 86,* 752–758.

Dunbar, J. (1977). Adherence to medication regimen: An intervention study with poor adherers. Unpublished doctoral dissertation, Stanford University.

Dunbar, J. (1985). Practical aspects of dietary management of hypertension: Compliance. *Canadian Journal of Physiologic Pharmacology, 64,* 831–835.

Dunbar, J. (1990). Predictors of patient adherence: Patient characteristics. In S. A. Shumaker, E. B. Schron, & J. K. Ockene (Eds.), *The Handbook of health behavior change* (pp. 348–360). New York: Springer.

Dunbar, J., Dunning, E. J., & Dwyer, K. (1993). The development of compliance research in pediatric and adolescent populations: Two decades of research. In N. Krasnegor, S. Johnson, L. Epstein, & S. Jaffe (Eds.), *Monograph on developmental aspects of health compliance behavior* (pp. 29–51). Bethesda, MD: National Institute of Child Health and Human Development and the Bureau of Maternal and Child Health and Resource Development.

Dunbar J., Dunning, E. J., Dwyer, K., Burke, L., & Snetselaar, L. (1991, March). *Influence of question type on self-reported compliance with dietary regimen*. Paper presented at the 12th annual meeting of the Society for Behavioral Medicine, Washington, DC.

Dunbar, J., & Waszak, L. (1990). Patient compliance: Pediatric and adolescent populations. In A. M. Gross & R. S. Drabman (Eds.), *Handbook of clinical behavioral pediatrics* (pp. 365–382). New York: Plenum Press.

Dunbar-Jacob, J., Dwyer, K., & Dunning, E. J. (1991). Compliance with antihypertensive regimens: A review of the research in the 1980's. *Annals of Behavioral Medicine, 13,* 32–39.

Dunbar-Jacob, J., Kwoh, C. K., Sereika, S., & Burke, L. (1995). [Patient preferences for social support.] Unpublished raw data.

Dunbar-Jacob, J., Kwoh, C. K., Starz, T. W., Sereika, S., McCall, M., Glaister, C., Burke, L. E., Dwyer, K., Rosella, J., & Holmes, J. (1992, July). *Adherence to arthritis medication.* Poster presented at the International Congress of Behavioral Medicine, Hamburg, Germany.

Dunbar-Jacob, J., Sereika, S., Burke, L. E., & Kwoh, C. K. (1993, November). *Do patients do what they say they do: Adherence in patients with rheumatoid arthritis.* Poster presented at the Friends of the National Institute for Nursing Research, Washington, DC.

Edmonds, D., Foester, E., Groth, H., Greminger, P., Siegenthaler, W., & Vetter, W. (1985). Does self-measurement of blood pressure improve patient compliance in hypertension? *Journal of Hypertension, 3*(Suppl. 1), 531–534.

Emery, C. F., Hauck, E. R., & Blumenthal, J. A. (1992). Exercise adherence or maintenance among older adults: One-year follow-up study. *Psychology and Aging, 7,* 466–470.

Engstrom, F. W. (1991). Clinical correlates of antidepressant compliance. In J. A. Cramer & B. Spilker (Eds.), *Patient compliance in medical practice and clinical trials* (pp. 187–194). New York: Raven Press.

Epstein, L. H., Beck, S., Figuero, J., Farkas, G., Kazdin, A. E., Daneman, D., & Becker, D. (1981). The effects of targeting improvements in urine glucose on metabolic control in children with IDDM. *Journal of Applied Behavioral Analysis, 14,* 365–375.

Ewart, C. K. (1989). Psychological effects of resistive weight training: Implications for cardiac patients. *Medicine and Science in Sports and Exercise, 21,* 683–688.

Fishbein, H. A. (1985). Precipitants of hospitalization in insulin-dependent diabetes mellitus (IDDM): A statewide perspective. *Diabetes Care, 8*(Suppl. 1), 61–64.

Fishbein, M., & Ajzen, I. (1975). *Belief, attitude, intention, and behavior: An introduction to theory and research.* Reading, MA: Addison-Wesley.

Fleece, L., Summers, M. A., Schnaper, H., Wilken, L. O., Yang, S., & Bradley, E. A. (1988). Adherence to pharmaco-therapeutic regimen: Assessment and intervention. *Alabama Journal of Medical Sciences, 25,* 389–393.

Geiss, S. K., Hobbs, S. A., Hammersley-Maercklein, G., Kramer, J. C., & Henley, M. (1992). Psychosocial factors related to perceived compliance with cystic fibrosis treatment. *Journal of Clinical Psychology, 48,* 99–103.

Gibbons, A. (1992, August 21). Exploring new strategies to fight drug-resistant microbes. *Science, 257,* 1036–1038.

Gilbert, B. O., Johnson, S. B., Silverstein, M., & Rosenbloom, A. (1982). The effects of a peer modeling film on children learning to self-inject insulin. *Behavior Therapy, 13,* 186–193.

Glanz, K. (1979). Dietitians' effectiveness and patient compliance with dietary regimens. *Journal of the American Dietetic Association, 75,* 631–636.

Glanz, K. (1980). Compliance with dietary regimens: Its magnitude, measurement, and determinants. *Preventive Medicine, 9,* 787–804.

Goodall, T. A., & Halford, W. K. (1991). Self-management of diabetes mellitus: A critical review. *Health Psychology, 10,* 1–8.

Gordon, D. D., Dolecek, T. A., Colman, G. G., Tillotson, J. L., Brown, H. B., Lenz-Litzow, K., Bartsch, G. E., & Grandits, G. (1986). Dietary intake in the Multiple Risk Factor Intervention Trial (MRFIT): Nutrient and food group changes over 6 years. *Journal of the American Dietetic Association, 86,* 744–751.

Greenan-Fowler, E., Powell, C., & Varni, J. W. (1987). Behavioral treatment of adherence to therapeutic exercise by children with hemophilia. *Archives of Physical and Medical Rehabilitation, 68,* 846–849.

Hackett, T. P., Cassem, N. H., & Wishnie, H. A. (1968). The coronary care unit: An appraisal of its psychologic hazards. *New England Journal of Medicine, 279,* 1365–1370.

Haynes, R. B. (1976). A critical review of the "determinants" of patient compliance with therapeutic regimens. In D. L. Sackett & C. B. Haynes (Eds.), *Compliance with therapeutic regimens* (pp. 26–50). Baltimore: Johns Hopkins University Press.

Haynes, R. B., Sackett, D. I., Gibson, E. S., Taylor, D. W., Hackett, B. C., Roberts, R. S., & Johnson, A. L. (1976). Improvement of medication compliance in uncontrolled hypertension. *Lancet, 1,* 1265–1268.

Hazzard, A., Hutchinson, S. J., & Krawiecki, N. (1990). Factors related to adherence to medication regimens in pediatric seizure patients. *Journal of Pediatric Psychology, 15,* 543–555.

Hicks, J. E. (1985). Compliance: A major factor in the successful treatment of rheumatic disease. *Comprehensive Therapy, 11,* 31–37.

Hyman, M. D., Insull, W., Palmer, R. H., O'Brien, J., Gordon, L., & Levine, L. (1982). Assessing methods for measuring compliance with a fat-controlled diet. *American Journal of Public Health, 72,* 152–160.

Iyriboz, Y., Powers, S., Morrow, J., Ayers, D., & Landry, G. (1991). Accuracy of pulse oximeters in estimating heart rate at rest and during exercise. *British Journal of Sports Medicine, 25,* 162–164.

Jacobson, A. M., Hauser, S. T., Wolfsdorf, J. I., Houlihan, J., Milley, J. E., Herskowitz, R. D., Wertlief, D., & Watt, E. (1987). Psychologic predictors of compliance in children with recent onset of diabetes mellitus. *Journal of Pediatrics, 110,* 805–811.

Joyce, C. R. B., Capla, G., Mason, M., Reynolds, E., & Mathews, J. A. (1969). Quantitative study of doctor–patient communication. *Quarterly Journal of Medicine, 38,* 183–194.

Kass, M. A., Meltzer, D., Gordon, M., Cooper, D., & Goldberg, J. (1986). Compliance with topical pilocarpine treatment. *American Journal of Ophthalmology, 101,* 515–523.

Keane, T. M., Prue, D. M., & Collins, F. I. (1981). Behavioral contracting to improve dietary compliance in chronic renal dialysis patients. *Journal of Behavior Therapy and Experimental Psychiatry, 12,* 63–67.

Kirscht, J. P., Kirscht, J. L., & Rosenstock, I. M. (1981). A test of interventions to increase adherence to hypertensive medical regimens. *Health Education Quarterly, 8,* 261–272.

Klopovich, P. M., & Trueworthy, R. C. (1985). Adherence to chemotherapy regimens among children with cancer. *Topics in Clinical Nursing, 7,* 19–25.

Korsch, B. M., & Negrete, V. F. (1972). Doctor–patient communication. *Scientific American, 227,* 66–74.

Kruse, W. H. (1991). Compliance with treatment of hyperlipoproteinemia in medical practice and clinical trials. In J. A. Cramer & B. Spilker, (Eds.), *Patient compliance in medical practice and clinical trials* (pp. 175–186). New York: Raven Press.

Kruse, W., Schlierf, G., & Weber, E. (1989). Continuous compliance monitoring—its utility for the interpretation of drug trials. *European Journal of Clinical Pharmacology, 36*(Suppl. A), 289.

LaPorte, R. E., Montoye, J. J., & Caspersen, C. J. (1985). Assessment of physical activity in epidemiologic research: Problems and prospects. *Public Health Report, 100,* 131–146.

Lemanek, K. (1990). Adherence issues in the medical management of asthma. *Journal of Pediatric Psychology, 15,* 437–458.

Leppik, I. E. (1991). Variability of antiepileptic medication concentrations and compliance. In J. A. Cramer & B. Spilker (Eds.), *Patient compliance in medical practice and clinical trial* (pp. 349–358). New York: Raven Press.

Levenson, J. L., Kay, R., Monteferrante, J., & Herman, M. V. (1984). Denial predicts favorable outcome in unstable angina pectoris. *Psychosomatic Medicine, 46,* 25–32.

Levenson, J. L., Mishra, A., Hamer, R. M., & Hastillo, A. (1989). Denial and medical outcome in unstable angina. *Psychosomatic Medicine, 51,* 27–35.

Leventhal, H., Meyer, D., & Nerenz, D. (1980). The common-sense representation of illness danger. In S. Rachman (Ed.), *Medical psychology* (pp. 7–30). New York: Pergamon Press.

Levine, D. M., Green, L. W., Deeds, S. G., Chwalow, J., Russell, R. P., & Finlay, J. (1979). Health education for hypertensive patients. *Journal of the American Medical Association, 241,* 1700–1703.

Litt, I. F., & Cuskey, W. R. (1981). Compliance with salicylate therapy in adolescents with juvenile rheumatoid arthritis. *American Journal of Diseases in Childhood, 135,* 434–436.

Logan, A. G., Milne, B. J., Achber, C., Campbell, W. P., & Haynes, H. B. (1979). Work-site treatment of hypertension by specially trained nurses: A controlled trial. *Lancet, 2,* 1175–1178.

Lucey, D., & Wing, E. (1985). A clinic based educational program for children with diabetes. *Diabetic Medicine, 2,* 292–295.

Martin, J. E., & Dubbert, P. M. (1987). Exercise promotion. In J. A. Blumenthal & D. C. McKee (Eds.), *Application in behavioral medicine and psychology: A clinician's sourcebook* (pp. 371–398). Sarasota, FL: Professional Resource Exchange.

Mason, J. O. (1992). Addressing the measles epidemic. *Public Health Reports, 107,* 241–242.

McCann, B. S., Brief, D. J., Follette, W. C., Walden, C. E., & Knopp, R. H. (1987, August). Spouse support and adherence in the dietary treatment of hyperlipidemia. Paper presented at the 95th Annual Convention of the American Psychological Association, New York.

McCann, B. S., Follette, W. C., Driver, J. L., Brief, D. J., & Knopp, R. H. (1988, August). Self-efficacy and adherence in the dietary treatment of hyperlipidemia. Paper presented at the 96th Annual Convention of the American Psychological Association, Atlanta, GA.

McCann, B. S., Retzlaff, B. W., Dowdy, A. A., Walden, C. E., & Knopp, R. H. (1990). Promoting adherence to low-fat, low-cholesterol diets: Review and recommendations. *Journal of the American Dietetic Association, 90,* 1408–1414.

McCann, B. S., Retzlaff, B. W., Walden, C. E., & Knopp, R. H. (1990). Dietary intervention for coronary heart disease prevention. In A. S. Shumaker, E. B. Schron, & J. K. Ockene (Eds.), *The handbook of health behavior change* (pp. 191–215). New York: Springer.

McCaul, K. D., Glasgow, R. E., & Schafer, L. C. (1987). Diabetes regimen behaviors: Predicting adherence. *Medical Care, 25,* 868–881.

McCulloh, D. K., Mitchell, R. D., Jambler, J., & Tattersall, R. B. (1983). Influence of imaginative teaching of diet on compliance and metabolic control in insulin dependent diabetes. *British Medical Journal, 287,* 1858–1861.

McDowell, J., Newell, C., & Rosser, W. (1989). A randomized trial of computerized reminders for blood pressure screening in primary care. *Medical Care, 27,* 297–305.

Meyer, D., Leventhal, H., & Gutmann, M. (1985). Common-sense models of illness: The example of hypertension. *Health Psychology, 4,* 115–135.

Minor, M. M. (1991). Physical activity and management of arthritis. *Annals of Behavioral Medicine, 13,* 117–124.

Mojonnier, M. L., Hall, Y., Berkson, D. M., Robinson, E., Wethers, B., & Pannbacker, B. (1980). Experience in changing food habits of hyperlipidemic men and women. *Journal of the American Dietetic Association, 77,* 140–148.

Morisky, D. E., Green, L. W., & Levine, D. M. (1986). Concurrent and predictive validity of a self-reported measure of medication adherence. *Medical Care, 24,* 67–74.

Morisky, D. E., Levine, D. M., Green, L. W., Shapiro, S., Russell, R. P., & Smith, C. R. (1983). Five-year blood pressure control and mortality following health education for hypertensive patients. *American Journal of Public Health, 73,* 153–162.

Myers, E. D., & Branthwaite, A. (1992). Out-patient compliance with antidepressant medication. *British Journal of Psychiatry, 160,* 83–86.

Nagy, V. T., & Wolfe, G. R. (1984). Cognitive predictors of compliance in chronic disease patients. *Medical Care, 22,* 912–921.

Nanada, Col., Fanale, J. E., & Kronholm, P. (1990). The role of medication noncompliance and adverse drug reactions in hospitalizations of the elderly. *Archives of Internal Medicine, 150,* 841–845.

Nessman, D. G., Carnahan, N. E., & Nugent, C. A. (1980). Increasing compliance: Patient-operated hypertension groups. *Archives of Internal Medicine, 140,* 1427–1430.

Norell, S. (1981). Monitoring compliance with pilocarpine therapy. *American Journal of Ophthalmology, 92,* 727–731.

Oldridge, N. B. (1982). Compliance with intervention and rehabilitation exercise programs: A review. *Preventive Medicine, 11,* 56–70.

Oldridge, N. B. (1988). Cardiac rehabilitation exercise programme: Compliance and compliance-enhancing strategies. *Sports Medicine, 6,* 42–55.

Paffenbarger, R. S., Jr., Hyde, R. T., & Wing, A. L. (1986). Physical activity, all-cause mortality and longevity of college alumni. *New England Journal of Medicine, 314,* 605–613.

Passero, M. A., Remor, B., & Solomon, J. (1981). Patient-reported compliance with cycstic fibrosis therapy. *Clinical Pediatrics, 20,* 264–268.

Perkins, K. A., & Epstein, L. H. (1988). In R. K. Dishman (Ed.), *Exercise adherence: Its impact on public health* (pp. 399–416). Champaign, IL: Human Kinetics Books.

Petitti, D. B., Friedman, G. D., & Kahn, W. (1981). Accuracy of information on smoking habits provided on self-administered research questionnaires. *American Journal of Public Health, 71,* 308–311.

Pietzcker, W. G. (1985). One-year outcome of schizophrenia patients—The interaction of chronicity and neuroleptic treatment. *Pharmacopsychiatry, 18,* 235–239.

Pollack, M. L., Carroll, J. F., Graves, J. E., Leggett, S. H., Braith, R. W., Limacher, M., & Hagberg, J. M. (1992). Injuries and adherence to walk/jog and resistance training programs in the elderly. *Medicine and Science in Sports and Exercise, 23,* 1194–1200.

Powell, K. E. (1988). Habitual exercise and public health: An epidemiological view. In R. K. Dishman (Ed.), *Exercise adherence: Its impact on public health* (pp. 15–39). Champaign, IL: Human Kinetics Books.

Rettig, B., Shrauger, D. G., Recker, R. R., Gallager, T. F., & Wiltse, T. H. (1986). A randomized study of the effects of a home diabetes education program. *Diabetes Care, 9,* 173–178.

Robertson, D., & Keller, C. (1992). Relationship among health beliefs, self-efficacy, and exercise adherence in patients with coronary artery disease. *Heart and Lung, 21,* 56–63.

Rosenstock, I. M. (1974). Historical origins of the health belief model. *Health Education Monographs, 2,* 328–335.

Rovelli, M., Palmeri, D., Vossler, E., Bartus, S., Hull, D., & Schweitzer, R. (1989). Noncompliance in organ transplant recipients. *Transplantation Proceedings, 21,* 833–834.

Rudd, P., Ahmed, S., Zachary, V., Barton, C., & Bonduelle, D. (1990). Improved compliance measures: Applications in an ambulatory hypertensive drug trial. *Clinical Pharmacology and Therapeutics, 48,* 676–685.

Saunders, E. (1985). Special techniques for the management of hypertension in blacks. In W. D. Hall, E. Saunders, & N. Schulman (Eds.), *Hypertension in blacks: Epidemiology, pathophysiology and treatment* (pp. 209–236). Chicago, IL: Year Book Medical Publications.

Saunders L. D., Irwig, L. M., Gear, J. S. S., & Ramushu, D. L. (1991). A randomized controlled trial of compliance improving strategies in Soweto hypertensives. *Medical Care, 29,* 669–678.

Schechtan, K. B., Barzilai, B., Rost, K., & Fisher, E. (1991). Measuring physical activity with a single question. *American Journal of Public Health, 81,* 771–773.

Schweitzer, R. T., Rovelli, M., Palmeri, D., Vossler, E., Hull, D., & Bartus, S. (1990). Noncompliance in organ transplant recipients. *Transplantation, 49,* 374–377.

Schwerin, H. S., Stanton, J. L., Riley, A. M., Schaefer, A. E., Leveille, G. A., Elliott, J. G., Warwick, K. M., & Brett, B. E. (1981). Food eating patterns and health: A re-examination of the Ten-State and HANES I surveys. *American Journal of Clinical Nutrition, 34,* 568–580.

Shea, S., Misra, D., Ehrlich, M. H., Field, L., & Francis, C. K. (1992). Correlates of nonadherence to hypertension treatment in an inner-city minority population. *American Journal of Public Health, 82,* 1607–1612.

Sherbourne, C. D., Hays, R. D., Ordway, L., DiMatteo, M. R., & Kravitz, R. L. (1992). Antecedents of adherence to medical recommendations: Results from the medical outcomes study. *Journal of Behavioral Medicine, 15,* 447–468.

Siconolfi, S. F., Lasater, T. M., Snow, R. C. K., & Carleton, R. A. (1985). Self-reported physical activity compared with maximal oxygen uptake. *American Journal of Epidemiology, 122,* 101–105.

Siscovick, D. S., Strogatz, D. S., Wagner, E. H., Ballard, D. J., James, S. A., Beresford, S., Kleinbaum, D. G., Cutchin, L. M., & Ibrahim, M. A. (1987). Provider-oriented interventions and management of hypertension. *Medical Care, 25,* 254–258.

Smith, D. M., Norton, J. A., Weinberger, M., McDonald., C. J., & Katz, B. P. (1986). Increasing prescribed office visits: A controlled trial in patients with diabetes mellitus. *Medical Care, 24,* 189–199.

Sohar, E., & Sneth, E. (1973). Follow-up of obese patients: 14 years after a successful reducing diet. *American Journal of Clinical Nutrition, 26,* 845–848.

Southam, M. A., & Dunbar, J. (1986). Facilitating patient compliance with medical intervention. In K. A. Holroyd & T. L. Greer (Eds.), *Self-management of chronic disease: Handbook of clinical interventions and research* (pp. 163–187). San Diego, CA: Academic Press.

Stason, W. B., & Weinstein, M. C. (1977). Allocation of resources to manage hypertension. *New England Journal of Medicine, 296,* 732–739.

Steckel, S. B., & Swain, M. A. (1977). Contracting with patients to improve compliance. *Journal of the American Hospital Association, 51,* 81–84.

Stevens, J., Burgess, M. B., Kaiser, D. L., & Sheppa, C. M. (1985). Outpatient management of diabetes mellitus with patient education to increase dietary carbohydrate and fiber. *Diabetes Care, 8,* 359–366.

Swain, M. A., & Steckel, S. B. (1981). Influencing adherence among hypertensives. *Research in Nursing and Health, 4,* 213–222.

Taylor, C. B., Bandura, A., Ewart, C. K., Miller, N. H., & DeBusk, R. F. (1985). Exercise testing to enhance wives' confidence in their husband's capability soon after clinically uncomplicated myocardial infarction. *American Journal of Cardiology, 55,* 635–638.

Taylor, C. B., Coffey, T., Berra, K., Jaffaidano, R., Casey, K., & Haskell, W. L. (1984). Seven day activity recall compared to a direct measure of physical activity. *American Journal of Epidemiology, 120,* 818–824.

Trueworthy, R. C. (1982, April 11). A new prognostic factor for childhood acute lymphoblastic leukemia: Drug absorption and compliance. Paper presented at the 4th annual pediatric hematology/oncology symposium, University of Kansas Medical Center, Kansas City.

Urquhart, J. (1991). Electronic monitoring of patient compliance. *Pharmaceutical Manufacturing Technology International.* New York: Sterling.

Velez, R., Anderson, L., McFall, S., & Magruder-Habib, K. (1985). Improving patient follow-up in incidental screening through referral letters. *Archives of Internal Medicine, 145,* 2184–2187.

Ward, A., & Morgan, W. (1984). Adherence patterns of healthy men and women enrolled in an adult exercise program. *Journal of Cardiac Rehabilitation, 4,* 143–152.

Webb, K. L., Dobson, A. J., O'Connell, D. L., Tupling, H. E., Harris, G. W., Moxon, J. A., Sulway, M. J., Leeder, S. R. (1983). Dietary compliance among insulin-dependent diabetics. *Journal of Chronic Disease, 37,* 633–643.

Weintraub, M., Au, W. Y. N., & Lasagna, L. (1973). Compliance as a determinant of serum digoxin concentration. *Journal of the American Medical Association, 224,* 481–485.

Wenerowicz, W. J. (1979). The use of behavior modification techniques for the treatment of hemodialysis patient non-compliance: A case study. *Journal of Dialysis, 3,* 41–50.

Wheeler, L. A., Wheeler, M. A., Ours, P., & Swider, C. (1985). Evaluation of computer based diet education in persons with diabetes mellitus and limited educational background. *Diabetes Care, 8,* 537–544.

White, K., Kolman, M. L., Wexler, P., Polin, G., & Winter, R. J. (1984). Unstable diabetes and unstable families: A psychosocial evaluation of diabetic children with recurrent ketoacidosis. *Pediatrics, 73,* 749–755.

Willett, W. C. (1990). Reproducibility and validity of food-frequency questionnaires. In W. C. Willett (Ed.), *Nutritional epidemiology* (pp. 92–126). New York: Oxford University Press.

Willett, W. C., Sampson, L., Sampfer, M. J., Rosner, B., Bain, C., Witschi, J., Hennekens, C. H., & Speizer, F. E. (1985). Reproducibility and validity of a semiquantitative food frequency questionnaire. *American Journal of Epidemiology, 122,* 51–65.

Williams, A., Stephans, R., McKnight, T., & Dodd, S. (1991). Factors affecting adherence of end-stage renal disease patients to an exercise programme. *British Journal of Sports Medicine, 25,* 89–93.

Wilson, D. P., & Endres, R. K. (1986). Compliance with blood glucose monitoring in children with Type I diabetes mellitus. *Journal of Pediatrics, 108,* 1022–1024.

Witschi, J. C., Singer, M., Wu-Lee, M., & Stare, F. S. (1978). Family cooperation and effectiveness in a cholesterol-lowering diet. *Journal of the American Dietetic Association, 72,* 384–389.

Wylie-Rosett, J., Wassertheil-Smoller, S., & Elmer, P. (1990). Assessing dietary intake for patient education planning and evaluation. *Patient Education and Counseling, 15,* 217–227.

Chapter

10

Death, Dying, and Bereavement

Sidney Zisook, Joanna J. Peterkin, Stephen R. Shuchter, and Anna Bardone

At some point in our lives, most of us will deal with the apprehension, fear, and devastation associated with our own demise, or with the death of those whom we love and hold dear. The realization that death is imminent is a stressful life event both for terminally ill people and for their survivors. Moreover, the grief experienced by survivors is often associated with intense suffering and disability and may lead to substantial psychological or medical morbidity.

Health psychologists may carry out several important functions in working with terminally ill patients. These include, but are not limited

We owe special thanks and appreciation to Arleen Goff.

to, evaluating psychological adjustment and the risk for suicide; providing therapy and support to the dying patient; serving as a liaison between the patient, the health care team, and the patient's family; and assisting family members and significant others with the process of bereavement. To deal with these ubiquitous and challenging clinical situations and to be able to provide effective care to bereaved and chronically and terminally ill people, clinicians must have adequate knowledge of what experiences to expect and the coping mechanisms used by dying or bereaved persons; the requisite skills to listen to and evaluate the psychosocial needs of patients, including the capability to manage these emotionally laden issues; and an open, accepting attitude that includes comfort with their own limitations and finitude. This chapter addresses various aspects of death, dying, and bereavement, including the meaning of death, the processes and stages involved in dying and bereavement, the prevalence and risk factors associated with suicide in terminally ill patients, and the care of dying and bereaved people.

Death and Acceptance of Death

Vital Statistics

The terms *death* and *dying* have no equivocal definitions. Death may be considered the absolute cessation of vital functions, and dying is the process of losing those functions. Dying may also be seen as a concomitant to living, each part of a birth-to-death continuum, overlapping developmentally (Weisman, 1988). From a more biological perspective, the American Bar and Medical Associations have joined forces to define death as being either the unrecoverable arrest of circulatory and respiratory functions or the unrecoverable arrest of neurologic function.

The leading causes of death are a reflection of how people live their lives in modern society (Kastenbaum, 1991). People often die as they have lived. Learning to drive more carefully, eat nutritionally, practice safe sex, limit the use of firearms, and reduce tobacco and alcohol intake would all contribute to a decline in the current death rates.

Alterations in lifestyles and technological advances during the past century have changed the most frequent causes of death and the life expectancy in the United States. In 1990, the average life expectancy was 47 years. It was 68 years in 1950, and 75 years in 1990. The age-adjusted rate of 515 deaths per 100,000 population in 1990 in the United States was at an all-time low (U.S. Department of Health and Human Resources, 1991). It is estimated that by the year 2050, the average life span will be 85 years, and barring major breakthroughs in genetic engineering, it may stabilize at this level. Thus, the task for future generations of clinicians will be to improve the quality of life rather than to pursue advances in quantity.

In 1990, 93% of deaths were attributable to illnesses or natural causes (U.S. Department of Health and Human Resources, 1991). In the United States, age-adjusted death rates for cardiovascular disease, cerebrovascular disease, and atherosclerosis have decreased, whereas the death rate for HIV has increased dramatically. In 1990, actual known deaths from HIV were 24,120, up 13% from 1989, which in turn was 29% higher than in 1988. The Centers for Disease Control has reported that the total number of deaths of men and women in the United States from HIV infection is now greater than 300,000. Overall, mortality rates are lower for the young than for the old, for women than for men, and for Whites than for Blacks. Deaths attributable to unnatural causes in 1990 were as follows: accidents, 4.3%; suicide, 1.4%; and homicide, 1.2%. Unnatural causes of death are particularly prevalent among the young. The leading cause of death in those aged 14 to 24 years is accidents, primarily vehicle accidents. A vast majority of fatal accidents, suicides, and homicides are related to alcohol.

Stages of Death and Dying

Clinicians must be aware of the magnitude of the psychological impact of dying on terminally ill patients, and the nature and range of the coping mechanisms used by patients to manage the many powerful and sometimes conflicting emotions elicited by the prospect of death (Schneidman, 1980). Kübler-Ross (1969) developed the concept that many patients confronted with the prospect of dying pass through five overlapping stages of coping from the time that they become aware of their prognosis to their actual death.

Denial. Commonly, the dying person's initial reaction is a refusal to believe that anything is wrong. Some may never pass through this stage. They may continue to seek someone to validate and support their position of denial. According to Kübler-Ross (1969), denial functions as a buffer after unexpected shocking news and permits patients to collect themselves while they begin to incorporate and integrate the new reality. However, she stresses that patients may still have the need to discuss the impending death when they are ready to face it. Talking about death a long while before it occurs gives the person time to process and deal with it. Time also gives the patient the opportunity to arrange business, interpersonal, and legal affairs.

Anger. Angry with their fate and frustrated with their inability to alter the ultimate prognosis, terminally ill people may be difficult to be with. Their anger is often displaced onto family members, friends, caregivers, and God. This stage is very difficult for family and friends to cope with, because every encounter with the patient may be distressing. This may cause avoidance by the support network, which only serves to create more discomfort for the patient. The key is to listen and to be tolerant and empathic without judging. The patient will generally realize that he or she will be listened to without the need for an argument.

Bargaining. Individuals in this stage attempt to negotiate for time and to postpone the inevitable. They may promise to become philanthropic, to donate money or body organs, or perhaps to reaffirm their relationship with God. According to Kübler-Ross (1969), "Bargaining is really an attempt to postpone; it usually includes a prize for good behavior, a self-imposed deadline and a promise that the patient will not ask for more if the postponement is granted" (pp. 83–84).

Depression. As dying persons come to terms with what will happen to them, depressive symptoms often emerge. Patients should be encouraged to express their sorrow. Just being there or a gentle touch often may mean more than any efforts to try to cheer the patient. If a true major depression occurs, it should be considered serious, and appropriate treatment should be instituted.

Acceptance. In this last stage, the dying person accepts his or her fate and realizes the imminence of death. This stage is reached after the patient has had time to mourn many losses and to envy those who will continue living. The family may require more support than the patient, and it is important to reassure the family that all that is possible will be done.

Coping

Kübler-Ross's (1969) five stages of coping should not be taken too literally or as prescriptions for the way one ought to die. Rather, they provide a general framework that may not explain the range of specific behavioral complexities that surface during the process of dying. Patients may exhibit other methods of coping, such as humor or becoming defensive. According to Avery Weisman (1972, 1974), the dying person experiences a dynamic tension between acceptance and denial. Weisman posited a clustering of intellectual and affective states that are set against a backdrop of one's personality and philosophy, noting the constant ebb and flow of interplay between hope and disbelief. Acceptance and denial play a game of tug of war, with armies of emotions such as anguish, rage, indifference, daring, terror, acquiescence, and even a yearning for death.

Coping strategies early in the dying process generally involve postponement and denial. As the disease becomes an established fact, coping strategies begin to incorporate the dying person's need to redefine himself or herself in terms of work, family, religion, economics, self-esteem, incapacity, and vulnerability. The person's illusions fluctuate between illusions of survival and fears of extinction, concomitant with various degrees of denial and acceptance (Schneidman, 1980). As decline and deterioration take over, increasing dependency becomes the norm. Assistance with living, more medication, less autonomy, and fewer alternatives signal decline (Weisman, 1972, 1974, 1988).

The dying do not use just a few stock coping mechanisms. As they do in the rest of life, patients may use diverse strategies to cope with the process of dying (Garfield, 1978). People may not deal with death much differently from the way they have previously dealt with life. They will continue to cope in the same ways when faced with dying. In the dying patient, one can easily observe denial, anger, depression, acting out, rationalization, projection, fantasy, avoidance, and withdrawal. Clinicians often need to guide patients toward the most adaptive styles of coping possible at a given time, but they should not forget that the living–dying interval is a time of repetitive stress, and toward the latter stages of the dying experience, the available repertoire of coping strategies may be reduced.

Cultural and Religious Beliefs

The cultural and religious background of patients may play an integral role in their interpretation of death and the coping mechanisms they use. Unfortunately, there is only a small collection of scientific literature on unique beliefs about life, dying, and death in North American subcultures. In the United States today, methods of dealing with death and dying are no doubt as mixed and as varied as the population itself (Zisook, 1995).

Pluralistic American society, with its many ethnic and racial groups, customarily demonstrates heterogeneous attitudes and behaviors about death. Any clinician working with such personal issues as death and dying must consider the broader sociocultural context of the individual and the family. If clinicians do not learn to function in a varied cultural milieu, the potential for miscommunication, incongruent expectations, and noncompliance of dying patients is enormous (Kearl, 1989).

In secular society, death is the final step in the walk of life. Many religious or spiritual people, however, view death as a transition rather than as an extinction. By explaining the unexplainable, religious or spiritual beliefs seem to serve the dual function of moderating the individual's anxieties about death and providing a means to reestablish the social order being shaken by death (Gonda & Ruark, 1984). Faith offers stability, security, and strength to those who are committed. Religion and spirituality influence one's concept of death and dying by offering a reason for being and a framework in which to interpret the inevitable.

Mainstream Christianity offers believers a future world of hope and eternal life through salvation. Death is the prelude to a glorious future in which the body is transformed and the soul lives on forever. Protestant America traditionally retains an equanimitous view of death. There are less clearly defined views of immortality in the Jewish religion. The Old Testament lacks specific references to a hereafter, despite the premise that heaven is a reward for living in accordance with God's laws. Hope of an afterlife is not at the core of modern Jewish life. Across denominational lines, a significant number of Americans accept the idea of reincarnation, drawing from the belief that they have had and will continue to have opportunities to grow.

Mourning behaviors and rituals must be understood within the bereaved individual's unique religious and cultural background. For example, members of the Church of Jesus Christ of Latter Day Saints (Mormons) are so resolute in their belief in an afterlife that bereaved survivors may actually be discouraged from active mourning. In contrast, Jewish Americans are strongly encouraged to participate in specific rituals of grief and mourning. They believe in expeditious burials and the prohibition of autopsy and cremation. Shiva, a 7-day period of full mourning after burial, is a traditional ritual practice in which the family and friends of the deceased mourn together. During the month following burial, partial mourning is exercised. Thereafter, normal life resumes with the repetition of specific memorial prayers for a period of 1 year. Mourning is finally concluded by the ceremonial unveiling of a tombstone. Similarly, the wake—a Roman Catholic ritual—provides the bereaved with an opportunity to verify the death, to bid farewell, and to pay tribute to the deceased. Graveside prayers are said and a mass is heard on the anniversary of the death. The Catholic Church generally accommodates the pious with the rituals (e.g., funeral), and the family provides the emotional support. In Catholic religion cremations are not permitted.

In addition to religious heterogeneity, the United States comprises a wide mix of other sociocultural subgroups whose unique views on mourning and the rituals surrounding death must be understood by clinicians entrusted with their care. For example, African Americans are more often resigned to the prospect of dying than are White Americans. They may express less fear of death, they may want to know if they are dying, they may grieve more openly, and they may be more likely to find solace in religion.

In a study conducted by Kalish and Reynolds (1976), Mexican American citizens were interviewed about their feelings toward death. Noting pervasive intergenerational influence and continuity, the investigators reported that this population had the strongest extended family associations and relied on the family for emotional support more than any other ethnic group studied. In addition, Mexican Americans were noted to intensely rely on complex Catholic rituals and to include children of all ages in grief and mourning processes.

Life and death as viewed by Native American cultures join together to constitute a continuous circle; therefore, death becomes a part of life. Because there are many different tribal ways of life, it is important to understand grief and bereavement within each unique Native American culture. A vast matrix of ceremonies and liturgies have been developed, often with the intent of regarding life after death as a reunion with deceased ancestors. The rites are both personal and social and are designed to ensure the appropriate mourning of the deceased and to restore harmony and equilibrium to life.

Care of the Dying

Largely attributable to the work of Elisabeth Kübler-Ross at the University of Chicago, public awareness and death education have grown exponentially over the past few decades. Kübler-Ross's pioneering work has led to the humane and sensitive treatment of terminally ill patients in medical settings, and her influence has fostered the well-accepted notion that death can be approached with dignity and independence.

Based on a comprehensive investigation of over 400 terminally ill patients, Kübler-Ross (1969) found that dying patients have an innate sense that they are dying and that they need to communicate their thoughts and feelings. Moreover, terminally ill people need to sustain hope despite no hope of a cure. Hope for recovery can be transformed into the courage required to face death. While providing consistent, compassionate, and humane support, caregivers should be careful not to avoid the truths of diagnosis, prognosis, and terminality. Patients need to be reassured that they will not be left abandoned. Perhaps the most important principle to abide by is to individualize treatment.

Before beginning to treat dying patients, it is important to consider one's goals. One essential goal enunciated by Hackett and Weisman (1962) is to help the patient achieve an "appropriate death" (Weisman, 1972, 1974, 1988). To achieve this end, the clinician must help patients to be as pain-free as possible, to operate on as effective a level as possible within the limits of their disability, to recognize and resolve residual conflicts, to satisfy remaining wishes that are consistent with their condition, and to be able to yield control to others in whom they have confidence. Kübler-Ross has suggested that clinicians help their patients complete the unfinished business of dying: reconciliations, resolution of conflicts, and pursuit of specific remaining hopes (Kübler-Ross, 1969). Dame Cecily Saunders (1978) stated that the goal of management is to help keep patients feeling like themselves for as long as possible. Others have recommended that clinicians focus not so much on dying, but on helping patients search for what they wish to accomplish in living (Le Shan, 1976). Stating that "there is no one best way to die," Cassem (1991, p. 343) emphasized the importance of individualizing treatment by getting to know the patient, responding to her or his unique needs and interests, proceeding at the patient's pace, and allowing the patient to shape the manner in which those in attendance behave.

A critical maxim that is highly valued by investigators who deal with terminally ill patients is to be honest with them. Honesty establishes trust. Many clinicians in the past, and even some now, advocate secrecy and silence when a patient is deemed terminal. Such clinicians refrain from informing their fatally ill patients of the prognosis in the belief that conveying bad news will precipitate faster health decline or hinder any chances for recovery. These beliefs are unfounded. The appropriate question is not whether to inform the patient, but rather how and when to do so. The news should be communicated in a sympathetic manner, be conveyed concisely and calmly but not bluntly, and unless otherwise contraindicated, be communicated in the presence of a spouse or partner (Cassem & Stewart, 1975). Questions from everyone involved with the patient should be encouraged. They should know that further and ongoing dialogue will be available to them. Patients should know what the next step will be and the general plan of action, and they should be strongly reassured that they will not be ignored, abandoned, or left alone. Moreover, it is important to note that simply telling patients the truth about their diagnosis and prognosis does not mean that they will completely accept it. Indeed, some degree of nonacceptance and denial is quite common, and perhaps even adaptive. Whenever possible, it is best to allow patients to accept their illness at their own pace.

Treatment of terminally ill patients almost always involves some palliative measures aimed at relieving such difficult symptoms as insomnia, diarrhea, or pain. There is no reason a dying person should suffer severe physical pain when the techniques to control or ameliorate it are now available. Patients may benefit a great deal from the reassurance that their care providers will not allow them to live or die in pain (Breitbart, Passik, & Levenson, 1992). In addition, it is important to identify troublesome side effects produced by therapeutic medications. Such side effects may include depressive symptoms and agitation. Treatment of concurrent psychopathology should always be considered. A major depression or persistent anxiety disorder may significantly hinder or disrupt adaptive coping processes. Just because one understands why a dying person may become depressed or anxious does not mean these reactions should not be treated aggressively. Clinicians should keep in mind that there comes a point when the focus of treatment should be the patient's comfort (Garfield, 1978). When possible, the patient's wishes should be respected, whether that means continuing aggressive intervention or resorting to palliative, comfort care—which means physical as well as psychological and social care. Keeping a terminally ill person comfortable requires constant contact by clinical staff and the family. The patient should be able to express her or his expectations of the care that is to be given, and both patient and family should be updated by treatment staff if the nature of that treatment needs to change.

Many individuals with a terminal illness decide to die at home. The family should be informed of services that are available for their assistance and how to obtain them. The family also needs to know all financial expenses that will be incurred. Ideally, if hospital contact is to be made from home, it should be available on a 24-hour basis, and someone on the other end of the telephone should be familiar with the patient's case.

Family members may need help on how to best aid and relate to their dying loved one. The task of coping with major changes in roles and relationships associated with the terminal stage of illness is compounded by a lack of preparation for knowing how to behave in the presence of someone who is dying. Family adaptation to the demands imposed by the dying requires variations in ordinary social roles, which can often create or increase strain on existing points of tension in interpersonal relationships (May, 1974).

Fatal illness destroys future hopes and plans, educational ambitions, established marital and parent–child adjustments, financial stability, and lifestyle. Extended illness puts excessive pressure on existing social support systems within and around the family, depleting financial and social resources as well as creating estrangement in interpersonal family relationships. Dobihal (1981) has offered the following suggestions to health professionals on how to assist the family: Train family members to participate in treatment; encourage them to provide emotional support and to anticipate the special needs of the patient; allow unlimited visiting so that the total family, including children, can spend time with the patient; and provide special hospital space for patient–family meetings as well as space for family members to live when the patient's death is imminent. Finally, special social and educational programs should be provided and should be continued, with the addition of clinician home visits, even after the patient has died. As is described below, many of these suggestions are incorporated in hospice care of the dying and their families.

Support Groups

In addition to the work of an individual clinician, it is often beneficial to take advantage of self-help groups and other agencies geared to support dying patients. Self-help programs allow patients the opportunity to share expertise and experience, offer practical health care and support, and provide a sense of belonging. Support groups are available specific to the disease diagnosis and type of treatment. For example, there are cancer support groups for cancer surgery patients and for cancer chemotherapy patients. Other examples of self-help groups include Reach-to-Recovery (for women with surgical procedure disfigurement) and Candlelighters (for families dealing with childhood cancer). The Wellness Community, which is nationwide, offers free weekly counseling, relaxation therapy, visualization techniques, and general support to both cancer patients and their families. Several other groups and programs, often working with professional medical services and hospital social workers, are available to supplement traditional medical and professional care (Kastenbaum, 1991).

Supportive interventions may enhance health and contribute to survivorship in some life-threatening illnesses. For example, in a prospective study of short-term group psychiatric intervention for patients with malignant melanoma, Fawzy et al. (1990) found that group treatment, consisting of health education, problem solving, stress management, and support, effectively reduced psychological distress and enhanced long-term effective coping. In a provocative and important 10-year follow-up study, Spiegel, Kraemer, Bloom, and Gottheil (1989) evaluated the effects of supportive group intervention in individuals with metastatic breast cancer. They demonstrated that patients who had weekly supportive group therapy and self-hypnosis for pain alleviation over the course of a year had a higher survival rate than those who did not. Survival time from the onset of intervention was 36.6 months in comparison with 18.9 months.

Hospice Care

The growth of the hospice movement and the availability of hospice care for terminally ill people have provided invaluable support for dying individuals and their families (Rhymes, 1990). Founded in London in 1967 by Dame Cecily Saunders, a *hospice* is a medically directed, nurse-coordinated program providing a continuum of home and in-patient care for the terminally ill patient and the family. It involves a multidisciplinary team acting under the direction of an autonomous hospice administration. The program provides palliative and supportive care to meet the various special needs that stem from physical, emotional, spiritual, social, and economic stresses experienced during the final stages of illness and during dying and bereavement (Zimmerman, 1986). Types of hospices available include those that provide home care, independent in-patient units, and units based within a hospital. Hospice care stresses the importance of pain relief, treating the patient and family as a unit, and an interdisciplinary team approach to care with active participation of the patient in all major decisions. The success of the hospice movement is evidenced by the fact that many of these principles have been integrated into routine medical care in many hospital and clinician practices.

HIV hospices (e.g., the Shanti groups, the San Francisco General Hospital model) continue to be too few in number, perhaps because of the enormous prejudice against AIDS patients, including children and babies. HIV patients in particular require more and better facilities for terminal care (Kübler-Ross, 1987). The needs of HIV patients are an important priority for present and future health care planning.

Advance Directives

As the movement for the protection of health care consumers gains credibility and as patients begin to realize that they have rights, more and more individuals are leaving advance directives (Ezekiel & Ezekiel, 1990). For example, living wills and medical directives are documents that detail patients' own guidelines and direct the level of care they would like if and when they become terminally ill and are unable to make decisions (Alexander, 1988). In addition, a durable power of attorney may be conferred on one whom the person designates as a health care proxy to help make decisions if that patient should become incompetent. The Self-Determination Act requires that all health care facilities provide admitted patients with written information about the right to refuse treatment, as well as keep written records of whether or not patients have directives or designated health care proxies. When there is doubt about the patient's wishes, common sense should prevail and the patient's next of kin should be consulted to provide a substituted judgment about what the patient would have wanted (Cassem, 1991).

Ethical Dilemmas and Euthanasia

Modern medical technology has created countless medical and ethical dilemmas that are now facing terminal patients, their caretakers, and society at large. For example, the ability of medicine to keep people alive for prolonged periods of time even after they have lost any reasonable hope for achieving an autonomous, meaningful existence raises serious questions regarding quality versus quantity of life. Increasingly, modern medicine has accepted the notion that patients have a right to say enough is enough and to refuse heroic or life-sustaining procedures, or to give others the right to make such choices for them. Even when these decisions have not been explicitly spelled out, there are times when family members, physicians, or clinicians make these choices or decide to pull the plug. Thus, passive euthanasia (not performing or withdrawing a procedure deemed necessary for continued life) is now an accepted part of medicine. Although much more controversial, clinicians have begun turning increased attention to the morality, feasibility, and desirability of active euthanasia (willfully and consciously performing a procedure with the purpose of ending a person's life). Guidelines for voluntary active euthanasia have been established and sanctioned in the Netherlands since the mid-1980s (de Wachter, 1989). The Netherlands' experience to date has had mixed reviews. Some have applauded the modern and compassionate care given to seriously ill patients by Dutch physicians, but others have pointed out abuses, noting that guidelines are not always followed (Muller, Van der Wal, Eijk, & Ribbe, 1994) and that involuntary euthanasia often occurs without the patient's or the family's request (Van Der Maas, Van Delden, Pijnenborg, & Looman, 1991). A similar debate is heating up in the United States. As of November 1994, Oregon has become the first state in the world to officially legalize physician-assisted suicide. Polls show that the majority of U.S. citizens (Blendon, Szalay, & Knox, 1992) and many physicians (Cohen,

Fihn, Boyko, Jonsen, & Wood, 1994) now favor legalizing active euthanasia and physician-assisted suicide, whereas others warn against inevitable abuses and misuses (Hendin & Klerman, 1993), arguing that attention should be focused on improving palliative care and patient comfort rather than on seeing death as the only solution to pain and suffering (Koenig, 1993). Opponents of physician-assisted suicide and active euthanasia point out that undiagnosed or inadequately treated depressions often are behind a patient's request for aid in dying (Conwell & Caine, 1991).

It is likely that many or most terminally ill patients who wish to die have a treatable depression (Conwell, 1994), and many patients may change their minds about such wishes (Chochinov, Wilson, Enns, Mowchun, & Levitt, 1993). The legality, morality, and advisability of physician-assisted suicide in patients, both with and without terminal illness, are contemporary issues that must be addressed, debated, and resolved (Conwell, 1994; Graber & Thomasma, 1990; Task Force on Ethics of the Society of Critical Care Medicine, 1990). Similar ethical and legal questions regarding such controversial issues as abortion on demand, rational suicide, alternative treatments, and cryonic suspension beg thoughtful answers. More complete discussion of these issues is beyond the scope of this chapter, but these vexing and unavoidable topics are beginning to be debated in sociopolitical arenas, symposia, and medical and psychological literature.

Management of Suicide

Since 1950, the rate of suicide in the United States has doubled. Over half a million attempted suicides each year are by young adults, especially those with untreated major depression (Rich, Young, & Fowler, 1986). In young adults both depression and substance abuse are often seen in individuals trying to take their own lives. In older individuals, major depression is even more prominent as a risk factor. Despite the rise of suicide in adolescence and young adulthood, the demographic group most at risk for successful suicide remains elderly people, especially older White men.

Blumenthal (1990) assigned suicide risk factors to five overlapping domains: psychosocial (support, life adversity, or medical illness), biological (age, access to alcohol and drugs, guns, or cognitive decline), psychiatric (affective, conduct, and organic mental disorders and schizophrenia), personality (hostility, impulsivity, depression, shame, and guilt), and genetic. Often, many of these factors coalesce, leading to a sense of hopelessness and helplessness in the person who makes a serious suicide attempt. Thus, an older White man with a chronic debilitating illness and major depression, who lives alone, has few friends, and owns a gun would be a prime suicide risk.

Although medical illness is a positive risk factor for elderly people, one illness that may predispose young adults to a high risk of suicide is HIV. Marzuk et al. (1988), for example, found the incidence of suicide was 36 times greater in men who were HIV positive than in others. McKegney and O'Dowd (1992) found a strikingly high percentage of suicide in HIV-positive patients who had not yet developed AIDS—even higher than in those with more advanced disease. In contrast, in a study of older, non-HIV-related cancer patients, Bolund (1987) found that 67% of cancer suicides occurred during the advanced stages of the disease.

Breitbart (1989) and Breitbart et al. (1992) have extensively studied the physical and psychiatric complications, including suicide, of terminal cancer and AIDS patients. The physical pain caused by these fatal illnesses, which is often poorly controlled, increases the risk of suicide. Suicidal ideation is common in patients with advanced illness who frequently experience pain, exhaustion, adjustment disorder, depression, and cognitive impairment. The risk of suicide is increased in terminal patients with preexisting psychopathology, a past history of attempts, and a positive family history. Breitbart (1989) emphasized the importance of helping terminally ill patients maintain as much control of their lives as possible and of providing comprehensive palliative care and effective pain management.

Discussion of the comprehensive care of suicidal patients is beyond the scope of this chapter. However, certain key principles are worth highlighting and are of particular relevance to individuals coping with the vast array of stressors associated with a life-threatening illness. First, although clinicians should be aware of risk factors, they should also remain humble regarding their ability to actually predict accurately who will attempt to kill themselves. Therefore, mental health clinicians should always be alert to the possibility and be sensitive to subtle hints. Second, because the vast majority of suicidal patients have a psychiatric disorder, especially a mood disorder, it is important to monitor the signs and symptoms of depression and treat the underlying psychiatric condition (Black & Winokur, 1990). When anxiety symptoms are present, it is important to treat them aggressively, as anxiety only increases the risk for suicide (Fawcett et al., 1990). If potentially lethal medications are prescribed, low doses and small numbers should be given at any one time. Third, even if the client does not address them directly, the therapist must ask about suicidal thoughts and plans. The outworn notions that such queries may suggest suicide to an otherwise nonsuicidal person are no longer tenable. Fourth, it is important to involve significant others, to educate and support them, and to enlist their help and support for the client, as well as to promote as supportive an environment and social milieu as possible. Fifth, although many therapists use nonsuicidal contracts, asking the client to sign a statement that she or he will come for an appointment or call before taking suicidal action, there are minimal published data confirming their utility. However, we feel it useful to attempt to extract such a commitment, at least verbally. It is imperative that the therapist honor his or her corresponding commitment and be reachable 24 hours a day, 7 days a week or to have suitable coverage arranged should the client call. Finally, patients benefit from the clinician's availability, consistency, perspective, determination, and hope. These verbal and nonverbal attributes can make the difference between life and death.

Bereavement and Grief

Family, friends, and caregivers can be profoundly affected by the death of a loved one. Indeed, bereaved individuals not only suffer from the torment and emotional upheaval that are part of acute grief, but may also be at high risk for prolonged suffering, social disorganization, impaired psychological or medical health, and even mortality (Jacobs, 1993; Klerman & Izen, 1977; Maddison & Viola, 1968; Parkes, 1972; M. Stroebe, Stroebe, & Hansson, 1993; Zisook, 1987).

Biological Consequences of Bereavement

Although the mechanisms of how grief adversely affects health are largely unknown, it is possible that it does so by perturbing the body's homeostatic mechanisms. Studies on neurohormonal and immunological consequences have been mixed. For example, some studies have found normal dexamethasone suppression tests in bereaved widows (Kosten, Jacobs, & Mason, 1984), whereas we have found nonsuppression in 16% of acutely bereaved individuals, with nonsuppression being related to the degree of separation anxiety (Shuchter, Zisook, & Kirkorowicz, 1986). Similarly, other indexes of endocrinologic abnormalities have been reported in some bereaved individuals, but not in others (Jacobs, Mason, et al., 1987). Studies on growth hormone (Kosten, Jacobs, Mason, et al., 1984) and prolactin levels (Jacobs et al., 1986) have supported possible alterations in relation to separation distress and coping strategies.

Several studies have found impaired immunological function in bereaved individuals (Bartrop, Luckhurst, Lazarus, Kiloh, & Penny, 1977; Irwin & Weiner, 1987; Schleifer, Keller, Camerino, Thorton, & Stein, 1983; Zisook, 1994). It is tempting to try to relate the impaired immunologic function reported in some bereaved individuals to the decline in health that also has been related to loss, but thus far no empirical data exist to support this hypothesis. Some of the reported alterations in T-lymphocyte response to mitogens or natural killer cell activity may be more related to depressive symptoms and advancing age than to bereavement per se (Irwin & Wiener, 1987). Finally, one study on sleep architecture found that elderly bereaved widows with depression have sleep EEG abnormalities that are found in patients with major depression but not in bereaved widows with "uncomplicated bereavement," suggesting that the depressions of bereaved individuals are biologically similar to other, non-bereavement-related major depressions (Reynolds et al., 1992).

Anticipatory Bereavement

When a person dies from a long-standing illness where death is expected, it is not uncommon for the bereavement process to begin before the loss has actually occurred. In such anticipatory grief, mourning begins with the acceptance that the loss will inevitably take place. The dying person, as well as the person to be bereaved, experience feelings of anticipation and awareness that alternate with periods of denial and not being able to accept that death will inevitably occur. Anticipatory grief may cushion the blow of death's reality, but in some instances, it may also lead to premature withdrawal and disconnection from the terminally ill person (Lundin, 1987). In order to provide beneficial counsel to patients and families prior to an anticipated loss, it is essential that there is a high degree of accurate communication and an understanding of anticipatory grief.

Tasks of Grief

The purposes, functions, and tasks of grief are not entirely clear. According to psychoanalytic theorists, the work of grief consists of the painful relinquishment of ties to the deceased—a necessary evil if bereaved people are going to end up free to invest emotional energy in new directions. As a result of undergoing this trial, bereaved people are eventually capable of loving another. Under certain circumstances, such as when the deceased person was an ambivalently loved object, the work can be obstructed; under such circumstances, melancholia rather than resolution of grief may result (Freud, 1957).

On the other hand, attachment theorists consider grief more in terms of its survival value, arguing that attachment behavior is instinctual and essential for the survival of the species (Bowlby, 1961). Breaking attachment bonds evokes powerful forms of attachment behaviors such as clinging, crying, and even angry outbursts. In bereavement, these behaviors are not successful because the deceased person does not reappear and the bond is not restored. Therefore, the searching behavior is eventually replaced by withdrawal, apathy, and despair—transient, normal behaviors that ultimately result in the formation of new attachments. Expanding this concept, Shuchter and Zisook (1987) have argued that one of the major tasks of grief is to successfully reconfigure a "continuing relationship" with the deceased person. Thus, modern theorists view grief more in terms of attachment behaviors than of separation (Bowlby, 1961, 1971).

Uncomplicated Bereavement and Grief

Beginning with Freud's "mourning and melancholia," several descriptions of uncomplicated grief and bereavement have appeared in the psychiatric literature over the past century. Freud (1957) described four distinguishing features of normal or uncomplicated mourning: a profoundly painful dejection, the loss of capacity to adopt new love objects, the inhibition of activity or turning away from activity not connected with thoughts of the loved person, and the loss of interest in the outside world insofar as it does not recall the deceased. Furthermore, Freud distinguished mourning from melancholia by the absence of ambivalent feelings about the deceased and the absence of significant disturbances in self-esteem in mourning.

Several investigators have proposed stages or phases of uncomplicated grief. Parkes (1972), for example, defined four phases of mourning: the period of numbness that occurs close to the time of the loss; the phase of yearning in which the bereaved yearns for the lost one to return and tends to deny the permanence of the loss; the phase of disorganization and despair, when the bereaved person finds it difficult to function in the environment; and, finally, the phase of reorganization when bereaved people begin to pull their lives back together. We have proposed similar stages of grief: an initial period of shock, disbelief, and denial; an intermediate acute mourning period of acute somatic and emotional discomfort along with social withdrawal; and a culminating period of resolution. In the resolution stage, the bereaved recognize what the loss has meant to them, that they have grieved, and that they can begin to shift their attention to the world around them. Memories and loneliness may be a part of that world, but the deceased, with his or her ills and problems, is not. The hallmark of the resolution stage is the ability of the bereaved to recognize that they have grieved and that they may now return to work, assume old roles, learn new ones, reexperience pleasure, and seek the companionship and love of others (Zisook, DeVaul, & Click, 1982; Zisook & DeVaul, 1985).

For some, bereavement provides an opportunity for personal growth that might not have otherwise occurred (Pollack, 1987; Shuchter & Zisook, 1993). One investigator has speculated that bereavement may lead to heightened creativity, noting that numerous successful artists, writers, and musicians have experienced painful losses (Solsberry, 1984). Yalom and Lieberman (1991) postulated that bereavement induces a heightened state of existential awareness. They suggested that bereaved individuals who examine their life deeply may have a different course of bereavement than those who do not. This is similar to positive changes reported by some terminally ill patients. Yalom and Lieberman also noted that bereaved individuals are challenged in many areas but, most important, they are confronted with major and mortal questions about existence, finitude, freedom, responsibility, isolation, and the meaning of life. According to their research, bereaved individuals who choose to attend or to respond to the challenge are very likely to undergo personal growth—a positive outcome of bereavement.

Total resolution of grief is more often a myth than a reality. In many ways and at various times, painful reminders of the lost relationship may affect the feelings, behavior, and functioning of the bereaved person for years, if not indefinitely (Zisook & Shuchter, 1985). Grief can suddenly reappear at specific times, such as during the anniversary of the death, as well as with other reminders of the deceased. Thus, all customary myths about approved mourning periods that generally allow a bereaved person months or up to a year to recover are often insufficient for the task. It is not the length of time, per se, that distinguishes complicated from uncomplicated grief, but the quality and quantity of reactions over time (Solsberry, 1984). Thus, a precise end point in time cannot be prescribed.

Complicated Grief

Many investigators have attempted to conceptualize or define the various complications of bereavement (e.g., Jacobs, 1993). Consequently, such terms as *unresolved, morbid, distorted, pathologic,* and *neurotic* have been proposed, and each is likely to capture different aspects of the grief response that potentially could go awry.

In general, most of these conceptualizations can be broken down into two major categories of complications. The first are complications of the process of grief itself, leading to variations in duration or intensity of the grief response (Lindemann, 1944; Parkes & Weiss, 1983; Raphael, 1983; Rynearson, 1990). Unfortunately, there are no empirical data to document how much is too much or too little. Pathological variants on which there is most agreement include grief that is too little (delayed grief); grief that is too long (chronic grief), and grief that is too intense (hypertrophic grief). Deutch (1937) wrote about the first of these complications, too little grief, suggesting that the absence of grief is abnormal and results in pathological problems later on. However, there has not been much empirical confirmation of her findings (Clayton, 1982; Parkes & Weiss, 1983; Wortman & Silver, 1989; Zisook, Shuchter, & Lyons, 1987). Alternatively, several investigators have found that hypertrophied grief, or grief that is very intense and distressing soon after the loss, may be a forerunner of chronic or enduring difficulties such as depression or anxiety (Clayton, 1982; Parkes & Weiss, 1983; Worden, 1991; Zisook & Shuchter, 1991; Zisook et al., 1987). Perhaps the best validated pathologic variant of the bereavement process is chronic grief—bereavement that is excessive in duration and never seems to come to a satisfactory conclusion. According to Parkes and Weiss (1983), chronic grief is more likely to occur when there is a close relationship between the bereaved and the deceased that is marked by dependence or ambivalence.

A second form of bereavement complications, which may or may not be related to the grief process itself, are pathologic outcomes to which bereaved individuals are vulnerable. These include, but are not limited to, depression (Clayton, 1990; Zisook & Shuchter, 1991), anxiety disorders (Jacobs et al., 1990; Zisook, Schneider, & Shuchter, 1990), chronic illness behavior, "grief-related facsimile illness," increased substance use and abuse (Zisook & DeVaul, 1977; Zisook & Shuchter, 1985), and possibly a number of medical problems, such as cerebral vascular disease in men and cirrhosis of the liver in women (Klerman & Clayton, 1984; Klerman & Izen, 1977; Maddison & Viola, 1968). To date, there is not uniform agreement that the mortality rate is higher in bereaved than in nonbereaved populations, but most of the evidence suggests that bereaved individuals are at an increased risk for premature death (Clayton, 1974; Kaprio, Koskenvuo, & Rita, 1987). Of all the pathological outcomes associated with bereavement, major depression has received the most attention.

Certainly, symptoms of depression are ubiquitous after any negative life event, including the death of a loved one. These symptoms are not only quite distressing but can be persistent. Not infrequently, several depressive symptoms cluster together and last for 2 or more weeks, thereby meeting criteria for a depressive syndrome. Acknowledging the frequency of depressive syndromes seen after the loss of a loved one, the *Diagnostic and Statistical Manual of Mental Disorders,* 4th edition (*DSM-IV;* American Psychiatric Association, 1994), refers to the depressive syndrome that begins and ends within 2 months of the death of a loved one as bereavement rather than major depression. Further, the *DSM-IV* states that suicidal ideation, morbid feelings of worthlessness, and psychomotor retardation are rare in bereavement; their presence suggests that the bereavement has been complicated by major depression. The *DSM-IV* uses a 2-month cutoff for bereavement because research has shown that depressive syndromes seen at that time often are persistent, are related to substantial and prolonged psychosocial impairment, and may be associated with protracted feelings of worthlessness and thoughts of suicide (Zisook & Shuchter, 1993). Moreover, it is not uncommon for major depressive episodes to begin after the first 2 months of bereavement, and bereaved individuals to be at risk for depression for at least 2 years (Zisook, Shuchter, Sledge, Paulus, & Judd, 1994). Unfortunately, clinicians may rationalize the depressive syndromes following bereavement as a normal aspect of grief and may therefore reassure rather than treat the patient. We believe that this frequently leads to the underrecognition or misdiagnosis and inadequate treatment of serious depressive disorders. Despite the fact that being depressed is understandable in the context of bereavement, we feel that when full *DSM-IV* criteria for a major depressive episode are met, particularly 2 or more months after the loss, the diagnosis of major depression should be made and bereavement should be noted on Axis IV. Decisions about when and how to treat are then made in the same way as in all other major depressions; that is, social support, intensity and duration of depression, past history, health, and suicidal ideation should all be taken into account when deciding if, when, and how the depression is best treated.

HIV-Related Bereavement

The surviving family members or lovers of individuals who have died from AIDS are uniquely impaired. The illness carries with it many stigmata, including caretakers' fear of contracting the illness, and it is most prevalent in people who are in the prime of life. Asymptomatic infection may permit the infected person and those close to him or her time to adapt to the diagnosis. But when an HIV-positive person begins to manifest symptoms of opportunistic infection or associated cancer, the illness again becomes a threat. Coping with the emotional reality is extremely arduous and complex. Often caretakers, as well as HIV-positive patients, wish for death, which can evoke feelings of guilt. According to Martin and Dean (1989), gay men who have lost lovers to AIDS are more depressed, consider suicide more often, are vulnerable to illicit drug use, and more often tend to seek professional help than other bereaved individuals.

Caregivers who observe the course of the fatal HIV illness that consumes their close friends and significant others are vulnerable to the consequences of intense stress. Lennon, Martin, and Dean (1990) have shown that caregivers of patients with AIDS who do not have adequate social support suffer more prolonged grief reactions after the death of AIDS patients they cared for than do caregivers who do not care for AIDS patients. A recent study conducted by Martin and Dean (1993) reported that the bereavement of a close friend or lover of an AIDS victim can lead to major depression, substance use, suicidal thoughts, and posttraumatic stress reactions. As in other forms of bereavement, anxiety is frequent; but in gay men with AIDS-related bereavement, the anxiety is highly specific to the AIDS epidemic as a stressful event and to their personal vulnerability to developing the disease. The likelihood of chronic and multiple bereavements also adds to the overall burden of AIDS-related grief reactions (Martin & Dean, 1993).

The treatment of bereavement reactions after a death due to AIDS is much like the treatment of other bereaved individuals. However, stigmatization of the illness, or of the gay community in general, must be dealt with. For some family members, guilt about the deceased person's sexual orientation or guilt about their own difficulty accepting the sexual preference are frequent themes. For bereaved lovers, their own HIV status, multiple losses, and other concurrent stressors complicate recovery. For the therapist, both gratification and frustration may be intensely felt. The treatment of HIV patients is inherently stressful and mobilizes strong reactions from health care providers. The therapist must confront fears of contamination, feelings of helplessness, and the news of loss (Novalis, Rojcewicz, & Peele, 1993). The clinician must be careful to keep things in perspective, avoid becoming the rescuer, and not become involved in setting up unrealistic goals; otherwise, he or she runs the risk of being severely stressed and therefore unable to render effective care.

Care of Bereaved Individuals

A variety of treatments are available for bereaved individuals; however, no one form of treatment has been proven superior to another, and there is no standard to be used for all patients. Some types of treatment that have been helpful with bereaved people include the following: self-help groups (e.g., Widows to Widows, They Help Each Other Spiritually [THEOS], and Compassionate Friends; Burnell & Burnell, 1989; Lieberman & Videka-Sherman, 1986; Vachon et al., 1980), volunteer services (Parkes, 1981), group psychotherapy (Parkes, 1981), supportive psychotherapy (Gerber, Weiner, Battin, & Arkin, 1975; Raphael, 1977; Weizman & Kamm, 1985), psychodynamic psychotherapy (Horowitz, Marmar, Weiss, De Witt, & Rosenbaum, 1984; Lazare, 1979), and antidepressant medication for bereavement-related depression (Jacobs, Nelson, & Zisook, 1987; Pasternak et al., 1991).

Although mutual support groups may fill a gap for those who have little or no social support, and there is some evidence to suggest that intervention programs help people move faster through the grieving process (Silverman, 1982; Vachon et al., 1980), not all bereaved people need or want formal intervention. Because of the paucity of outcome data on the efficacy of interventions, it is not entirely clear which programs are appropriate for whom and when. However, the Institute of Medicine Committee has offered some guidelines about the appropriateness of the general approaches under various circumstances. For example, it is felt that most bereaved individuals are not generally ready to seek help outside their immediate social network or to benefit from it for at least several weeks after the loss (Osterweis, 1984). Some evidence indicates that a formal intervention program during the very early period of crisis can be helpful for people at high risk (i.e., because of multiple or traumatic loss, stigmatized loss, unsupportive social environment, an ambivalent relationship with the deceased, past history of depression, substance abuse, poor health, multiple losses, and other concomitant life stresses; Raphael, 1977, 1983; Rynearson, 1990) or for mothers who lose newborns (Zeanah, 1989) but that for the general bereaved population such immediate intervention will have little impact. Therefore, for most bereaved people who are not regarded as being at a particularly high risk for the adverse consequences of bereavement, the support of family and friends, if available, is generally sufficient. If such support is not available, then mutual support groups can be quite beneficial.

Dimond, Lund, and Caserta (1987) noted that the positive aspects of bereavement support groups included self-expression, contact, shared confidences, closeness, and mutual helping. Strategies used by most bereavement groups include education about the grief process; having each survivor tell his or her story; explaining the psychological, cognitive, and physical symptoms of grief; and exploring how each person copes with memories of the deceased. Thus, sharing, group cohesion, education, support, and normalization are key elements in bereavement group treatment (Colburn & Malena, 1988; Yalom & Vinagradov, 1988).

Although natural restorative and healing processes can help most people get through their grief without professional assistance, there are circumstances that may warrant professional mental health intervention. For example, unexpected losses have been associated with a greater risk of psychological and physical disability during bereavement than losses after a long-term illness, especially immediately after the loss. Sanders (1983) found that survivors of sudden death experienced more anger and somatic symptoms than survivors who had lost a loved one from a chronic illness. Parkes (1972, 1990) and Parkes and Weiss (1983) discovered factors that contributed to a poor resolution of the grief process: a short duration of terminal illness (sudden loss), death not attributable to cancer, and not having had the chance to discuss the imminent death with the dying person. Parkes (1972) coined the term "unexpected loss syndrome" for a cluster of behaviors that become apparent after experiencing a sudden loss: social withdrawal, bewilderment, and protest. The presence of this syndrome may result in a complicated recovery. When counseling survivors of sudden loss, clinicians may need to "help survivors actualize the loss" (view the body and keep the focus on the death); use the words *death* and *dead* in an effort to help bring the situation into reality for the survivors; explore any guilt, blame, and feelings of abandonment; help the survivors deal with any anger; correct denial and distortions; and discuss the impact that the loss will have in the future.

In working with bereaved individuals, we favor an integrative approach that uses aspects of psychodynamic, cognitive, behavioral, supportive, and educative psychotherapies. This approach is problem specific and uses the following therapeutic tasks: development of the capacity to experience, express, and integrate painful affects; use of the most adaptive means of modulating painful affects; integration of the continuing relationships with the deceased; maintenance of health and continued functioning; successful reconfiguration of altered relationships; and integration of a healthy self-concept and a stable worldview.

These tasks reflect the key dimensions of the bereavement process and run the gamut of changes initiated by the death of a loved one. People may deal with several of these dimensions simultaneously. The time courses for the dimensions might be quite different and variable. Thus, we have arrived at a view in which individuals go through parallel dimensions proceeding in highly variable, idiosyncratic ways and in time frames often extending far beyond commonly ascribed periods for grief experiences. The clinician's task at any one moment is the careful assessment of each of these dimensions to see how well the survivor is managing.

The series of tasks may be worked through over years. Interventions are based on specific problems that are defined at a given point in time. They are focused, practical, and time limited, but with an understanding that other difficulties in the future may require further intervention. Some effort is directed at education, including references to reading material about the grief process (Shuchter, 1986; Shuchter & Zisook, 1986, 1990).

Tasks of Bereavement

1. Development of the capacity to experience, express, and integrate painful affects. Bereaved individuals may experience some of the most disturbing and disruptive symptoms of their lives. Acute aspects of grief are both physically and psychologically painful. Symptoms include depression, anxiety, anger, fear, and guilt (Sanders, 1989). There are many ways in which the therapist can facilitate the survivor's grief experience and expression of affects. If the bereaved are not able to simply express their feelings, the therapist may help them overcome the barriers by helping them realize that those feelings are normal. By inquiring about specific feelings, the therapist provides perspective and understanding. At times, specific evocative techniques may help. For example, the therapist may use powerful, direct, or even blunt language or may have the bereaved bring in a photograph, videotapes, clothing, letters, or other symbols of the deceased. The clinician may also ask the bereaved to write letters to the deceased, to keep a journal with drawings or pictures, to role-play, or to use directed imagery. The purpose of these techniques is to encourage the fullest expression of thoughts and feelings regarding the loss, including regrets and disappointments. It is important to remember, however, that the therapist should never assume that certain affects such as guilt or anger are inevitable concomitants of grief and consequently insist that the patient express these feelings that may not fit.

2. Adaptive modulation of affects. It is important to assess the bereaved person's customary and present coping strategies. Faced with the onset of recurrent, often unpredictable, and usually disruptive emotional and cognitive upheavals, people find ways to protect themselves from the distress. Survivors will ultimately use their customary defenses when possible, or they may resort to more primitive ones or to the use of multiple defenses when overwhelmed by acute grief. Frequently seen coping mechanisms during bereavement include distraction (such as watching television), rationalization (he's better off this way than to be suffering), faith, indulgence in food or alcohol, and dissociation. It is clear that no one can tolerate all of the painful effects associated with grief all of the time and that some "dosing" becomes a necessary component of work with the bereaved. In other words, therapists must help bereaved individuals find a workable balance between helping them to face the painful feelings that are an integral part of grief and encouraging protective mechanisms to ward off excess pain over and above what can be tolerated. The balance is fluid, and shifts from time to time and situation to situation. In general, it is advisable to respect the adaptive aspects of the bereaved person's customary coping strategies. To the extent that the bereaved may need help in eliciting more direct affective responses, the evocative techniques mentioned above may be useful. Alternatively, often-bereaved individuals may experience too much distressing affect, which may overwhelm their ability to function. In such cases, the dosing requires helping the bereaved find ways to modulate their affect, such as by encouraging displacement or distractions. The therapists' major task is to support the more adaptive coping mechanisms while actively discouraging the more maladaptive ones, such as alcohol use, excessive eating, or impulsive acting out.

3. Integration of the continuing relationship with the deceased. One of the most powerful means of coping with the death of a loved one is coping that mitigates completely against the loss, that is, the ability of the survivor to keep the dead alive. Obviously, this does not occur in a literal sense, but through a variety of psychological mechanisms that permit survivors to maintain their ties to the deceased. Continuing contact can be experienced in several ways, such as symbolic representation, belief in an afterlife, carrying on discussions with the deceased, hallucination, identification phenomena, living legacies, social and cultural rituals, tributes, visitations, and memories. The thread that is contained in each of these psychological phenomena is the effort to keep the person alive in whatever way this can be accomplished. Bereaved individuals must somehow find a way to continue their relationship with the deceased person, which allows them to appropriately experience grief and to continue their involvement in grieving. A natural way for the therapist to assist with this task is to systematically explore all aspects of the relationship that existed between the survivor and the deceased person, both as it has evolved over time before the death and as it has evolved since the death. The therapist can use normalization to sanction the development of any of the many forms of continuing relationships to the survivor as a means of mitigating against the intense affect associated with realization of the loss.

4. Maintenance of health and continued functioning. Bereaved individuals are vulnerable to dysfunction in many ways: Problems may develop with physical health, psychological health, work performance, and social adjustment. As therapists, our goals are to identify those factors and help prevent or minimize the impact of any of their complications. Especially for elderly people, regular medical checkups are advisable, in particular after prolonged caretaking, when medical needs may have been neglected. Depression should always be suspected and appropriate evaluation performed. If major depression or other psychiatric conditions are present, prompt treatment should be instituted. Treating depression or anxiety does not interfere with grief. Conversely, untreated depression blocks any attempts to adapt to stress, restore functional capacity, or complete grief work.

5. Successful reconfiguration of altered relationships. One of the inevitable consequences of bereavement is that survivors experience significant changes in other relationships. There may be greater closeness, a different meaning, an altered role or dynamic, or other changes in relationships with people in their lives, many of whom have also been affected by the loss. For example, when a spouse dies, the surviving parent will have to face the responsibility of helping the children with their grief, as well as the reality of single parenthood and the shifting roles that follow in regard to gratification and discipline. At the same time, the bereaved may be expected to provide support to older parents or in-laws. Initially, friends may be quite supportive. However, in time the bereaved may find themselves becoming avoided or rejected. New romances may offer both the hope and the fear of intimacy and sexuality, as well as precipitate conflict associated with companions. Feelings of betrayal, the culture shock of dating, and the conflicts inherent in all relationships are all highly probable scenarios. Thus, there are many kinds of dilemmas that can arise out of changing relationships, which may take new forms and new courses of development. Therefore, thorough assessment is essential.

6. Integration of a new identity and worldview. Some of the most profound changes that occur in bereaved individuals are those that reflect their personal identity. For many people, bereavement is likely to be the most disruptive, threatening, and challenging experience they will ever face in their lives. Under such circumstances, it is not surprising that there is a potential for dramatic change. At first, bereaved people often experience an intense regression to what Horowitz, Wilner, Marmar, and Krupnick (1980) described as the emergence of "latent negative self-images." These are perceptions of the self as being helpless, inadequate, incapable, childlike, or personally bankrupt. Over time, these may give way to more positive self-images—by-products of the bereaved finding themselves able to tolerate their grief, carry on their tasks, and learn new ways of dealing with the world. There may be a growing sense of strength, autonomy, independence, assertiveness, and maturity.

Similarly, bereaved individuals may experience a change in their worldview. Initially, they may be struck by the unfairness of death or perhaps their own impotence in preventing it. In time, these beliefs may be replaced by new ones, and the fragility and finiteness of life, as well as the limits of its control, become more understandable. The end result is that bereaved people often become more patient, accepting, and giving, and more appreciative of daily living. They may develop new careers or change career direction. They enjoy themselves with more gusto, and find new outlets for creativity. Alternatively, some people stagnate or wither and are unable to experience personal growth or to meet life's challenges.

The roles of the psychotherapist in the bereaved person's evolving identity are numerous. Therapists must recognize early regression for what it is, and they must be able to maintain a conviction about the bereaved person's adaptive capacities. Contained in such a conviction are both the belief and knowledge that the bereaved person can survive and will feel better. As survivors venture out to try something new, they may find themselves stymied by old conflicts that can be examined in a psychotherapeutic fashion.

Case Illustration: Bereavement-Related Depression

Bob was a 46-year-old artist and writer with two grown children: a 20-year-old daughter and an 18-year-old son. He had lost his wife, Jane, 8 months before therapy, after her second heart attack. They had been married for more than 20 years. He described the marriage as warm, mutually supportive, and secure.

Jane had recovered from her first heart attack 4 years before her death. Several months before her death she began feeling more fatigued, run down, and ill. While in a restaurant with Bob, she suddenly developed ventricular fibrillation. Bob kept her alive while waiting for the paramedics by performing cardiopulmonary resuscitation. She was taken to the hospital, but immediately lapsed into a coma and died approximately a week after admission. Bob was with her constantly during her hospitalization and had to make the difficult decision to allow Jane's life supports to be discontinued.

Bob's immediate grief was mild. He continued to work effectively and he began to date an attractive, outgoing woman about 6 weeks after his wife's death. While the relationship was going well, he felt good. However, Bob began suffering anxiety and depressive symptoms when he became aware of his girlfriend's inability to make a commitment to him. Whenever he perceived or was threatened by separation from his new girlfriend, his depressive symptoms intensified and he became anxious. His symptoms became increasingly frequent and severe over the several months prior to his initial appointment with a therapist.

The clinician saw Bob weekly for 5 weeks, then every other week for another 2 months. They discussed the nature of his new relationship, and he began to understand that he had started the relationship in order to avoid dealing with some of his feelings about his dead wife. They also talked about his intense guilt feelings related to his "being unfaithful." He directly related his guilt feelings to transient fantasies of women and of being attracted to a nurse at Jane's bedside immediately after he made the decision to discontinue life supports. He talked about other losses he had experienced in his life. For example, both his parents had died within a few weeks of each other 10 years earlier. He also discussed some of his disappointments in his marriage, particularly in that although he and his wife had maintained a very close and supportive friendship, their sexual relationship had essentially ceased after her first heart attack.

Bob experienced much catharsis followed by relief during his third session while watching home videotapes he had taken of his family and wife before she was ill. However, Bob continued to express fears of an imminent depression if his girlfriend were to break up with him. Within a few months, he felt much better and discontinued regular psychotherapy. He agreed to come in on an as-needed basis.

Approximately 6 months later, Bob began feeling more depressed. These feelings revived on what would have been his 25th wedding anniversary and worsened on the anniversary of his wife's death. It also seemed that his depressed feelings were related to his beginning to date other women, which made him feel unfaithful to his present girlfriend. The therapist and Bob talked about how these feelings paralleled those he had concerning his wife and how the girlfriend was symbolically replacing Jane. Soon, Bob reported feeling normal again.

Bob did not return until the following year, when he began feeling depressed with some suicidal ideation, which related to an imminent breakup with his girlfriend. He then began pining for his wife. Because of his increased depression, which had become more persistent and which was associated with suicidal ideation, antidepressant medication was started.

During the next two sessions, Bob talked more about his relationship with his wife, how much he missed her, and how neither he nor the children had actively grieved after she died. He felt better between sessions, but he still believed that he had not yet "let go" and that his grief festered like an abscess. To "lance the abscess," Bob and his therapist began focusing on concrete representations of his wife that he kept in the house, such as her favorite shawls, purses, and underwear. This led to Bob's describing intense guilt feelings about not doing more to get his wife to see a physician during the last 6 months of her life when she was obviously "going downhill." He described the last time he was with his wife, at her bedside when she died, saying good-bye to her at that time, staying with her, cradling her in his arms, kissing her, talking to her, and then separating himself from her, which Bob said he literally and symbolically did by pulling the curtain around her, walking away, and "feeling that now she is dead, there's nothing more I can do." He cried during much of that session and ended by stating, "I'm not sure I'll ever be able to give her up." At the next session Bob talked more about his guilt and came to see that he had done all that he could.

At the next session, Bob reported feeling better. He talked about how much he missed his wife and his "feeling as though she were still alive and wanting to hug her." He stated that he was feeling much better and that he felt a major part of his improvement was putting "my new girlfriend in perspective." Bob came to the next session stating he was feeling "back to normal."

Bob returned to the therapist a year later, as it was important for him to "touch bases." He stated that he was doing well, although there were some isolated periods lasting a day when he experienced depression, loneliness, despondency, and decreased energy. In general, he was eating and sleeping well and feeling good about himself. He had stopped taking the antidepressant 6 months earlier, but continued to take an anxiolytic intermittently when he felt particularly anxious or alone. He was in the process of breaking up with the woman he had begun dating shortly after his wife's death, saying "I find her cold and unemotional." He was dating several other women at this time and felt comfortable about his social life. He agreed to call should he feel more anxious and depressed or if he wanted to talk.

Discussion of Case Illustration

Bob experienced two forms of pathologic grief: The first involved an inhibition of the grief process and the second was the development of an autonomous depression. At various points throughout his treatment, methods were used to help Bob overcome his avoidance of painful affects relating to Jane's death. As a result of this avoidance, he had been unable to process aspects of this loss cognitively or emotionally, and as a result, he remained psychologically frozen. Through the use of emotional triggers (her belongings, photographs, and home movies), Bob was able to bring her death to life and integrate this loss and his continued relationship with Jane, freeing himself from the guilt he felt for abandoning her and becoming available for other relationships. Bob's depressive symptoms responded ostensibly to a combination of psychotherapy and pharmacology. Often the major depressive syndromes seen in bereavement require pharmacologic intervention. Bob's psychiatrist remained available to him over time to help Bob deal with multiple issues as they became relevant and disabling. We have referred to this form of treatment as "hovering over the bereaved" (Shuchter & Zisook, 1990).

The Future

Despite the recent efforts and knowledge gained from studies by investigators on dying and bereavement, a need for continuing work remains. For instance, conclusions about the applicability or effectiveness of specific interventions cannot be drawn from the current data available. Furthermore, there is a paucity of good outcome data regarding the efficacy and indications, if any, of the major types of bereavement interventions; that is, mutual supports, hospices, psychotherapy, and medication therapy. The Institute of Medicine has outlined several research opportunities for the future, such as research on the processes and outcomes of bereavement, including intervention strategies, and finding those individuals who are the most vulnerable and at highest risk of experiencing negative outcome (Committee for the Study of Health Consequences of the Stress of Bereavement, 1984).

The psychosocial impact on mental health professionals working with bereaved individuals, and in particular HIV patients, needs to be explored. What situational factors in HIV infection and AIDS are most stressful for care providers, and what types of provider psychotherapeutic interventions are the most helpful? Does personality of caregiver or recipient alter the perception of group effectiveness? Moreover, what is the morbidity associated with the cumulative effects of caregiving for patients in general, as well as for HIV patients? To date, most research studies have concentrated on the bereaved person during the first year of bereavement. More longitudinal studies are necessary for the bereaved and their care providers.

Additional research is required concerning the impact of bereavement on the family. What types of coping are the most beneficial to the family as a unit, not just to the patient who is terminally ill? Along similar lines, research studies need to be conducted to determine whether coping from previous losses affects coping with a current loss. Attention should also be focused on the consequences of the death of a sibling, a child, and parents during adult life, as well as to the type of loss; that is, suicide, homicide, abortion, and so forth.

Cross-cultural and minority studies are also indicated. The effects of bereavement, the types of coping mechanisms, and the biology of grief need to be explored in ethnic minorities: Asian, Hispanic, and African American individuals; people in nontraditional conjugal relationships; children; and HIV-positive individuals. A final note to consider is that now that more is known about the natural history of AIDS and how to treat the disease, the impact of these new factors on AIDS-related bereavement should be reevaluated. In essence, there is a lot more work to be done.

REFERENCES

Alexander, G. J. (1988). *Writing a living will.* New York: Praeger.

American Psychiatric Association. (1994). *Diagnostic and statistical manual of mental disorders* (4th ed.). Washington, DC: Author.

Bartrop, R., Luckhurst, E., Lazarus, L., Kiloh, L. G., & Penny, R. (1977). Depressed lymphocyte function after bereavement. *Lancet, 1,* 834–836.

Black, D., & Winokur, G. (1990). Suicide and psychiatric diagnosis. In S. Blumenthal & D. Kupfer (Eds.), *Suicide over the life cycle* (pp. 135–153). Washington, DC: American Psychiatric Press.

Blendon, R. J., Szalay, U. S., & Knox, R. A. (1992). Should physicians aid their patients in dying? *Journal of the American Medical Association, 267,* 2658–2662.

Blumenthal, S. J. (1990). An overview and synopsis of risk factors, assessment, and treatment of suicidal patients over the life cycle. In S. J. Blumenthal & D. Kupfer (Eds.), *Suicide over the life cycle* (pp. 685–733). Washington, DC: American Psychiatric Press.

Bolund, C. (1987). Suicide and cancer: II. Medical and care factors in suicides by cancer patients in Sweden. *Journal of Psychosocial Oncology, 48,* 33–38.

Bowlby, J. (1961). Processes of mourning. *International Journal of Psychoanalysis, 42,* 317.

Bowlby, J. (1971). *Attachment and loss: 1. Attachment.* Harmondsworth, England: Pelican Books.

Breitbart, W. (1989). Psychiatric management of cancer pain. *Cancer, 63,* 2336–2342.

Breitbart, W., Passik, S., & Levenson, J. (1992). Terminally ill cancer patients. In W. Bretibart & J. Holland (Eds.), *Psychiatric aspects of symptom management in cancer patients* (pp. 203–268). Washington, DC: American Psychiatric Press.

Burnell, G. M., & Burnell, A. L. (1989). *Clinical management of bereavement: A handbook for professionals.* New York: Human Sciences Press.

Cassem, N. H. (1991). The dying patient. In N. H. Cassem (Ed.), *The Massachusetts General Hospital handbook of general hospital psychiatry* (p. 343). St. Louis, MO: Mosby.

Cassem, N. H., & Stewart, R. S. (1975). Management and care of the dying patient. *International Journal of Psychiatry in Medicine, 6,* 293–304.

Chochinov, H., Wilson, K., Enns, M., Mowchun, N., & Levitt, M. (1993, May). *Depression among the terminally ill.* Symposium held at the 146th annual meeting of the American Psychiatric Association, San Francisco.

Clayton, P. J. (1974). Mortality and morbidity in the first year of bereavement. *Archives of General Psychiatry, 30,* 747–750.

Clayton, P. J. (1982). Bereavement. In E. S. Paykel (Ed.), *Handbook of affective disorders* (p. 403). London: Churchill Livingstone.

Clayton, P. J. (1990). Bereavement and depression. *Journal of Clinical Psychiatry, 51,* 34.

Cohen, J. S., Fihn, S. D., Boyko, E. J., Jonsen, A. R., & Wood, R. W. (1994). Attitudes toward assisted suicide and euthanasia among physicians in Washington State. *New England Journal of Medicine, 331,* 89–94.

Colburn, K., & Malena, D. (1988, September–October). Bereavement issues for survivors of Persons with AIDS. *American Journal of Hospice Care,* 20–25.

Committee for the Study of Health Consequences of the Stress of Bereavement. (1984). Conclusions and recommendations. In M. Osterwies, F. Solomon, & M. Green (Eds.), *Bereavement: Reactions, consequences and care* (pp. 283–295). Washington, DC: National Academy Press.

Conwell, Y. (1994). Suicide in the elderly: Diagnosis and treatment of depression in the elderly. In L. S. Schneider, C. F. Reynolds, B. Lebowitz, & A. Friedhoff (Eds.), *Diagnosis and treatment of depression in later life* (pp. 397–418). Washington, DC: American Psychiatric Press.

Conwell, Y., & Caine, E. D. (1991). Sounding Board: Rational suicide and the right to die. *New England Journal of Medicine, 325,* 1100–1102.

Deutch, H. (1937). Absence of grief. *Psychoanalytic Quarterly, 6,* 12–22.

de Wachter, M. A. M. (1989). Active euthanasia in the Netherlands. *Journal of the American Medical Association, 262,* 3316–3319.

Dimond, M. F., Lund, D. A., & Caserta, M. S. (1987). The role of social supports in the first two years of bereavement in an elderly sample. *Gerontologist, 27,* 599–604.

Dobihal, E. F. (1981). *When a friend is dying: A guide to caring for the terminally ill and bereaved.* Nashville, TN: Abingdon Press.

Ezekiel, E., & Ezekiel, L. (1990). Living wills: Past, present and future. *Journal of Clinical Ethics, 1,* 9–19.

Fawcett, J., Scheftner, W. A., Foff, L., Clark, D. C., Young, M. A., Hedeker, D., & Gibbons, R. (1990). Time-related predictors of suicide in major affective disorder. *American Journal of Psychiatry, 147,* 1189–1194.

Fawzy, F. I., Cousins, N., Fawzy, N. W., Kemeny, M. E., Elashoff, R., & Morton, D. (1990). A structured psychiatric intervention for cancer patients. *Archives of General Psychiatry, 47,* 720–725.

Freud, S. (1957). Mourning and melancholia. In J. Strachey (Ed.), *Standard edition of the complete psychological works of Sigmund Freud* (Vol. 14, pp. 237–260). London: Hogarth Press.

Garfield, C. (1978). *Psychosocial care of the dying patient.* New York: McGraw-Hill.

Gerber, I., Weiner, A., Battin, D., & Arkin, A. M. (1975). Brief therapy to the aged bereaved. In B. Schoenberg & I. Gerber (Eds.), *Bereavement: Its psychosocial aspects* (pp. 310–313). New York: Columbia University Press.

Gonda, T. A., & Ruark, J. E. (1984). *Dying dignified: The health professional's guide to care.* Reading, MA: Addison-Wesley.

Graber, G., & Thomasma, D. (1990). *Euthanasia: Toward an ethical social policy.* New York: Continuum Press.

Hackett, J., & Weisman, A. D. (1962). The treatment of dying. *Current Psychiatric Therapy, 2,* 121.

Hendin, J., & Klerman, G. (1993). Physician-assisted suicide: The dangers of legalization. *American Journal of Psychiatry, 150,* 143–145.

Holland, J. (1991). Progress and challenges in psychosocial and behavioral research in cancer in the twentieth century. *Cancer, 67,* 676–773.

Horowitz, M. J., Marmar, C., Weiss, D. S., De Witt, K. N., & Rosenbaum, R. (1984). Brief psychotherapy of bereavement reactions: The relationship of process to outcome. *Archives of General Psychiatry, 41,* 438–448.

Horowitz, M. J., Wilner, N., Marmar, C., & Krupnick, J. (1980). Pathological grief and the activation of latent self-images. *American Journal of Psychiatry, 137,* 1157.

Irwin, M. R., & Weiner, H. (1987). Depressive symptoms and immune function during bereavement. In S. Zisook (Ed.), *Biopsychosocial aspects of bereavement* (pp. 141–155). Washington, DC: American Psychiatric Press.

Jacobs, S. (1987). Psychoendocrine aspects of bereavement. In S. Zisook (Ed.), *Biopsychosocial aspects of bereavement* (pp. 141–155). Washington, DC: American Psychiatric Press.

Jacobs, S. C. (1993). *Pathological grief: Maladaptation to loss.* Washington, DC: American Psychiatric Press.

Jacobs, S. C., Brown, S. A., Mason, J., Wahby, V., Kasl, S., & Ostfeld, A. (1986). Psychological distress, depression, and prolactin response in stressed persons. *Journal of Human Stress,* 113–118.

Jacobs, S. C., Hansen, F., Kasl, S., Ostfeld, A., Berkman, L., & Kim, K. (1990). Anxiety disorders during acute bereavement: Risk and risk factors. *Journal of Clinical Psychiatry, 7,* 269–274.

Jacobs, S. C., Mason, J., Kosten, T., Kasl, S. V., Ostfeld, A. M., & Wahby, V. (1987). Urinary free cortisol and separation anxiety early in the course of bereavement and threatened loss. *Biological Psychiatry, 22,* 148–152.

Jacobs, S. C., Nelson, J. C., & Zisook, S. (1987). Treating depression of bereavement with antidepressants: A pilot study. *Psychiatric Clinics of North America, 10,* 501–510.

Kalish, R., & Reynolds, D. (1976). *Death and ethnicity.* Los Angeles: University of Southern California Press.

Kaprio, J., Koskenvuo, M., & Rita, H. (1987). Mortality after bereavement: A prospective study of 95,647 widowed persons. *American Journal of Public Health, 77,* 283–287.

Kastenbaum, R. J. (1991). *Death, society and human experience* (2nd ed.). New York: Macmillan.

Kearl, M. (1989). *Endings: A sociology of death and dying.* New York: Oxford University Press.

Klerman, G. L., & Clayton, P. (1984). Epidemiologic perspectives on health consequences of bereavement. In M. Osterweis, F. Solomon, & M. Green (Eds.), *Bereavement: Reactions, consequences and care* (pp. 15–44). Washington, DC: National Academy Press.

Klerman, G. L., & Izen, J. (1977). The effects of bereavement and grief on physical health and general well-being. *Advanced Psychosomatic Medicine, 9,* 63.

Koenig, J. G. (1993). Legalizing physician-assisted suicide: Some thoughts and concerns. *Journal of Family Practice, 37,* 171–179.

Kosten, T., Jacobs, S. C., & Mason, J. (1984). The DST in depression during bereavement. *Journal of Nervous and Mental Disease, 172,* 359–360.

Kosten, T., Jacobs, S. C., Mason, J., Brown, S., Atkins, S., Gardner, C., Schneiber, S., Wahby, V., & Ostfeld, A. (1984). Psychological correlates of growth hormone response to stress. *Psychosomatic Medicine, 46,* 49–58.

Kübler-Ross, E. (1969). *On death and dying.* London: Macmillan.

Kübler-Ross, E. (1987). *AIDS: The ultimate challenge.* New York: Macmillan.

Lazare, A. (1979). Unresolved grief. In A. Lazare (Ed.), *Outpatient psychiatry, diagnosis and treatment* (pp. 498–512). Baltimore: Williams & Wilkins.

Lennon, M. C., Martin, J. L., & Dean, L. (1990). The influence of social support on AIDS-related grief reaction among gay men. *Social Science and Medicine, 31,* 477–484.

Le Shan, E. (1976). *Learning to say good-bye: When a parent dies.* New York: Macmillan.

Lieberman, M. A., & Videka-Sherman, L. (1986). The impact of self-help groups in the mental health of widows and widowers. *American Journal of Orthopsychiatry, 56,* 435–449.

Lindemann, E. (1944). Symptomatology and management of acute grief. *American Journal of Psychiatry, 101,* 141.

Lundin, T. (1987). The stress of unexpected bereavement: Psychology of stress. *Stress Medicine, 3,* 109–114.

Maddison, D., & Viola, A. (1968). The health of widows in the year following bereavement. *Journal of Psychosomatic Research, 12,* 297.

Martin, J. L., & Dean, L. (1989). Risk factors for AIDS-related bereavement in a cohort of homosexual men in NY City. In B. Cooper & T. Helgason (Eds.), *Epidemiology and the prevention of mental disorders* (pp. 170–184). London: Routledge & Kegan Paul.

Martin, J. L., & Dean, L. (1993). Effects of AIDS-related bereavement and HIV-related illness on psychological distress among gay men: A 7-year longitudinal study, 1985–1991. *Journal of Consulting and Clinical Psychology, 61,* 94–103.

Marzuk, P. M., Tierney, H., Tardiff, K., Gross, F. M., Morgan, E. B., Hsu, M. A., & Mann, J. (1988). Increased risk of suicide in persons with AIDS. *Journal of the American Medical Association, 259,* 1333–1337.

May, W. (1974). The metaphysical plight of the family. *Hastings Center Studies, 2,* 19–30.

McKegney, F. P., & O'Dowd, M. A. (1992). Suicidality and HIV status. *American Journal of Psychiatry, 149,* 396–398.

Muller, M. T., Van der Wal, G., Eijk, J. T. M, & Ribbe, M. W. (1994). Voluntary active euthanasia and physician-assisted suicide in Dutch nursing homes: Are the requirements for prudent practice properly met? *Journal of the American Geriatrics Society, 42,* 624–629.

Novalis, P., Rojcewicz, S., & Peele, R. (1993). *Clinical manual of supportive psychotherapy.* Washington, DC: American Psychiatric Press.

Osterweis, M. (1984). Bereavement intervention programs. In M. Osterweis, F. Solomon, & M. Green (Eds.), *Bereavement: Reactions, consequences and care* (pp. 239–279). Washington, DC: National Academy Press.

Parkes, C. M. (1972). *Bereavement studies of grief in adult life.* New York: International Universities Press.

Parkes, C. M. (1981). Evaluation of a bereavement service. *Journal of Preventive Psychiatry, 1,* 179–188.

Parkes, C. M. (1990). Risk factors in bereavement: Implications for the prevention and treatment of pathologic grief. *Psychiatric Annals, 20,* 308–313.

Parkes, C. M., & Weiss, R. S. (1983). *Recovery from bereavement.* New York: Basic Books.

Pasternak, R. E., Reynolds, C. F., Schlernitzauer, M., Hoch, C. C., Buysse, O. J., Houck, P. R., & Perel, J. M. (1991). Acute open-trial Nortriptyline therapy of bereavement-related depression in late life. *Journal of Clinical Psychiatry, 52,* 307–310.

Pollack, G. (1987). The mourning-liberation process in health and disease. In S. Zisook (Ed.), *Psychiatric clinics of North America: Grief and bereavement* (Vol. 10, pp. 345–354). Philadelphia, PA: W. B. Saunders.

Raphael, B. (1977). Preventive intervention with the recently bereaved. *Archives of General Psychiatry, 34,* 1450–1454.

Raphael, B. (1983). *The anatomy of bereavement.* New York: Basic Books.

Reynolds, C. F., Hoch, C. C., Buysse, D. J., Houck, P. R., Schlernitzauer, M., Frank, E., Mazumdar, S., & Dupfer, D. J. (1992). Electroencephalographic sleep in spousal bereavement and bereavement-related depression of late life. *Biological Psychiatry, 31,* 69–82.

Rhymes, J. (1990). Hospice care in America. *Journal of the American Medical Association, 264,* 369–372.

Rich, C., Young, D., & Fowler, R. (1986). San Diego suicide study: Young vs. old subjects. *Archives of General Psychiatry, 43,* 577–582.

Rynearson, E. K. (1990). Pathologic grief: The Queen's croquet ground. *Psychiatric Annals, 20,* 295–303.

Sanders, C. M. (1983). Effects of sudden versus chronic illness death on bereavement outcome. *Omega, 11,* 227–241.

Sanders, C. M. (1989). *Grief: The mourning after.* New York: Wiley.

Saunders, C. (1978). *The management of terminal illness.* Chicago: Year Book Medical Publishers.

Schleifer, S. J., Keller, S., Camerino, M., Thorton, J. C., & Stein, M. (1983). Suppression of lymphocyte stimulation following bereavement. *Journal of the American Medical Association, 259,* 374–377.

Schneidman, E. S. (1980). *Voices of death.* New York: Harper & Row.

Shuchter, S. R. (1986). *Dimensions of grief: Adjusting to the death of a spouse.* San Francisco: Jossey-Bass.

Shuchter, S. R., & Zisook, S. (1986). Treatment of spousal bereavement: A multidimensional approach. *Psychiatric Annals, 16,* 295–305.

Shuchter, S. R., & Zisook, S. (1987). A multidimensional model of spousal bereavement. In S. Zisook (Ed.), *Biopsychosocial aspects of bereavement* (pp. 35–47). Washington, DC: American Psychiatric Press.

Shuchter, S. R., & Zisook, S. (1990). Hovering over the bereaved. *Psychiatric Annals, 20,* 327–333.

Shuchter, S. R., & Zisook, S. (1993). The course of normal grief. In S. Stroebe, W. Stroebe, & R. Hansson (Eds.), *Handbook of bereavement* (pp. 23–43). Cambridge, England: Cambridge University Press.

Shuchter, S. R., Zisook, S., & Kirkorowicz, C. (1986). The dexamethasone suppression test in acute grief. *American Journal of Psychiatry, 143,* 879–881.

Silverman, P. R. (1982). Transitions and models of intervention. *Annals of the Academy of Political and Social Sciences, 464,* 174–187.

Solsberry, M. (1984). Adults' reactions to bereavement. In M. Osterweis, F. Solomon, & M. Green (Eds.), *Bereavement: Reactions, consequences and care* (pp. 47–68). Washington, DC: National Academy Press.

Spiegel, D., Kraemer, H., Bloom, J., & Gottheil, E. (1989, October 14). Effect of psychosocial treatment on survival of patients with metastatic breast cancer. *Lancet*, 888–891.

Stroebe, M., Stroebe, W., & Hansson, R. (1993). *Handbook of bereavement*. Cambridge, England: Cambridge University Press.

Task Force on Ethics of the Society of Critical Care Medicine. (1990). Consensus report on the ethics of foregoing life-sustaining treatments in the critically ill. *Critical Care Medicine, 18,* 1435–1439.

U.S. Department of Health and Human Resources. (1991). *Vital Statistics Report of the United States*. Washington, DC: Author.

Vachon, M. L. S., Lyall, W. A. L., Rogers, J., Freedman-Letofsky, K., & Freeman, S. J. J. (1980). A controlled study of self-help intervention for widows. *American Journal of Psychiatry, 137,* 1380–1384.

Van Der Maas, P. J., Van Delden, J. J. M., Pijnenborg, L., & Looman, C. W. N. (1991). Euthanasia and other medical decisions concerning the end of life. *Lancet, 338,* 669–674.

Weisman, A. D. (1972). *On dying and denying: A psychiatric study of terminality*. New York: Behavioral Publications.

Weisman, A. D. (1974). *The realization of death*. New York: Jason Aronson.

Weisman, A. D. (1988). Thanatology. In H. I. Kaplan & B. J. Sadock (Eds.), *Comprehensive textbook of psychiatry: IV* (pp. 1748–1758). Baltimore: Williams & Wilkins.

Weizman, S. G., & Kamm, P. (1985). *About mourning: Support and guidance for the bereaved*. New York: Human Sciences Press.

Worden, J. W. (1991). *Grief counseling and grief therapy: A handbook for the mental health practitioner* (2nd ed.) New York: Springer.

Wortman, C. B., & Silver, R. C. (1989). The myths of coping with loss. *Journal of Consulting and Clinical Psychology, 57,* 349–357.

Yalom, I. D., & Lieberman, M. A. (1991). Bereavement and heightened existential awareness. *Psychiatry, 54,* 334–345.

Yalom, I. D., & Vinagradov, S. (1988). Bereavement groups. *International Journal of Group Psychotherapy, 38,* 419–457.

Zeanah, C. H. (1989). Adaptation following perinatal loss: A critical review. *Journal of the American Academy of Child and Adolescent Psychiatry, 28,* 467–480.

Zimmerman, J. M. (1986). *Hospice complete care for the terminally ill*. Baltimore: Urban & Schwatrzenber.

Zisook, S. (Ed.). (1987). *Grief and bereavement*. Philadelphia, PA: W. B. Saunders.

Zisook, S. (1994). Bereavement, depression and immune function. *Psychiatry Research, 52,* 1–10.

Zisook, S. (1995). *Death and dying: Comprehensive textbook of psychiatry*. Baltimore: Williams & Wilkins.

Zisook, S., & DeVaul, R. A. (1977). Grief-related facsimile illness. *International Journal of Psychiatric Medicine, 7,* 329–336.

Zisook, S., & DeVaul, R. (1985). Unresolved grief. *American Journal of Psychoanalysis, 45,* 370–379.

Zisook, S., DeVaul, R. A., & Click, M. A. (1982). Measuring symptoms of grief and bereavement. *American Journal of Psychiatry, 139,* 1550–1593.

Zisook, S., Schneider, D., & Shuchter, S. R. (1990). Anxiety and bereavement. *Psychiatric Medicine, 8,* 83–96.

Zisook, S., & Shuchter, S. R. (1985). Time course of spousal bereavement. *General Hospital Psychiatry, 7,* 95–100.

Zisook, S., & Shuchter, S. R. (1991). Depression through the first year after the death of a spouse. *American Journal of Psychiatry, 148,* 1346–1352.

Zisook, S., & Shuchter, S. R. (1993). Uncomplicated bereavement. *Journal of Clinical Psychiatry, 54,* 365–373.

Zisook, S., Shuchter, S. R., & Lyons, S. E. (1987). Adjustment to widowhood. In S. Zisook (Ed.), *Biopsychosocial aspects of grief and bereavement* (pp. 51–74). Washington, DC: American Psychiatric Press.

Zisook, S., Shuchter, S. R., Sledge, M., Paulus, M., & Judd, L. L. (1994). The spectrum of depressive phenomena after spousal bereavement. *Journal of Clinical Psychiatry, 55*(Suppl.), 29–36.

Author Index

Page numbers in italics refer to listings in reference sections.

Subject Index

About the Editors

Perry M. Nicassio is Professor of Psychology and Director of Health Psychology Programs at the California School of Professional Psychology and an Associate Adjunct Professor in the Department of Psychiatry at the University of California, San Diego School of Medicine. He graduated Phi Beta Kappa from the University of Southern California in 1969 and, from Northwestern University, received his master's in 1971 and PhD in 1973 in clinical psychology.

A Fellow of Division 38 of the American Psychological Association (APA), Nicassio has authored numerous scholarly articles on health psychology and behavioral medicine and has been actively involved in research on the treatment of sleep and stress-related disorders, the role of culture change in the health of immigrant groups, and the psychosocial adjustment of patients with rheumatic disease. Nicassio has served on the board of *Health Psychology,* as a consultant to various agencies within the National Institutes of Health, and as senior adviser to the American Psychiatric Association on the revision of code for the *Diagnostic and Statistical Manual of Mental Disorders* (4th ed.). For several years, he was Chair of the Health Services Committee of Division 38.

Timothy W. Smith is Professor of Psychology and Director of Graduate Training Programs in Clinical and Health Psychology at the University of Utah. He received his PhD in Clinical Psychology from the University of Kansas in 1982 and was a predoctoral intern and postdoctoral Fellow in the Brown University Program of Medicine. He has received Early Career Awards from Division 38 and from the American Psychonomic Society. An associate editor of both *Health Psychology* and the *Annals of Behavioral Medicine,* Smith has authored over 100 articles and chapters on clinical and health psychology. He has also coauthored two books—*Coronary Heart Disease: A Behavioral Perspective* (with A. S. Leon) and *Anger, Hostility, and the Heart* (with A. W. Siegman).